LAPAROSCOPIC SURGERY

An Atlas for General Surgeons

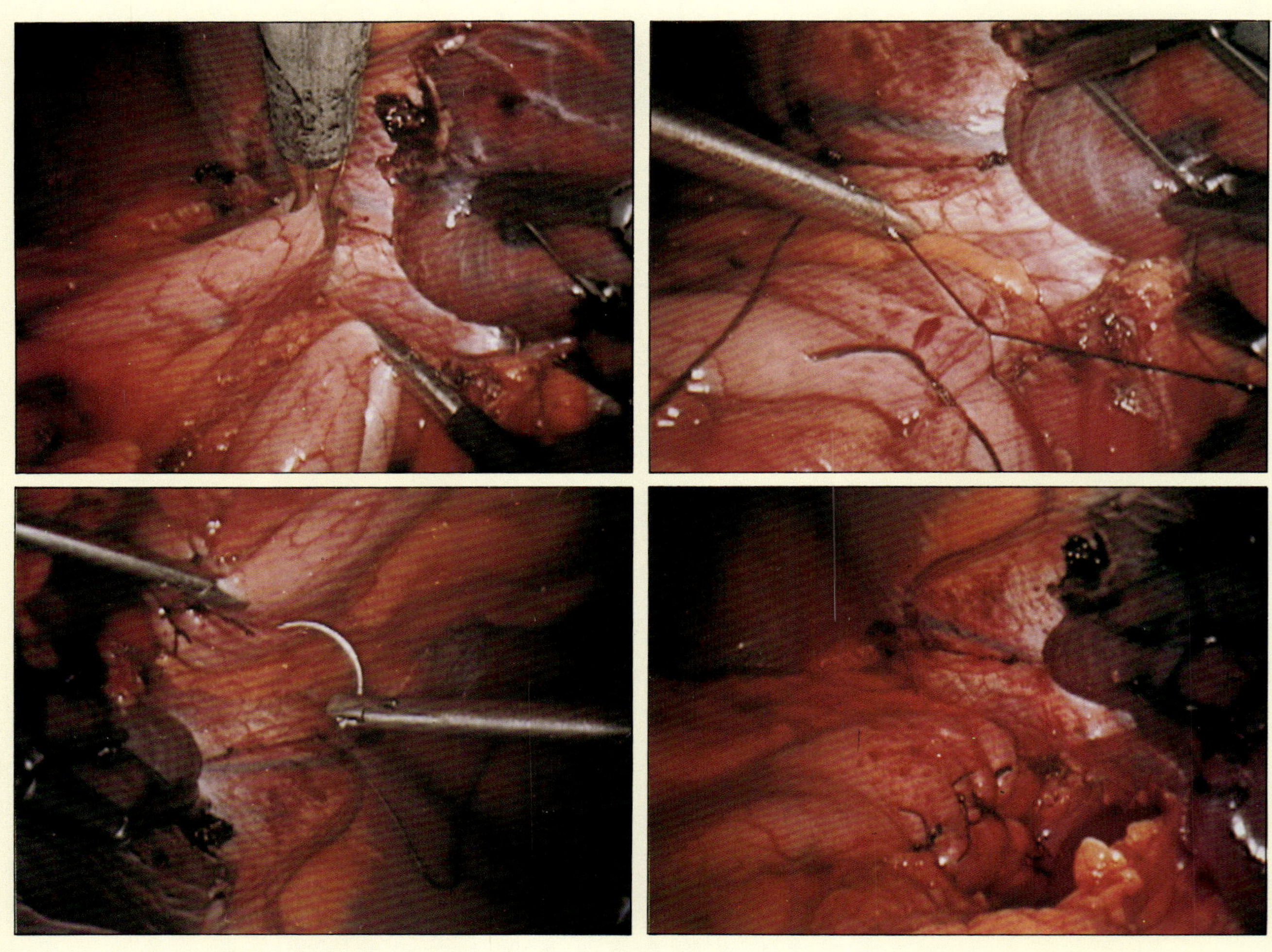

Suturing of the gastric fundus during the performance of a laparoscopic Nissen fundoplication.

LAPAROSCOPIC SURGERY

An Atlas for General Surgeons

EDITED BY

Gary C. Vitale, MD
Associate Professor of Surgery
University of Louisville School of Medicine
Louisville, Kentucky

Joseph S. Sanfilippo, MD
Professor of Obstetrics and Gynecology
Director of Endocrinology
University of Louisville School of Medicine
Louisville, Kentucky

Jacques Perissat, MD
Professor
Centre Hospitalier et Universitaire de Bordeaux
Bordeaux, France

With 26 Contributors

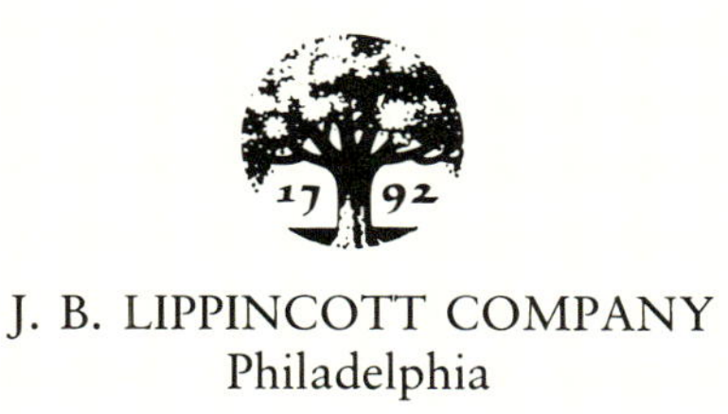

J. B. LIPPINCOTT COMPANY
Philadelphia

Acquisitions Editor: Lisa McAllister
Developmental Editor: Paula Callaghan
Project Editor: Bridget C. Hannon
Indexer: Holly Campbell Lukens
Designer: Doug Smock
Cover Designer: Richard Merchán
Production Manager: Caren Erlichman
Senior Production Coordinator: Kevin P. Johnson
Compositor: Achorn Graphic Services, Inc.
Printer/Binder: Walsworth Publishing Company
Pre-Press: Jay's Publishers Services, Inc.

Cover illustration: Suturing of the gastric fundus during the performance of a laparoscopic Nissen fundoplication.

6 5 4 3 2 1

Library of Congress Cataloging-in-Publication Data

Laparoscopic surgery : an atlas for general surgeons / edited by Gary C. Vitale, Joseph S. Sanfilippo, Jacques Perissat.
p. cm.
Includes bibliographical references and index.
ISBN 0-397-51268-6 (alk. paper)
1. Abdomen—Endoscopic surgery—Atlases. I. Vitale, Gary C.
II. Sanfilippo, J. S. (Joseph S.) III. Perissat, J.
[DNLM: 1. Surgery, Laparoscopic—atlases. WO 517 L299 1995]
RD540.L2777 1995
617.5'5059—dc20
DNLM/DLC
for Library of Congress 94-42336
CIP

♾ This Paper Meets the Requirements of ANSI/NISO Z39.48-1992 (Permanence of Paper).

The authors and publisher have exerted every effort to ensure that drug selection and dosage set forth in this text are in accord with current recommendations and practice at the time of publication. However, in view of ongoing research, changes in government regulations, and the constant flow of information relating to drug therapy and drug reactions, the reader is urged to check the package insert for each drug for any change in indications and dosage and for added warnings and precautions. This is particularly important when the recommended agent is a new or infrequently employed drug.

Dedication

The authors would like to dedicate this book to their parents, Anthony M. and Marie J. Vitale, Elena T. and Joseph P. Sanfilippo, and Fernande and Georges Perissat, with gratitude and appreciation for their inspiration, leadership and love.

Contributors

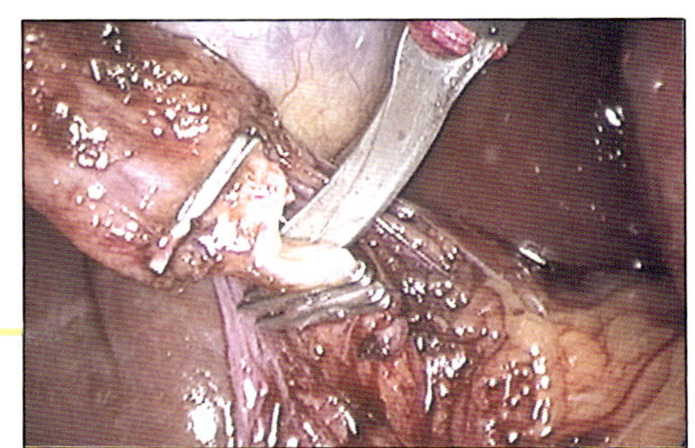

Eleanor F. Asher, MD
Department of Anesthesiology
University of Louisville School of Medicine
Louisville, Kentucky

E.L. Bokey, MD
Professor, Colon and Rectal Unit
University of Sydney
Concord Hospital
Concord, New South Wales
Australia

José Camps, MD
Laparoscopic Research Fellow
Creighton University School of Medicine
Omaha, Nebraska

William G. Cheadle, MD
Associate Professor
Department of Surgery
University of Louisville School of Medicine
Louisville, Kentucky

Denis Collet, MD
Centre Hospitalier et Universitaire de Bordeaux
Cliniques Chirurgicales
Service de Chirurgie Générale et Digestive
Centre de Chirurgie Laparoscopique
Bordeaux, France

Alfred Cushieri, MD
Department of Surgery and Centre for Surgical Skills
Ninewells Hospital and Medical School
University of Dundee
Dundee, Scotland

I.P. Davis, MD
Professor, Colon and Rectal Unit
University of Sydney
Concord Hospital
Concord, New South Wales
Australia

Michael Edye, MD
Centre Hospitalier et Universitaire de Bordeaux
Cliniques Chirurgicales
Service de Chirurgie Générale et Digestive
Centre de Chirurgie Laparoscopique
Bordeaux, France

Robert J. Fitzgibbons, Jr., MD
Professor of Surgery
Creighton University School of Medicine
Omaha, Nebraska

P. Hewitt, MD
Professor, Colon and Rectal Unit
University of Sydney
Concord Hospital
Concord, New South Wales
Australia

Paul D. Indman, MD
Clinical Associate Professor
Department of Gynecology and Obstetrics
Stanford University
Senior Consultant in Gynecologic Endoscopic Surgery
Santa Clara Valley Medical Center
Los Gatos, California

Gerald M. Larson, MD
Professor
Department of Surgery
University of Louisville School of Medicine
Louisville, Kentucky

Claude L. Liguory, MD
Clinique Medico-Chirurgical
de l'Alma
Paris, France

Thom E Lobe, MD
Professor of Surgery and Pediatrics
Chairman, Section of Pediatric Surgery
University of Tennessee
Memphis, Tennessee

Linda F. Lucas, MD
Department of Anesthesiology
University of Louisville School of Medicine
Louisville, Kentucky

Dan C. Martin, MD
Department of Surgery
University of Tennessee, Memphis
Memphis, Tennessee

Jacques Perissat, MD
Professor
Centre Hospitalier et Universitaire de Bordeaux
Bordeaux, France

Edward H. Phillips, MD
Clinical Associate Professor of Surgery
USC/Los Angeles County Medical Center
Attending Surgeon
Cedars-Sinai Medical Center
Los Angeles, California

Marcello Pietrantoni, MD
Assistant Professor
Division of Maternal-Fetal Medicine
Department of Obstetrics and Gynecology
University of Louisville School of Medicine
Louisville, Kentucky

Harry Reich, MD
Wyoming Valley Gyn-Ob Associates
Kingston, Pennsylvania

Benjamin M. Rigor, MD
Professor and Chairman
Department of Anesthesiology
University of Louisville School of Medicine
Louisville, Kentucky

Joseph S. Sanfilippo, MD
Professor of Obstetrics and Gynecology
Director of Reproductive Biology
University of Louisville School of Medicine
Louisville, Kentucky

Julia A. Schroder, MD
Department of Anesthesiology
University of Louisville School of Medicine
Louisville, Kentucky

Kurt Semm, KRCOG
Direktor dere Abteilung, Frauenheilkunde
Im Kliniku, der Christian-Albrechts-Universität
Und Michaelis-Henammenschule
Kiel, Germany

Steven R. Smith, JD
Dean and Professor of Law
Cleveland State University College of Law
Cleveland, Ohio

Pierre J. Testas, MD
Professor of Digestive Surgery
Paris Sud University
Paris, France

Thierry G. Vancaillie, MD
Center for Gynecologic Endosurgery
San Antonio, Texas

Gary C. Vitale, MD
Associate Professor of Surgery
University of Louisville School of Medicine
Louisville, Kentucky

Jean-Christophe De Watteville, MD
Assistance Hôpiteaux Publique de Paris
Assistant des Hôpiteaux
Service de Chirurgie
Générale et Digestive
Paris, France

Foreword

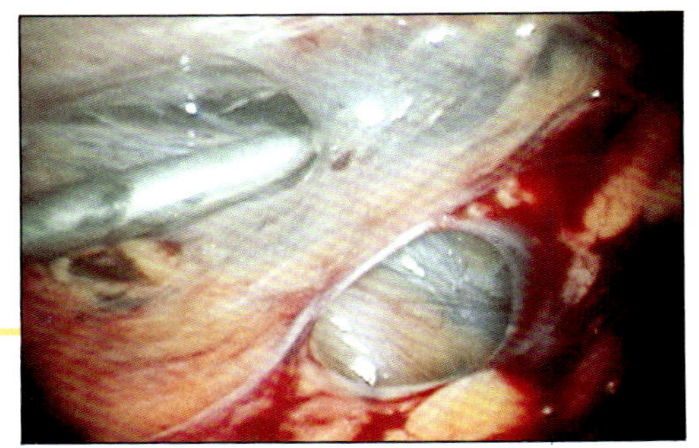

Futuristic laparoscopic innovations and imaginative endoscopic procedures are no longer symbols of the latest fads in medicine, but have assumed mainstream status in the care of patients in leading hospitals and medical centers all over the world. But does even this progression of stature justify yet another major text and atlas focusing on what many of us had assumed was 21st century technology? A hurried thumb-through of this excellent new treatise will yield a positive answer and a detailed study will evoke an enthusiastic endorsement of the volume, its prose and illustrations. To some degree, this effort provides a compelling glimpse of what will be the present and future of surgical practice.

This book appears at a time when the overwhelming controversies of the early years have become less strident and the warm maturity of both endoscopic and laparoscopic approaches has replaced the circus atmosphere of weekend courses; the techniques illustrated in this important book have assumed a major role in postgraduate medical curricula around the modern medical world.

- To what extent should upper gastrointestinal endoscopy and its retinue of beguiling interventions in the biliary tract be the primary province of the gastroenterologist as opposed to the surgeon?
- How short can a weekend course be and still provide primitively safe laparoscopic skills for the gynecologist or surgeon?
- To what extent does devious cost-shifting permit the raft of new (and often disposable) technical innovations and devices to consume the putative savings of shortened hospitalization?
- What are the educational minima versus desirable standards for conduct of the growing number of seemingly safe laparoscopic and thorascopic operations?
- Given the presumed safety and defined lowering of morbidity of many abdominal operations with less invasive approaches, what are the bases of traditional indications for an operation? Does half an indication justify half an operation?
- To what extent does ease of access to certain body cavities permit the tedious, expensive, and possibly dangerous conduct of massive intracavity procedures, certainly best exemplified by Whipple's operation for cancer? Dr. Alfred Cuschieri of Dundee, Scotland, suggests that where access is a major cause of morbidity, then less invasive methods become ideal; when the procedure per se contributes dominantly, then the patient is likely best served by more conventional approaches.[1]

Interested observers can answer most of these queries when thay have consumed and assimilated this exceptional book. The growing tendency of both certifying and accrediting bodies to focus on the numbers of specific operations and their routes of approach provides clear examples of these educational trends in the United States. Even so, clinical credentialing has yet to match the pace of evolving laparoscopic and thoracoscopic operations. Even now, we are replacing opinions[2] with interesting and seemingly valid data,[3,4] which will soon define the basic skills and educational climate that creates the best possible environment for the individual who matters most, the patient.

Indeed, this book's authorship is a product of those kinds of relationships and deserves a word so that all its readers can appreciate this volume's birth process. Dr. Joseph Sanfilippo is Professor of Obstetrics and Gynecology at the University of Louisville, the doctor many faculty call upon for their own family, and a popular president of the medical staff of one of our leading hospitals. A contemporary and friend, Dr. Gary Vitale, was a young surgeon with strong hepatobiliary interests nurtured by a research fellowship in Dundee with Alfred Cuschieri. Those career interests were being consumed by a flourishing but unfocused career as a much sought after young general surgeon in our medical center. Dr. Vitale enlisted the aid of Professor Maurice Mercadier in getting one of the most sought after posts as an assistant to the renowned endoscopist, Professor Claude Liguory. His, and his family's mastery of the language and lifestyle of their hosts at the Clinique de l'Alma and Bicetre Hospital in Paris ripened into a friendship and the most productive mastery of basic and interventional endoscopic skills, often the missing link in the surgeon's laparoscopic approach to the biliary tract. Professor Jacques Perissat's warm invitations to Bordeaux led to another flourishing friendship. As the master and innovator, Professor Perissat's imagination has produced a second generation of professional exchanges that culminated in the decision to do this book right and many of the insights and little tricks are his.

Thus the volume produces the best of Franco-American scholarship, technical advances, and particularly clear illustrations that are an invitation to both the present and the future of less invasive techniques in medical care. The limits to progress have always been our imagination, and this is a stimulating expression of how those limits have yielded to interdisciplinary progress.

References

1. Collet D, Cadiere GB: FDCL Group for Gastro-Esophageal Reflux Disease: Conversions and complications of laparoscopic treatment of gastro-esophageal reflux disease: a survey conducted by FDCL. Am J Surg (in press).
2. Altman LK: Surgical injuries from new operation lead New York to demand improved training. New York Times. June 14, 1992; section 1:1.
3. Grundfest WS: Credentialing in an era of change [Editorial]. JAMA 1993;270:2725.
4. See WA, Cooper CS, Fisher RJ: Predictors of laparoscopic complications after formal training in laparoscopic surgery. JAMA 1993;270:2689.

Hiram C. Polk, Jr., MD

Preface

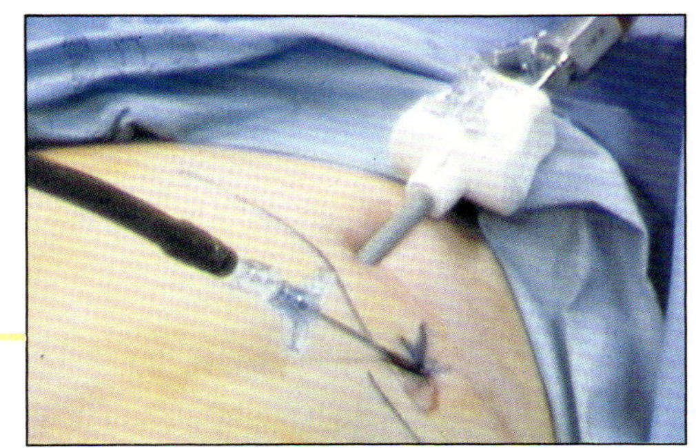

The Babylonian Talmud (Niddah-Treatise, Section 65b) describes the first endoscopic surgery, which used a lead funnel with a bent mouthpiece and a wooden drain pipe to allow direct visualization of an internal organ—in this case the vagina and uterine cervix.

From the strict sense of historical perspective, the first laparoscopic inspection took place in Germany in 1902, at which time the abdomen of a dog model was used to facilitate application of diagnostic laparoscopy. The first recorded evaluation of intra-abdominal organs in the human was in 1911 by the Swedish surgeon, Jacobaeus. As time progressed and technological advances such as cold fiberoptics (1963) took place, new and innovative laparoscopic procedures continued to be reported. Although laparoscopic surgery traditionally has been ascribed to the realm of the gynecologic surgeon, it is now also an integral part of the general surgeon's armamentarium. The first endoscopic appendectomy was performed in 1980.

General surgeons were not always very quick to take advantage of interventional endoscopic techniques at their advent. Notably, surgeons left the development of ERCP and endoscopic sphincterotomy to the gastroenterologists in the 1970's. It is interesting that gastroenterologists also made the best early use of laparoscopy for gastrointestinal diseases. Many gastroenterologists were trained in diagnostic laparoscopy in the 1970's, but gradually abandoned it as interventional endoscopic and radiologic techniques allowed collection of the same or similar diagnostic information without the need for general anesthesia.

Once the revolution began, surgeons did not make the same mistake they initially made with interventional endoscopy. This revolution took most surgeons by surprise, and even the innovators could not have predicted the explosion of interest and rapidity of dissemination worldwide of this new technique. It is also of interest historically that a good part of the motivation to move forward with this technique was patient-driven. It became clear to surgeons that if they didn't learn to perform laparoscopic cholecystectomy, they would soon not be doing many cholecystectomies at all. The ability of today's rapid communication and the media to inform and generate enthusiasm among the public is unprecedented. Even without this fanfare, which clearly contributed to the rapid spread of laparoscopy, it was clearly an idea whose time had come given the recent advances in videoendoscopy. In fact, it is surprising when one reviews the history of gynecologic advances in laparoscopy, particularly the work of Kurt Semm, that general surgeons did not embrace the movement at the start. The ideas were hovering about in the early 1980's, but it took the catalyst of French laparoscopic cholecystectomy to move things forward.

Our mission with the current textbook is to provide the most recent laparoscopic surgical advances from international authorities, and to convey to the reader an orderly sequence of learning and application of knowledge. Once the general surgeon has acquired basic laparoscopic skills, the reasoning and understanding behind technological advances in laparoscopic surgery should allow one to take the next step and thus broaden his or her horizons with respect to laparoscopic skills, ability to avoid and manage complications, acquire new skills such as intra- and extracorporeal knot-tying, and a host of additional aspects including operative laparoscopy in the pediatric patient, the pregnant patient, abdominal emergencies and an increasing realm of new and innovative concepts.

As the exponential growth of laparoscopic surgery continues to evolve, both in the United States as well as internationally, this textbook is designed to provide the surgeon with the principles, direction and expertise to perform specific laparoscopic surgical procedures well when coupled with adequate laboratory and clinical training.

Gary C. Vitale, MD
Joseph Sanfilippo, MD
Jacques Perissat, MD

Acknowledgments

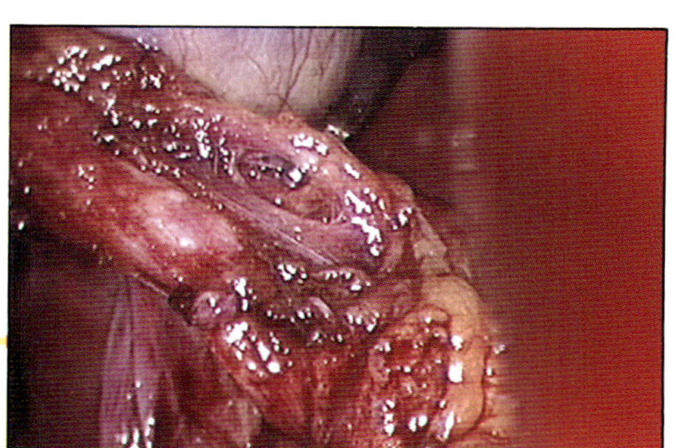

We would first like to thank Dr. Hiram Polk, Jr., for his vision and encouragement throughout the planning of this book. His enthusiasm for the proper training of the next generation of surgeons has exemplified the high quality we strive for in surgical education. The editors appreciate the assistance of many people who helped in preparing the book. Shirley Cook and Norma Braver, in particular, were invaluable. Lisa McAllister, Paula Callaghan, Bridget Hannon, and Kevin Johnson with J.B. Lippincott have been superb to work with, and we have benefitted from their professional expertise. Ms. Helen Stewart's personal dedication to the many details in coordinating the project proved indispensable. We are greatly indebted to her. We appreciate the fine quality drawings rendered by Bud Hixson. We are very thankful to our assistants, Ms. Leta Weedman and Ms. Pam Slusher, for their continuing help. Finally, we would like to thank our wives and families for their forbearance in the time dedicated to the challenge of completing the book. Their patience allowed us to pursue our goal: producing a book beneficial to clinicians.

Contents

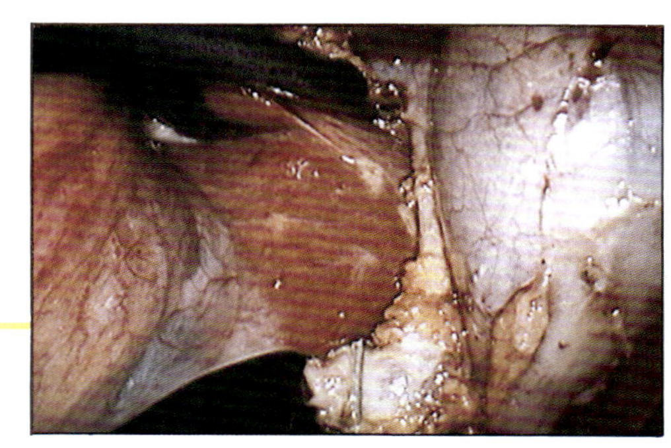

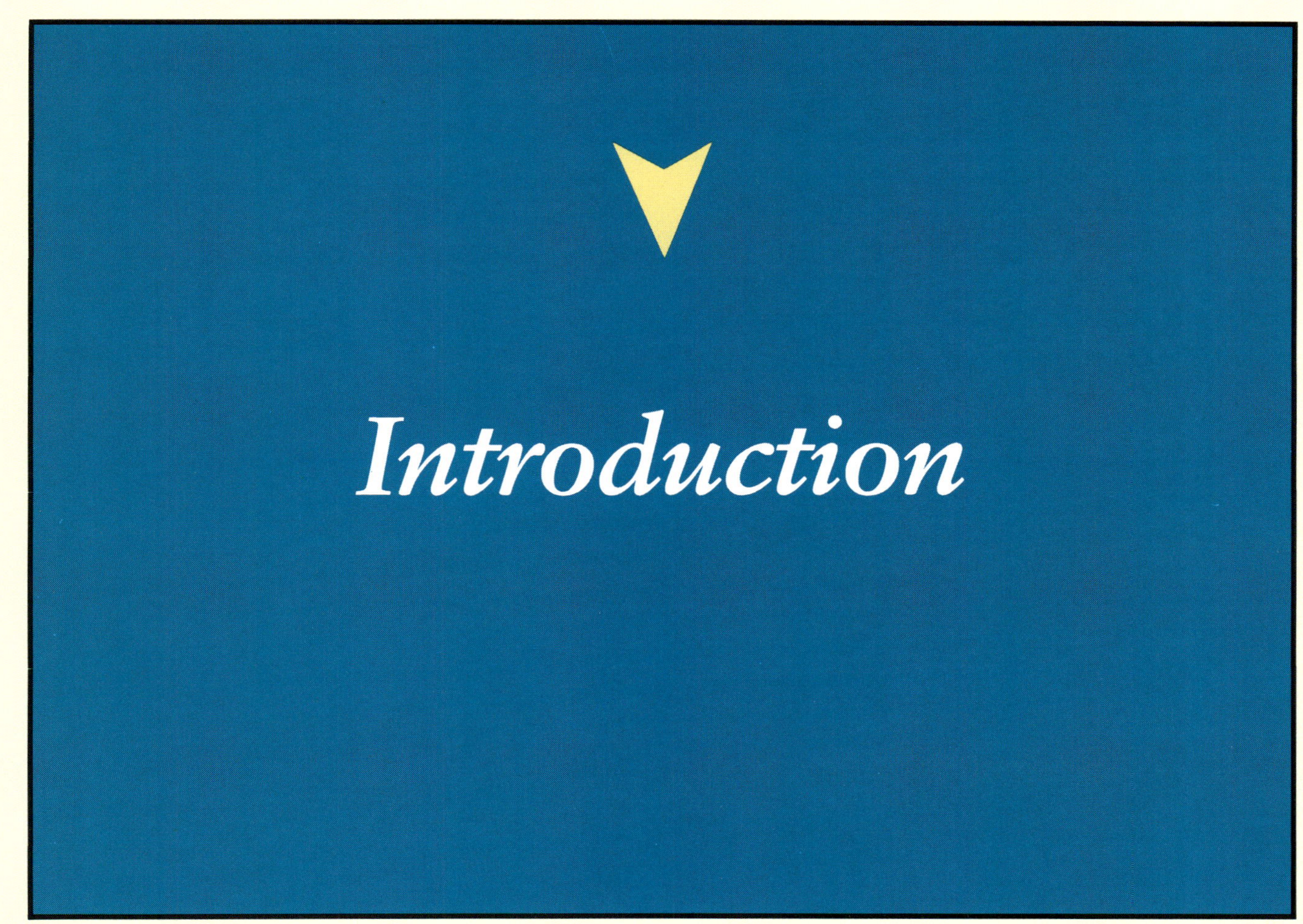

Introduction

Chapter 1

Laparoscopic Surgery: An Atlas for General Surgeons, edited by Gary C. Vitale, Joseph S. Sanfilippo, and Jacques Perissat. J. B. Lippincott Company, Philadelphia, © 1995.

The History of Endoscopy

Kurt Semm

The history of endoscopy dates back to the Talmud of Babylon. It contains a description of a lead siphon, named Siphophert, with a mouthpiece, which was bent inward and held a mechul (wooden drain). All of this apparatus was introduced into the vagina and was used to differentiate between vaginal and uterine bleeding. This was the first endoscopic examination. Although the term "endoscopein" is attributed to Avicenna (980–1037 A.D.), the procedure was first practiced by an Arab, Albulassim (912–1013 A.D.). By placing a mirror in front of the exposed vagina, he became the first to use reflected light as a source of illumination for observation of the body's inner recesses. Tulio Caesare Aranzi developed the first endoscopic light (Venice, 1587). He employed the Benedictine monk Don Panuce's principle of the "camera obscura" for medical purposes: the rays of the sun coming through a hole in the window shutter were concentrated by a glass jar filled with marbles and then projected into the nostrils.

It was Bozzini (Fig. 1-1) who gave birth to modern endoscopy in 1805, when he developed the first "light cable." This construction allowed rays of light to be projected into the body's cavities, which were then reflected back to the eye of the observer. The historical development of endoscopy was made complete by Desormeaux (1843), when he devised the portable endoscope (Fig. 1-2).

Foremost in the further development of abdominal endoscopic surgery are photography and video monitors, which began with Stein in Frankfurt as he presented his "photo-endoscope" in 1874 (Fig. 1-3).[1]

The true pioneers of endoscopic methods are the gynecologists Boesch, Power and Barnes, Palmer, Frangenheim, Fikentscher, and Semm, but the first line of technical development was accomplished in the field of cystoscopy.[2–8] The achievement primarily reflects the work of Nitze (Fig. 1-4), who developed an endoscope with a small bulb at its tip that presented no danger of burning the bladder because the water used for distention provided a cooling effect.

In 1902, Kelling first observed a dog's abdominal cavity through an air-filled abdomen and, after performing this on humans, named this procedure "coelioscopy."[9] This procedure became routine in humans in 1914 by a Swede, Jacobaeus, who named it "laparoscopy."[10] In the years following, this method was reinvented twice—first by Steiner (a Swiss) in 1924 as abdominoscopy and then by the Italian Redi in 1935 as splanchnoscopy.[11,12] Korbsch wrote the first textbook of laparothoracoscopy in Munich, Germany (1927).[13]

To reduce the risks involved in performing a blind puncture of the abdominal wall, Goetze (Fig. 1-5) developed the automatic needle in 1918 and promoted the ideal practice of initially establishing a pneumoperitoneum using oxygen.[14] With Fikentscher in 1955, Semm developed the Universal Tubal-Gas Insufflation Apparatus (Fig. 1-6) for the purpose of diagnosis in tubal disorders.[6] Palmer used coelioscopy primarily for the presurgical diagnosis of sterile female patients.[4] Gynecologic laparoscopy, as initially presented in 1955 at the German university level, was completely dismissed as ludicrous, owing to a number of serious complications. This was followed by the development of the first automatic CO_2 gas insufflator, according to Semm, for "internists."[15] This work was based on the flow principles learned from prior experience performing tubal insufflation (Fig. 1-7).[6]

As the practice of automatically creating a pneumoperitoneum under physiological pressure control became routine at the First Medical Clinic in Munich, laparoscopy as a diagnostic procedure for gynecology became the rule at the University Women's Clinic in Munich.[7] It was also at this time that a cold light source was developed (Fig. 1-8), whereby the extracorporeal light is transmitted through a glass fiber bundle. These innovations decreased the occurrence of the two great dangers

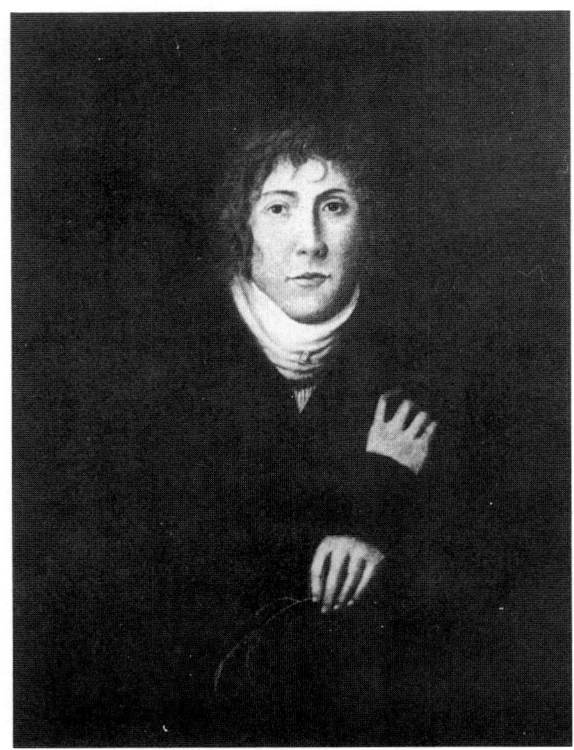

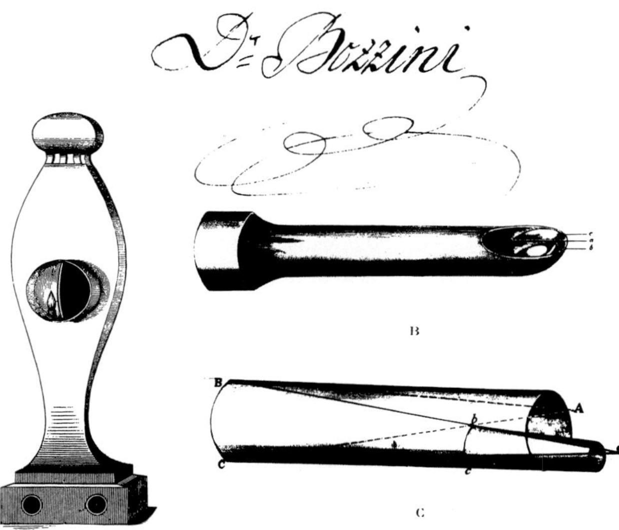

FIGURE 1-1. Endoscope developed by Philipp Bozzini (1805) and self-portrait (Philipp Bozzini, 25 May 1773 in Mainz and April, 1809 in Frankfurt a. Main, Germany).

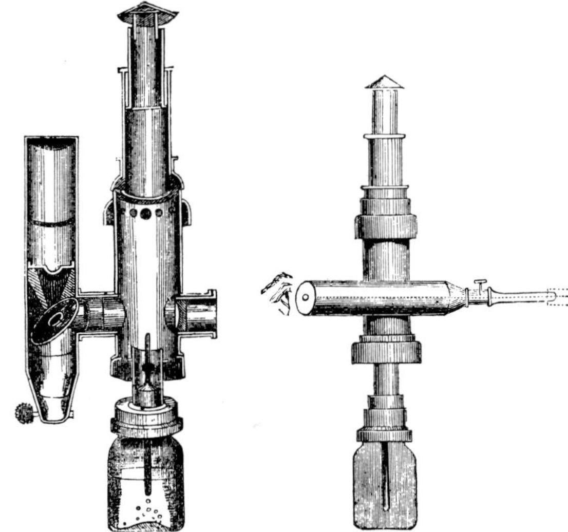

FIGURE 1-2. Endoscope developed by Antonin Jean Desormeaux (1815–1894); presented to the Academie Imperiale de Medicine, Paris, July 20, 1883.

of using laparoscopy in gynecology (ie, burning the bowel of the patient or causing a gas embolism).[7]

The practice of gynecologic laparoscopy as a diagnostic procedure was viewed skeptically and dismissed by many surgeons; therefore, the word "pelvioscopy" was chosen to address the surgical procedures that were developed.

These techniques were first described in the United States by Power and Barnes in 1941.[3] After demonstrating the CO_2-Pneu (Fig. 1-9) during the American Fertility Congress, 1967, by Semm, Melvin Cohen published this accomplishment.[16,17] Almost immediately, repelvioscopy became widely accepted in America, after the foundation of the American Association of Gynecological Laparoscopists in 1972. More than 95% of the laparoscopies performed in the United States were tubal sterilization procedures by HF-current coagulation. In Europe in the mid-1960s and early 1970s, pelvioscopy was almost exclusively used as a diagnostic procedure for infertility evaluation and treatment.

The actual history of advanced pelvioscopic surgery may be categorized as follows:

1. The development of instruments and apparatuses required for operative pelvioscopy (Fig. 1-10)
2. The development of the steps involved in the pelvioscopic operative procedure:
   A. A laparotomy was required to achieve hemostasis when it was not obtained during pelvioscopy
   B. The capability of providing adequate hemostasis with endocoagulation (Fig. 1-11), endoloops, sutures, or ligatures (1965–1991; Table 1-1)
3. The introduction of simultaneous display of diagnostic and operative pelvioscopy on video monitors

As the range of operations that could be performed pelvioscopically increased, so did the risk of hemorrhage increase, which could not be controlled by standard coagulation methods. The subsequent emergencies that resulted forced the development of the endoligature and subsequently the endosuture. With the increase in the number of instruments available (see Fig. 1-10) and the

(text continues on page 9)

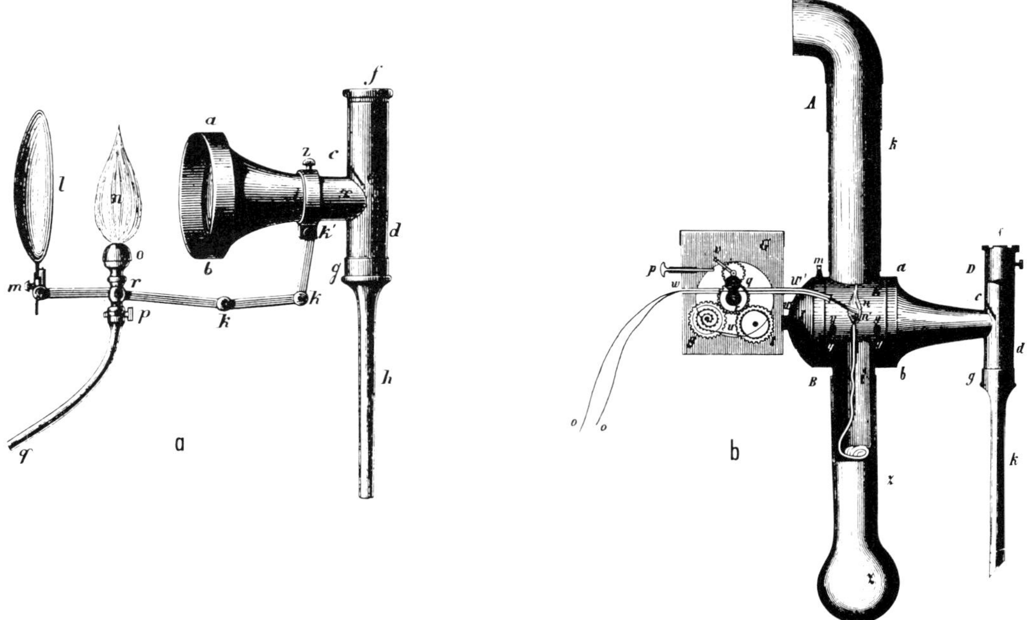

FIGURE 1-3. (**A**) Photo-endoscope, and (**B**) endo-camera developed by Theodore S. Stein of Frankfurt, Germany (1874).

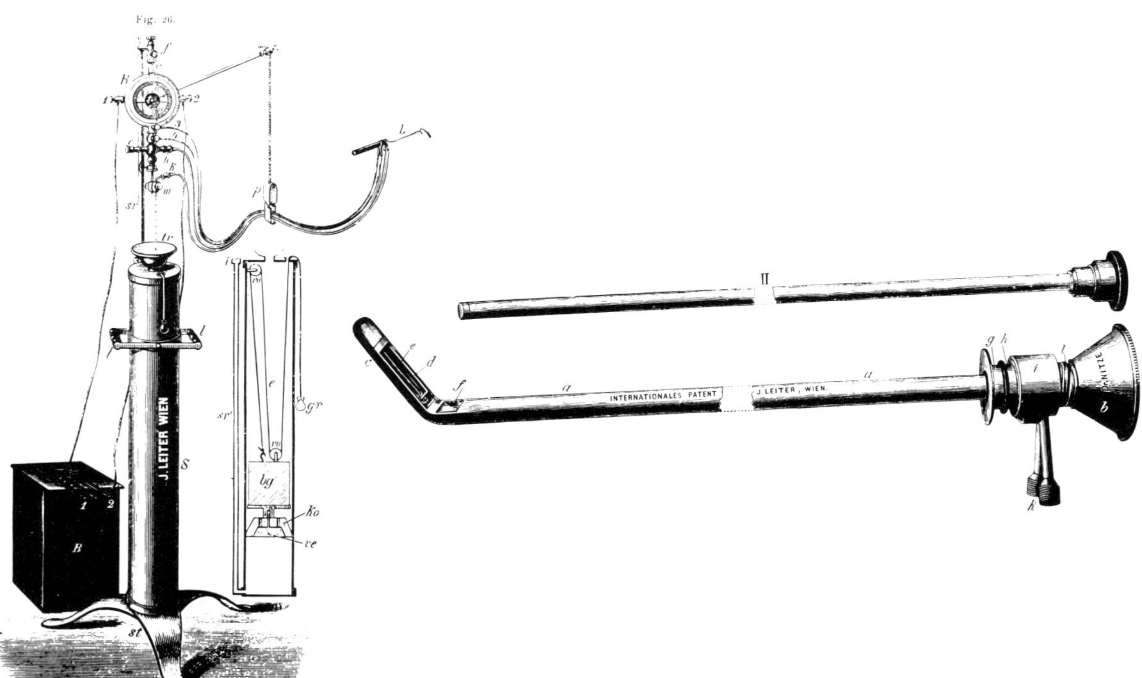

FIGURE 1-4. Cystoscope developed by Max Nitze (1879), Dresden, Germany, with an electric bulb for illumination.

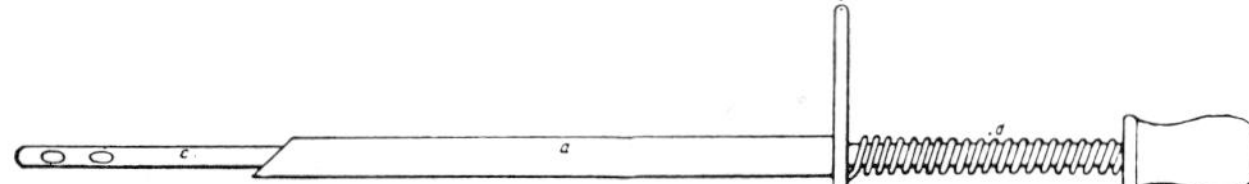

FIGURE 1-5. Automatic needle for insufflation, developed by Otto Goetze (1918).

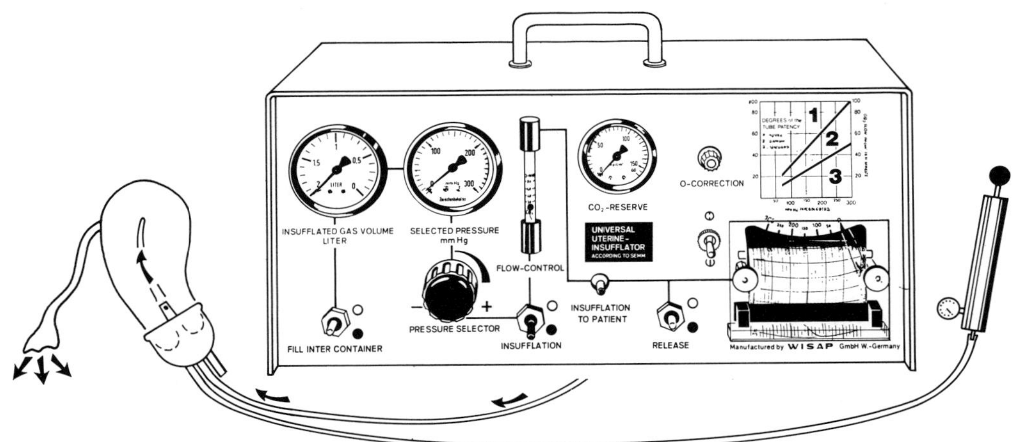

FIGURE 1-6. Universal uterine insufflator developed by Fikentscher and Semm (1955, Munich, Germany).

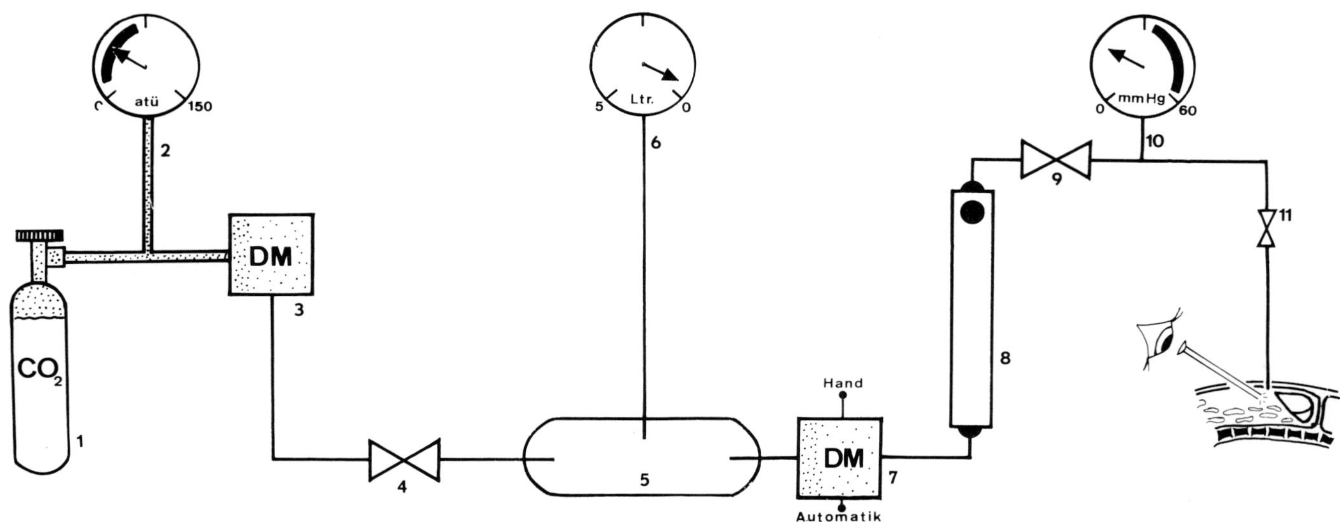

FIGURE 1-7. Physical principles of riskless intracorporeal gas insufflation developed by Semm (1955).

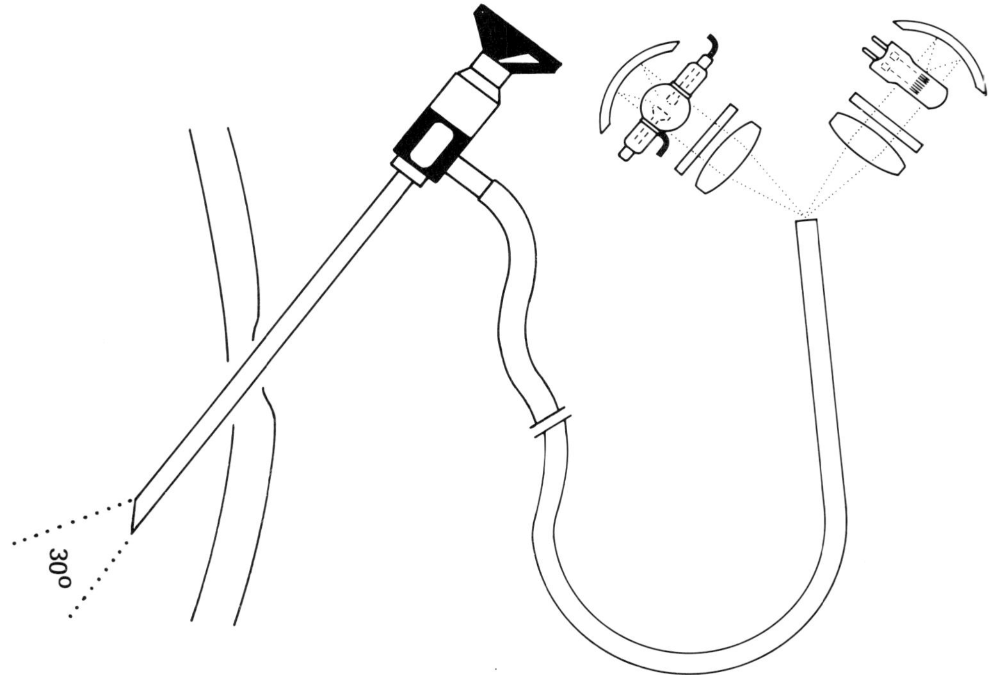

FIGURE 1-8. Intraabdominal cold light illumination, using external combined halogen and flash light source and glass-fiber light conduction.

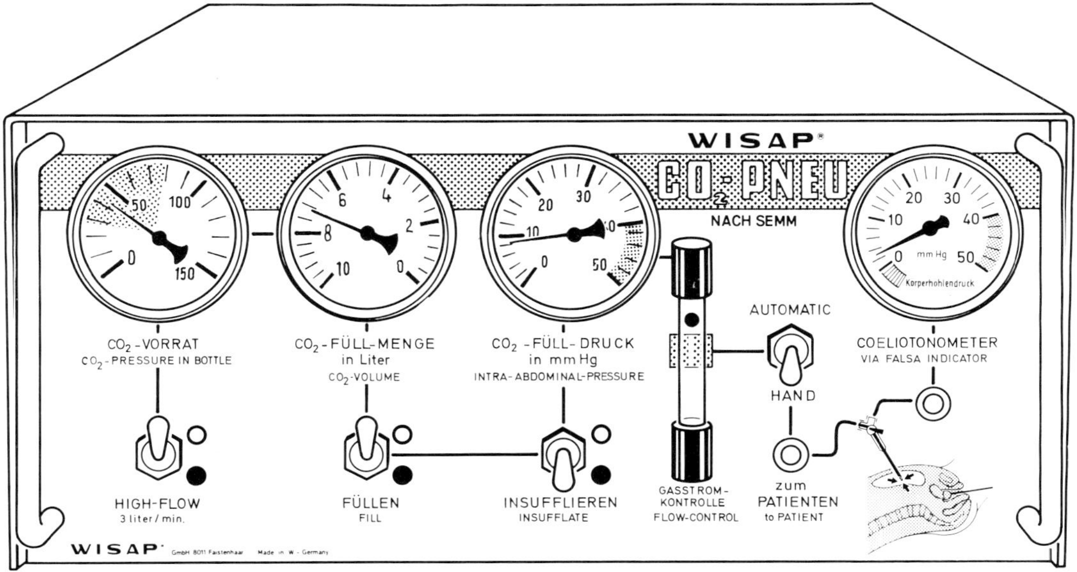

FIGURE 1-9. First CO_2-Pneu developed by Semm with the "Quadro-Test" (1964 to 1988), using adapted coeliotonometer by Goetze-Semm insufflation needle.

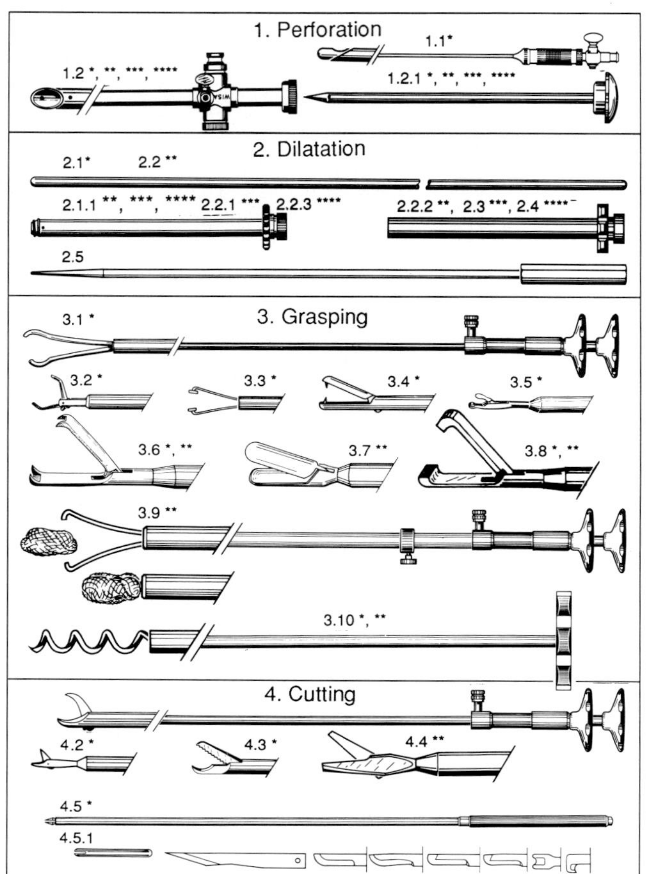

A

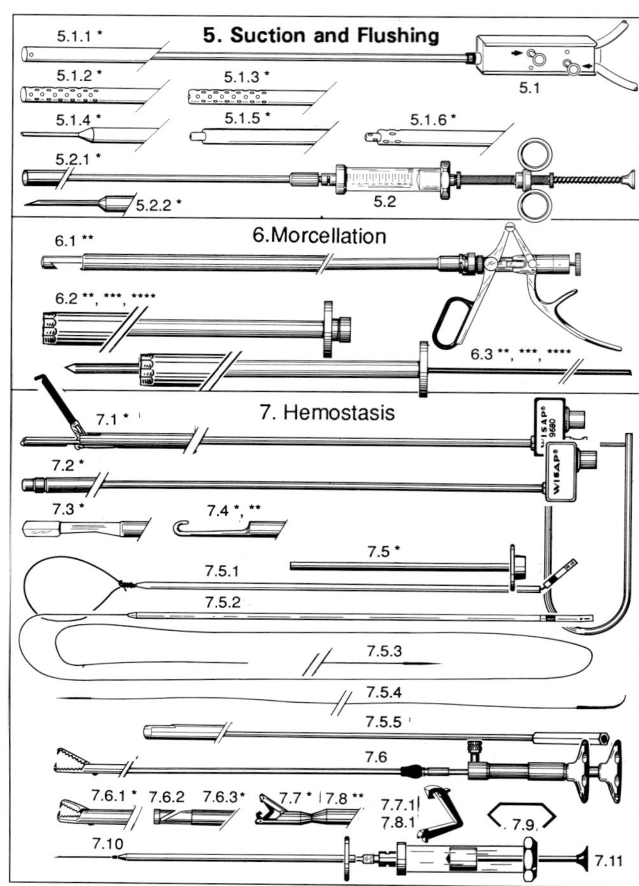

B

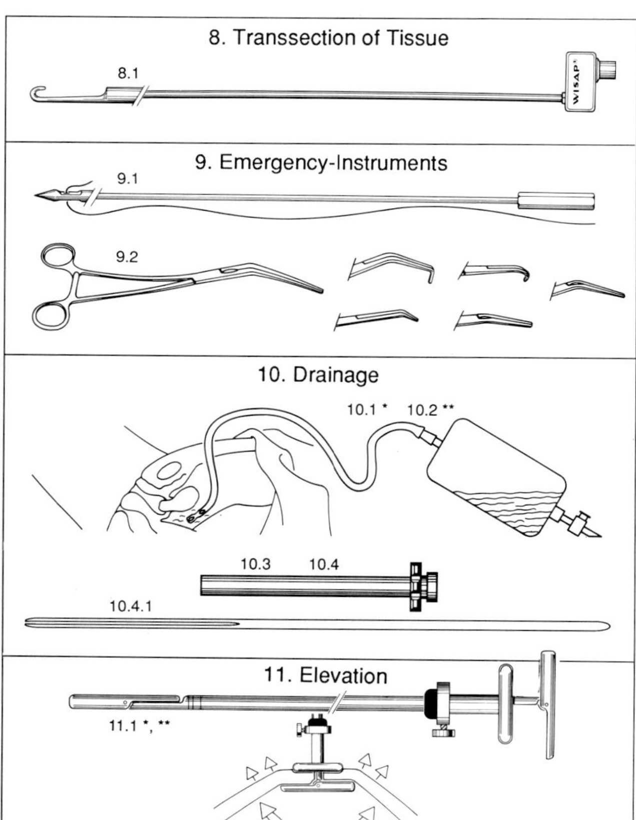

C

FIGURE 1-10. Basic instruments developed by Semm for surgical pelvioscopy.

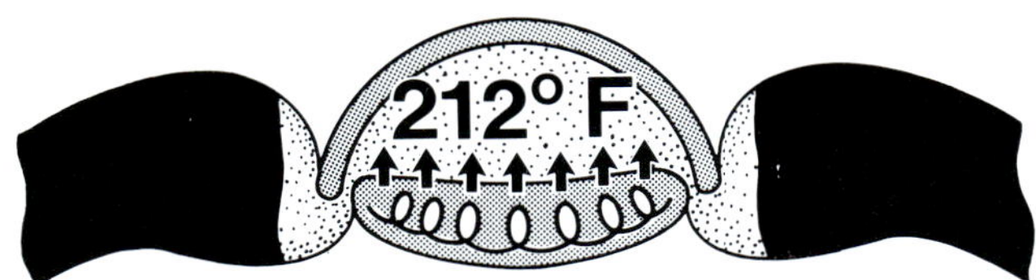

FIGURE 1-11. Principles of endocoagulation developed by Semm; only heat waves (not high-frequency current) coagulate the protein.

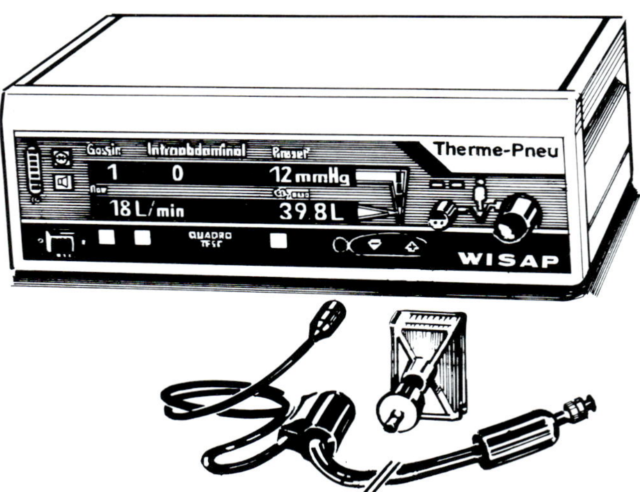

FIGURE 1-12. Computerized Therme-Pneu by Semm (1991), with integrated "Quadro-Test" and heated CO_2-gas.

various innovative ways they were used, new procedures were also developed. When loss of the CO_2 pneumoperitoneum occurred, which could not be replaced quickly enough by the CO_2-Pneu, the Op-Pneu-Electronic and the Pelvi-Pneu "Quadro-Test" were developed, which now deliver 20 L per minute by maximal pressure of 40 mm Hg (WISAP computerized model) (Fig. 1-12).

A particularly important advancement came with the Pelvi-Trainer (Fig. 1-13).[18] Since its development, all operative steps may first be practiced on models, thus ensuring ultimate safety for the patient.

With further advancements in both instrumentation and devices required for operative pelvioscopy, the array of laparoscopic operations steadily increased. This expansion unfolded in two steps. The first was characterized by the fact that in the case of large bleeding vessels (which could not be controlled by monopolar or bipolar coagulation high frequency current or a laser), laparotomy had to be performed. Because of this, the range of pelvioscopic operations was limited to lysis of filmy adhesions, fimbriolysis, and ovarian biopsy. Pelvioscopy became popular throughout the world because it was an effective and simple way to perform tubal ligations by HF-current mono- (and later) bipolar coagulation.

After the advent of safe and secure methods of accomplishing hemostasis, the number of operations that could be performed endoscopically increased greatly (Table 1-2). After tubal ligation came the first procedures for the correction of distal tubal occlusion. In 1972, after better means of achieving adequate endocoagulation were developed by 110°C, it became possible for the first time to remove small pedunculated myomas endoscopically, with minimal blood loss.[19] Operative endoscopy as we know it began in 1976 when the Roeder loop was introduced, making omental adhesiolysis and resection possible. This device served as an endoligature, which allowed tissue to be ligated easily and successfully, making it possible to replace a broad spectrum of classic abdominal surgical procedures with laparoscopic techniques.

Laparoscopic appendectomy was first performed by Semm in 1980 and published in the English literature in 1982.[20] Twelve months later, a German editor returned the manuscript, stating that the "journal would look ridiculous to publish such nonsense." The first German account appeared in 1983 by an Austrian publisher in Vienna.[21]

Pelvioscopic cholecystectomy was the next step in this progression. Mouret, a French general surgeon who was highly skilled in gynecologic surgery and laparoscopic technique, developed this procedure in Lyon in 1987.[22] In 1988 in Paris, Dubois tried this new technique, liked

TABLE 1-1
Development of Diagnostic/Surgical Tools by Semm for Pelvi-Laparoscopy

1965	Thermo-coagulator
1965	Cold-light
1966	CO_2-Pneu
1967	CO_2-Pneu-Automatic
1968	Pelvioscope Hook-Scissors
1969	Uterus Mobilizer by vacuum
1971	High-Frequency-Coagulator/bipolar
1972	Endocoagulator
1974	Crocodile-Forceps-Coagulation
1976	Applicator for Loop Litigation
1978	Op-Pneu-Electronic
1979	Endo-Ligation
	Tissue Morcellator
1980	Endo-Suture Aquapurator
1982	Myoenucleator
1985	Pelvi-Trainer
	Operations-Optic-Set
1986	Emergency-Needle
1988	CO_2-Pelvi-Pneu
	Serrated Edged Macro Morcellator (SEMM-Set)
1989	Abdominal Cavity Expander (ACE)
1991	Calibrated Uterine Resection Tool (CURT)
	Ery-Stop with Haemostaser
1992	Auto-Moto-Drive for CURT
	Pneu-Therme
1994	Computer Therme-Pneu (20 L/min)
	Aqua Purator "GIGA Washer"

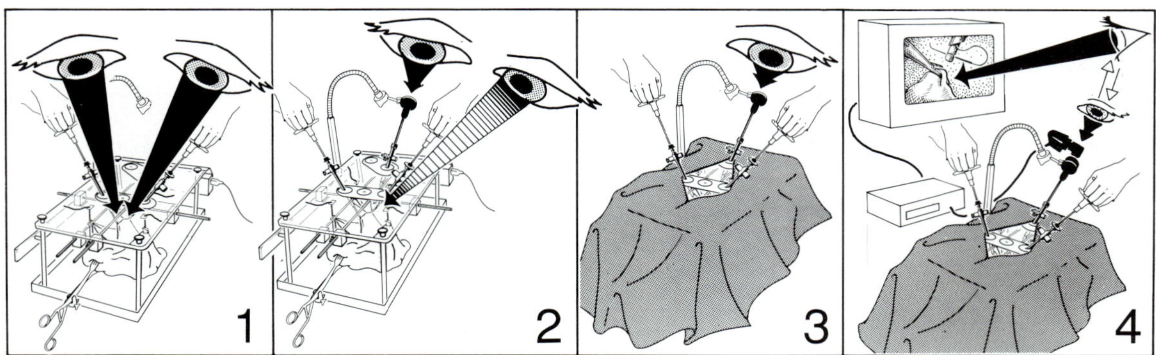

FIGURE 1-13. Pelvi-Trainer model developed by Semm for self-training program (four-step program).

it, expanded on it, and performed it routinely. When reports of this procedure were first published in 1989, they too were received with criticism and skepticism in some circles.[23]

Pelvioscopic surgery has been the pacesetter for the concept of minimally invasive surgery. All surgical specialties are using the basic techniques and instruments developed between 1963 and 1994 by Semm, a gynecologist.[24–28] For reducing pains after laparoscopic surgery the insufflation of heated gas for pneumoperitoneum has been developed.[29] Also, "gasless" laparoscopy is in discussion.

Prolonged hospitalizations are minimized, as is long postoperative convalescence. At the end of the 20th century, surgery will have taken on a new dimension. Terms such as operative laparoscopy and pelvioscopy are rapidly being incorporated into a more encompassing term: minimally invasive surgery.

TABLE 1-2
Development of Diagnostic/Surgical Procedures for Pelviscopy

	Year
DIAGNOSTIC	
Hysteroscopy	1843
Colposcopy	1874
Laparoscopy	1946
Douglascopy (culdoscopy)	1954
Cervicoscopy	1954
Fetoscopy	1954
Pelvioscopy	1967
Tubaloscopy	1968
Myomascopy	1991
SURGICAL	
Laparoscopy (tubal sterilization)	1934
Coelioscopy (tubal sterility)	1946
Hysteroscopy	1954
Pelvioscopy	
Endocoagulation	1972
Myoma enucleation	1975
Endoligation	1976
Tubal pregnancy	1976
Omentum adhesiolysis	1977
Salpingostomy	1978
Endosuture	1979
Laser	1979
Appendectomy	1980
Bowel suture	1983
Vasopressin	1985
Laparoscopic Assisted Hysterectomy (LAVH)	1989
CASH/Classic Abdominal SEMM Hysterectomy	1991
TUMA (Total Uterine Mucosa Ablation)	1992
IVH (Intrafascial Vaginal Hysterectomy)	1993

References

1. Stein TS: Das Photoendoskop. Berl Klin Wochenschr H3, 1874.
2. Boesch PF: Laparoskopie. Schweiz Z Krankenh U Anstaltsw 1936;6:62.
3. Power FH, Barnes AC: Sterilization by means of peritoneoscopic tubal fulguration; preliminary report. Am J Obstet Gynecol 1941;41:1038.
4. Palmer R: Coelioscopie gynecologie. Rapport du Professor Moquot. Acad de Chir 1948;72:363.
5. Frangenheim H: Die Bedeutung der Laparoskopie fur die gynaekologische Diagnostik. Fortschr Med 1958;76:451.
6. Fikentscher R, Semm K: Beitrag zur Methodik der uterotubaren Pertubation. Geburtshilfe Frauenheilkd 1955; 15:313.
7. Semm K: Die Laparoskopie in der Gynakologie. Geburtshilfe Frauenheilkd 1967;27:1029.
8. Semm K; Rice AL, trans: Atlas of gynecologic laparoscopy and hysteroscopy. Philadelphia: WB Saunders, 1977.
9. Kelling G: Ueber die Oesophagoskopie. Gastroskopie und Coelioskopie. Muench Med Wochenschr 1902;49:21.
10. Jacobaeus HC: Konnen durch die Laparoskopie Indikationen zu chirurgischen Eingriffen gewonnen werden? Nord Med Ark 1914;14:1.
11. Steiner OP: Abdominoskopie. Schweiz Med Wochenschr 1924;54:84. Surg Gynecol Obstet 1924;38:266. (In translation.)
12. Redi R: Ueber ein neues endoskopisches chirurgisches Instrument, das Splanchnoskop. Zentralbl Chir 1935; 62:558.
13. Korbsch R: Lehrbuch und Atlas der Laparoskopie und Thorako-skopie. Muenchen: Lehmann, 1927.

14. Goetze O: Die Rontgendiagnostik bei gasgefullter Bauchhohle. eine neue Methode. Munch Med Wochenschr 1918; 65:1275.

15. Eisenburg J: Ueber eine Apparatur zur schonenden und kontrollierbaren Gasfullung der Bauchhohle fur die Laparoskopie. Klin Wochenschr 1966;44:593.

16. Semm K: Das Pneumoperitoneum mit CO_2. Visum 1967;6:1.

17. Cohen MR: Laparoscopy, culdoscopy and gynecography; technique and atlas. Philadelphia: WB Saunders, 1970.

18. Semm K: Pelvi-Trainer, ein Ubungsgerat fur die operative Pelviskopie zum Erlenen von edoskopischer Ligatur und Nahttechniken. Geburtshilfe Frauenheilkd 1986;46:60.

19. Semm K: Gynaecologic pelvisopy. Obstet Gynecol Digest 1972;14:21.

20. Semm K: Advances in pelviscopic surgery (appendectomy). In Current problems in obstetrics and gynecology. Chicago: Year Book Medical Publishers, 1982;54.

21. Semm K: Die gyneakologische Appendektomie. Gyneakol Prax 1983;7:26.

22. Cuschieri A, Dubois F, Mouiel J, et al: The European experience with laparoscopic cholecystectomy. Am J Surg 1991;161:385.

23. Dubois F, Berthelot G, Levard H: Cholecystectomie par coelisocopie. Presse Med 1989;18:980.

24. Semm K, Mettler L: Technical progress in pelvic surgery via operative laparoscopy. Am J Obstet Gynecol 1980; 138:121.

25. Semm K: Slide atlas for pelviscopy, hysteroscopy and fetoscopy (incl. 240 slides). Keil 1980.

26. Semm K: Die endoskopische intraabdominelle Naht. Geburtshilfe Frauenheilkd 1982;42:56.

27. Semm K; Friedrich ER, trans-ed: Operative manual for endoscopic abdominal surgery. Chicago: Year Book Medical Publishers, 1987.

28. Semm K: Hysterektomie per laparotomiam oder per pelviskopiam. Ein neuer Weg ohne Kolpotomie durch CASH. Geburtshilfe Frauenheilkd 1991;51:996.

29. Semm K: Schmerzreduzierung nach pelvi/-laparoskopischen Eingriffen durch Einblasen von körperwarmem CO_2-gas (Flow-Therme). Gerburtsh u Fravenheilk 1994; 54:300.

Chapter 2

Laparoscopic Surgery: An Atlas for General Surgeons, edited by Gary C. Vitale, Joseph S. Sanfilippo, and Jacques Perissat. J. B. Lippincott Company, Philadelphia, © 1995.

Surgical Endoscopy and the Law

Steven R. Smith

Legal principles influence the practice of endoscopy. The purposes of the various forms of legal regulation are (1) to protect patients from unnecessary injuries by preventing unqualified persons from performing endoscopic procedures and by eliminating faulty equipment; (2) to provide compensation to those injured as a result of the carelessness of physicians, nurses, and others; and (3) to protect the patient's right to make fundamental decisions for themselves (autonomy). Among the legal issues related to all forms of endoscopy are qualifications for practice, professional liability (malpractice), hospital practice, informed consent to treatment, equipment failure, treatment of minors, and confidentiality.

ETHICAL AND LEGAL CONSIDERATIONS

Legal issues raised in endoscopy generally follow legal principles applicable to other areas of medical practice. In some instances, however, special attention is required. For example, the development of a number of new techniques and the special skills they require imply that some formal specialty training should be completed before they are undertaken.[1]

The legal principles discussed in this chapter may not fully describe the law in a particular state for two reasons. First, most of the issues discussed are matters of state law and the law varies somewhat from state to state. Although most states follow the same general principles of law, there are some important differences. For example, several states have modified malpractice principles by statute, and some vary in their approach to minors' consent to treatment.[2] Thus, in any state, there are exceptions or nuances to general legal principles. A second reason for caution is the speed with which the law is changing. Generally, the law related to medicine is in flux, particularly in areas affecting new technology.

The variations in legal principles from state to state and the speed with which the law is changing mean that those practicing endoscopy should pay particular attention to the variations and changes in the law in their own state. It may require that practitioners establish continuing relationships with attorneys. Certainly, institutions such as hospitals should have their policies and practices relating to endoscopy reviewed by an attorney who is competent in the area of health law. It is an area of the law where some early "preventive" activity can avoid future legal problems.

In one technical sense, the M.D. or D.O. degree (as part of a license to practice medicine) may be the only qualification legally required to use endoscopy on humans. A state license permits the holder to practice virtually all kinds of medical or surgical procedures. This broad statement of authority to practice is misleading, however. There are substantial ethical and legal limits on physicians practicing in areas in which they are not fully competent, even if the state license permits a full range of practice—for example, a physician "shall . . . obtain consultation . . . when indicated."[3] The practitioner who practices endoscopy without formal training also risks malpractice liability if the practitioner's quality of care does not conform to that of a well-qualified professional. Such a professional is "holding himself or herself out" as an expert and probably will be held to the standard of care of an expert.[4] The emphasis should be on some kind of *formal* training in endoscopy.[5] Simply reading about new procedures or hearing them described is not sufficient. There should be a period of supervised clinical training in the new techniques. Even a practitioner who has had some formal training in endoscopy should undertake additional training before performing a new technique. Again, the element of adequate supervision by existing experts in the field is of great importance.[6]

In addition to the ethical imperative and liability avoidance value of obtaining good training before endoscopic surgery is undertaken, such training is generally necessary before these procedures are performed in hospitals or other institutions. Indeed, institutions should have policies and procedures in place to ensure that only those properly trained are permitted to perform endoscopic surgical laparoscopic procedures within their institution.

Hospitals have taken on new roles in ensuring the quality of health care. (*Hospitals* is used here broadly to refer to the wide range of institutions in which health care may be practiced.) Hospital accreditation rules, state regulations, and legal liability principles have imposed greater obligation on hospitals.[7] It is important that hospitals take seriously these obligations in surgical endoscopy in terms of the qualifications of those practicing, staff qualifications and training, and equipment acquisition and maintenance.[8] Hospitals have an obligation to ensure that practitioners who undertake complicated diagnosis and treatment within the institution are qualified to do so.[9] The process of granting hospital privileges to practitioners is an important part of this limitation on practice. It is important that hospitals use any existing formally adopted professional standards for determining adequate training.[10] They should also determine that their grant of privileges to practitioners is sufficiently specific to limit practice to those areas in which the physician is adequately trained. Carelessness in the process of granting privileges to a practitioner who turns out to be negligent may result in liability for the hospital.[8]

Hospitals also have a responsibility to review continuously the work of practitioners to ensure that they are competent in the use of new technology and knowledge. The usual range of hospital committees and peer review mechanisms should be adequate for this process if those reviews are meaningful in terms of quality and if they are used to make changes in staff privileges when it appears that a member of the staff is no longer at a reasonably high level of competence in some areas.[11] Actually, privilege adjustment (removing authority to undertake some procedures) is probably the "weak link" in hospital privilege qualification reviews. The competition for patients, the economic pressures caused by Diagnosis Related Groups and similar reimbursement mechanisms, and the closer ties between physicians and hospitals occasioned by delivery systems such as Preferred Provider Organizations may make it more difficult for hospitals to impose these practice limits on otherwise good practitioners.[12] Nevertheless, the hospital that does not make these privilege adjustments is inviting liability for this failure. Fortunately, accrediting standards are helping hospitals undertake such privilege reviews.

In addition, hospitals should determine that practitioners are practicing only within the limits of their privileges and competence. Those who are not privileged to perform specific endoscopic procedures must not be permitted to perform them, and hospitals should not permit physicians without staff privileges in these areas of practice to schedule the procedures.[13] Moreover, nurses and other professionals who see unauthorized practice or practices occurring should report them to supervisors or otherwise try to stop them.[14]

Hospitals have considerable responsibility for the equipment they purchase and maintain for any and all procedures.[15] A hospital should be aware that it has a particularly strong obligation to provide medical equipment that is in proper working order.

Civil liability, or malpractice, may arise from the improper application of surgical endoscopic procedures.[16] Most commonly, these cases are associated with the tort of negligence (a civil action based on the absence of reasonable care), although in rare instances, liability may be based on an intentional tort (eg, battery or intentional infliction of emotional distress) or on a contract (a physician guaranteeing a cure or good result).

Negligence may arise from a number of acts or failure to act. Major sources of medical negligence are:

1. Failure to conduct adequate examinations and tests
2. Careless execution of medical and surgical procedures
3. Inappropriate prescription or administration of drugs
4. Inadequate monitoring of the patient
5. Failure to refer patients to other specialists as needed
6. Unethical conduct that harms a patient

Put most simply, a person is required to act as a reasonably prudent person would under the circumstances. This general obligation is refined for professionals. A physician is expected to act as a reasonably prudent physician would act under the circumstances.

The level of care that is required is not one of perfection. Not every mistake is negligence. A mistake is negligence only if it is an error that a reasonably careful practitioner (or specialist) would not have made under the circumstances.[17] Negligence focuses on a single incident rather than on the general competence or reputation of a practitioner. Just as an outstanding driver may infrequently be negligent by missing a stop sign, an outstanding physician may be negligent in providing a particular medical service to a specific patient on a given day. Finally, note that the level of care that is expected is defined to include the circumstances under which it is given. The law considers circumstances, such as emergency conditions, in determining what a reasonable person would do. In short, malpractice is based on actions that would be considered by the profession itself to be bad practice.[18]

The level of care expected of someone increases as he or she becomes more expert (or in any way claims to be more expert) through special training or experience. Thus, a specialist is expected to have a greater expertise and maintain a higher level of competence in the area of specialty.[19]

In some instances, a practitioner performing certain procedures is treated as though he or she were specially trained in that area of practice because (1) it would be negligent to undertake this procedure without specialty training, (2) it was negligent to not refer the patient to another physician, or (3) the physician had in effect held him- or herself out as being proficient in the procedure. This principle has special relevance in endoscopic surgery because it is likely that any practitioner performing those procedures would be held to a standard of care of someone adequately trained and proficient in them.

Although there are no guarantees that any practitioner can avoid malpractice claims, there are several ways to reduce the risk of a successful claim.[20]

- The most important factor is to engage in good quality, careful medical practice. You should adhere to the highest professional standards.
- Be sure that you are adequately trained before undertaking a diagnostic procedure or treatment. The areas of endoscopic surgery require formal training.[21] Be careful not to claim (directly or indirectly) training or qualifications that you do not have; do not present yourself as being an expert in an area in which you do not have adequate training or experience.
- Refer a patient to other physicians for care or consultation if the required care is not within your area of expertise.
- Maintain the currency of knowledge in your areas of practice. This point is especially important in endoscopic and laser surgery, in which knowledge is advancing rapidly. Establish mechanisms to ensure that you stay current with the changes in your field.
- Be sure that the facility in which care is provided is adequately equipped to provide good emergency care if an unanticipated bad event occurs during treatment. Feel confident in the level of training of the staff at the facility.[22] If you select personnel for your office, do so with care because you will probably be responsible for their negligence.
- Use great caution in undertaking a "nonstandard" treatment (ie, a treatment not generally accepted and used by the rest of the medical community).[23] At the same time, it is important that the most suitable or accepted treatment be provided to a patient and that the practitioner not use outdated techniques or equipment.[24]
- Obtain adequate informed consent (as described in this chapter). Informed consent should be obtained for procedures that are physically invasive. Moreover, in at least an informal way, consent should also be obtained for use of prescription drugs.[25]

The above suggestions for avoiding malpractice are directed toward providing good quality medical service. They help avoid professional negligence. The following suggestions do not reduce the possibility of negligence but they may reduce the odds that a liability claim will be made if negligence occurs. Only a small proportion of negligent treatment results in a legal claim. These suggestions are for avoiding malpractice claims (or for managing them if filed) rather than for avoiding malpractice.

- Avoid unrealistic expectations by the patient and the patient's family. Unrealistic expectations suggest that someone is at fault if anything goes wrong. The informed consent process can be used to develop realistic expectations about the diagnostic procedure or treatment.
- Maintain good communication with patients.[26] Keep them informed. Let them know what to expect in terms of their conditions and their treatments. Except for good medical reasons, do not avoid delivering news, even if it is bad. If something does not go as expected, explain the problem and describe what can be done next.[16] There is considerable debate about whether a physician should tell a patient when the physician has made an error. There is much to be said for being open with patients about error without saying that the error was careless. Others, especially some insurance companies, oppose this form of openness that admits mistakes. In any case, communicate to the patient that you care about them.
- Maintain good records. The records should be as complete an account as possible in explaining why you did something (or did not do it) in addition to what you did. Be aware that others may read these files, so you do not want to put confessions of negligence in them. *Under no circumstances try to alter records*. This alteration is likely to be discovered and will subsequently make you look dishonest.[27]
- If something goes wrong, contact your insurance company immediately. Your insurance contract probably requires that you notify the company of possible claims.
- If something goes wrong, discuss the course of action with your insurance company and others involved (such as the hospital) to determine what should be done regarding the patient. Issues include what to tell the patient and whether to offer a settlement. I believe that it is best to be relatively straightforward and not to charge the patient. Although it is true that in some cases this tactic may give the patient information that could be used against you, it also is likely to reduce the chance that a claim will be filed.

INFORMED CONSENT

The primary purpose of the ethical and legal requirement of informed consent is to implement an important personal interest: the right of patients to determine what is to be done to their bodies (autonomy privacy).[28] Informed consent is essentially a legal doctrine but it may also have medical benefits by preparing the patient for medical or surgical procedures or increasing trust in physicians.[29] It can be used to (1) lower the patient's unrealistic expectations that a procedure is foolproof or guaranteed, (2) increase the patient's feelings of participation in his or her health and health care, and (3) encourage patients to discuss expectations and concerns about treatment.[30] In short, it is an opportunity to improve communication with patients. As such, the process of obtaining informed consent should not be merely a dry legalistic exercise but an important part of the total treatment plan.[31]

Endoscopic and laser surgery are within the group of procedures that require specific informed consent.[32] Other treatments, including some prescription medications, also require some form of informed consent.[33] Although in most states informed consent need not be in writing, a written document or notation helps to prove that information was given and that the patient did indeed consent.

Informed consent is intended to give the patient sufficient information to permit an intelligent decision on whether to accept the proposed treatment or diagnostic procedures.[34] The information generally considered to be essential to informed consent includes the following:[35]

1. Description of the procedure or treatment to be undertaken.
2. Review of the benefits and the risks or hazards of the treatment or procedure
3. Statement of the alternatives to the proposed treatment or procedure
4. Consideration of the consequences and risks of rejecting treatment or diagnosis

Although the specific information changes, depending on the procedure to be performed (or the drug to be prescribed), the basic question is always the same: what information would a person in the patient's position need to make a well-informed decision?

The obligation to provide information about the consequences of refusing the proposed procedure should not be neglected. This obligation is significant when a patient is rejecting or delaying treatment (or a diagnostic process) and the delay may significantly harm the patient. An example of the importance of this obligation is the case in which a patient refused a Papanicolaou smear, developed cancer that went undetected until a cure was impossible, and sued the physician who had recommended the test for failure to warn her of the potentially fatal consequences of her refusal.[36,37] Although this case goes further than most in suggesting liability (it is reasonable to assume that the patient could have been aware of the risk she was taking), it underlines the importance of disclosing the risks of refusal.

There are few widely accepted exceptions to the informed consent requirement.[38] The two major exceptions are commonly referred to as the "emergency exception" and the "therapeutic privilege." Both of these labels are somewhat misleading if taken literally.

The emergency exception is the common sense rule that when someone is incapable of providing consent and immediate treatment is necessary to avoid death or serious injury, the treatment may be undertaken without informed consent.[39] This exception does not apply every time emergency medical treatment is necessary but only when there is a real emergency and there is no way to obtain informed consent (or refusal). It is important to emphasize that there are two requirements for using the emergency exception: the absence of any way of obtaining informed consent and the existence of a health emergency. Ordinarily, when a patient is incompetent to give or refuse consent, the next of kin or guardian gives or refuses it. The emergency exception generally does not apply when it is possible to contact the next of kin or guardian. Also, the emergency exception does not apply when a competent patient refuses consent to important treatment. In such cases, the physician or hospital may seek a court order to provide treatment.[40]

The exception of therapeutic privilege permits information to be withheld from patients if that information would significantly and adversely affect their health. For example, if a patient is likely to become extremely agitated as a result of hearing about certain risks associated with surgery, the information about those risks may be withheld. The decision to withhold information in many circumstances should be made in consultation with the patient's family. Great caution should be exercised in claiming the therapeutic privilege. The physician invoking it should be prepared to demonstrate clearly the necessity of withholding the information and that serious harm is likely to ensue from giving the information to the patient. That the patient would refuse treatment if given the information is not an adequate reason to invoke the privilege.[41]

The concept of informed consent assumes that the patient is legally competent to make decisions relating to his or her medical care. In some circumstances, patients are not competent to make their own decisions because of their age (minors) or mental condition.[42] If a patient is incompetent, the law provides for a substitute decision-maker in the form of a guardian or next of kin.[43]

Traditional common law principles hold that minors are not legally able to consent to treatment for themselves. Minors are generally those younger than the ages of 18 or 21 years (or somewhere between in some states) as defined by state law.[44] A few minors are considered "emancipated" from their parents because of early marriage or a permanent separation from the parental home. They are treated as adults for the purpose of consenting to medical care.[45] Despite considerable evidence that adolescents are able to be effective decision-makers well before the age of 21 (or 18) years, generally, the decision to consent is still vested in the parents or guardians of minors.[46–50] There are exceptions to this general rule, however.

Ideally, the informed consent process should include a written document that sets out the basic information needed by the patient to make a decision to undergo the proposed procedure plus—in instances of serious or risky procedures—at least two oral conversations with the patient (and in most cases the patient's family). One conversation is used to present the information concerning the proposed procedure and to invite questions; the second is used to answer questions and secure consent. It is also desirable for the physician to document these events as soon as possible by summarizing the conversations with the patient, with the family, or both in the patient's chart.

It is not always possible or necessary to undertake this formal "two conversations plus written consent" process. When there is a need for immediate action or the procedure proposed is not risky or invasive, a more informal consent process is in order. Even in these circumstances, where consent is obtained more quickly and informally, the information necessary to make a decision should be imparted to the patient or the substitute decision-maker. Again, it is desirable to make notes of these conversations.

Special consent must be obtained if the patient will be a research subject or will not be receiving generally accepted (standard) medical care. Special consent should be considered if the patient is to be used in teaching.

An example of a consent document that may be used for surgical endoscopy is presented in the appendix of this chapter. No single document can be universally relied on as an informed consent document for all occasions, and consent must be undertaken with the law of the state in which the procedure will be performed kept in mind.[51]

Although there are differing views on this issue, it is wise to develop informed consent documents tailored to specific procedures.[52]

The failure to obtain informed consent may result in civil liability (malpractice). Negligence is usually the tort resulting from the absence of informed consent, although battery is a remote possibility.

The Federal Food and Drug Administration's (FDA) regulation of medical equipment and the liability associated with the equipment are complicated matters that could (and do) fill volumes.[53,54] Liability (as opposed to FDA regulations) is an area that state law generally controls. Therefore, there is diversity in the way states handle it.

The careless design, manufacture, or maintenance of equipment may result in negligence liability. A high degree of care is expected of those who provide medical equipment because they know that any defects are likely to do serious harm to patients. The law requires care not only by the manufacturer of the equipment but also by those who maintain and use it.[55]

A product defect may result from an error in manufacturing or packaging, from an error in designing the product, or from defective labeling (notably, a failure to give adequate warnings or instructions concerning the product).[56] Determining what constitutes a "defect" has caused difficulty, and defining a "design defect" has been particularly troublesome.[43,57] That someone was injured by a product is not sufficient to prove that the product was defective in a legal sense.

From the law, some gross generalizations can be made. Where strict liability is imposed for medical devices or equipment, as a practical matter, the manufacturer is usually responsible for any defect in design or manufacture or for a failure to label or warn properly. The hospital is responsible for failing to pass on to the physician any warning and for defects caused by its mistreatment of the product. Physicians are usually not part of the chain of distribution through which strict liability is passed. Physicians may be negligent, however, for not selecting the proper instrument or equipment, for misusing it, or for failure to inspect it; this liability usually results in negligence rather than in strict liability.[58]

Both physicians and patients probably overestimate the degree to which the confidentiality of information about treatment can be maintained.[59] The protection of confidentiality that the law has given with one hand has often been removed by the other. This suggests that physicians should be cautious in promising absolute confidentiality to information obtained during treatment.[60] At the same time, physicians should be careful not to disclose any patient information without legal justification.[61]

Traditionally, parents must consent to treatment for their minor children.[62] In many states, this rule has been modified somewhat by statute or court decision for some kinds of treatment but as a general matter, consent to treatment is the obligation of parents rather than minor children.[63–72] The Supreme Court has recognized a constitutional right to privacy that includes the right of a "mature" minor to decide to have certain medical treatment.[64,65] A mature minor is one capable of understanding the nature and consequences of a decision (eg, to have an abortion).[66] At the same time, the Court has upheld as being constitutional the state laws that require parental consent, so long as the minor can go to court to obtain consent to treatment that is in his or her "best interest."[67] These issues most often arise in the areas of contraception and abortion.

State statutes allowing minors to consent to treatment may permit or require that the parents be notified of the treatment.[68,69] Where such notification is required, the practitioner should inform the minor at the beginning of the treatment of this requirement.[68] This is an area of the law that practitioners who treat minors should watch closely for changes.

When patients are used as research subjects (eg, in clinical trials of new drugs), special care must be exercised to ensure that they are protected from harm.[73] After the disclosure of Nazi atrocities committed in the name of research, attention was focused on the risks of experimentation.[74] Much human experimentation is controlled by federal law, institutional regulations, and ethical principles. Almost any experimentation undertaken should be first examined by a review body, such as an ethics committee or Institutional Review Board. Institutional Review Board approval is required by the federal government for government-funded studies and human trials of new drugs and devices.[75]

Institutional Review Boards and other review committees should ensure that the potential benefits of the study outweigh the potential risks, that there is adequate informed consent, and that the risks are as limited as possible.[76] This review is intended to protect the patient, but indirectly it also helps to protect the physician by avoiding unnecessary experimental risks.[77]

As the use of surgical endoscopy continues to expand, it is likely to be the subject of increased liability if it is misused and liable to increased regulation by government entities and institutions (eg, a hospital). It is especially important that increasingly sophisticated endoscopic techniques be performed only by those practitioners well trained to perform them and that equipment be carefully maintained. It is also important that the medical profession not "oversell" the value of the technique or suggest that it is risk-free. Such high expectations could lead to the view that if something goes wrong there must have been some negligence.

Finally, the caveat at the beginning of the chapter is crucial to remember: the law relevant to surgical endoscopy varies from state to state and will be in considerable flux during the next decade.

The appendix shows an example of a fairly complete informed consent form for an endoscopic procedure. Because it is tailored to one type of endoscopic surgery, it would not be usable, as is, for all endoscopic procedures. It does provide, however, a general approach that could be readily adapted to fit any occasion. Note particularly that the form assumes that it will be accompanied by a complete discussion(s) with the patient. The form contains several blanks that the physician should complete before providing it to the patient.

References

1. Cullado MJ, Porter JA, Slezak FA: The evolution of surgical endoscopy training. Meeting the American Board of Surgery requirements. Am Surg 1991;57:250.
2. Smith SR: Legal rights of minors. In: Lavery JP, Sanfilippo J, eds. Pediatric and adolescent obstetrics and gynecology. New York: Springer-Verlag, 1985:338.
3. Revised principles of medical ethics. Chicago: American Medical Association, 1980.
4. MacDonald MG, Meyer KC, Essig B: Health care law. A practical guide. New York: Matthew Bender, 1985.
5. Rodning CB, Zingarelli WJ, Webb WR, Curreri PW: Postgraduate surgical flexible endoscopic education. Ann Surg 1986;203:272.
6. Rogers DW: Two simple models for teaching fiberoptic choledochoscopy techniques. Surg Gynecol Obstet 1986; 162:584.
7. Comment: Hospital corporate negligence based on a lack of informed consent. Suffolk Univ Law Rev 1985;19:835.
8. Miller RD: Problems in hospital law. Rockville, MD: Aspen Publications, 1990.
9. Mulholland D III: The evolving relationship between physicians and hospitals. Tort Ins Law J 1987;22:295.
10. Sanfilippo JS, Indman PD: Photo documentation. In: Vitale GC, Sanfilippo JS, Perissat J, eds. Laparoscopic surgery: an atlas for general surgeons. Philadelphia: JB Lippincott. In press.
11. Dent TL: Training, credentialling, and granting of clinical privileges for laparoscopic general surgery. Am J Surg 1991;161:399.
12. Furrow B: Medical malpractice and cost containment: tightening the screws. Case Western Reserve Law Rev 1986;36:985.
13. Murphy EK: Liability for noncompliance with hospital policies, national standards. AORN J 1990;52:1060.
14. Darling v Charleston Community Memorial Hospital, 33 I112d 326, 211 NE2d 253 (1965), cert denied, 383 US 946 (1966).
15. Goerth CR: Failure to comply with industry standards can spell negligence. Occup Health Saf 1986;55:50.
16. Shiffman MA: Medical malpractice—handling general surgery cases. Colorado Springs, CO: Shepard's/McGraw-Hill, 1990.
17. Ficarra BJ, Corso FM: Iatrogenic surgical liability. Leg Med 1985;236.
18. Perdue J: Medical malpractice: new faces, new facts, new fundamentals. St. Mary's Law J 1987;18:955.
19. Michand GL, Hutton MB: The emergence of a specialty standard of care. Tulsa Law J 1979;16:720.
20. Shapiro DL: A clinician's guide to reducing the risk of malpractice. Psychother Priv Prac 1987;5:31.
21. Satava RM: Establishing an endoscopy unit for surgical training. Surg Clin North Am 1989;69:1129.
22. Bailey RW, Imbembo AL, Zucker KA: Establishment of a laparoscopic cholecystectomy training program. Am Surg 1991;57:231.
23. Epstein RA: Legal liability for medical innovation. Cardozo Law Rev 1987;8:1139.
24. Prillaman HL: A physician's duty to inform of newly developed therapy. J Contemporary Health Law Policy 1990;6:43.
25. Brest AN: Malpractice liability and drug therapy. Clin Ther 1987;9:138.
26. Adamson TE, Gullion DS, Tschann JM: Educational implications of the relationship between patient satisfaction and medical malpractice claims. Proc Annu Conf Res Med Educ 1985;24:38.
27. Miller PJ: Documentation as a defense to legal claims. J Am Optom Assoc 1986;57:144.
28. Studer M: The doctrine of informed consent: protecting the patient's right to make informed health care decisions. Montana Law Rev 1987;48:85.

29. Rose RM: Informed consent: history, theory and practice. Am J Otol 1986;7:82.
30. Dodson T: Medical malpractice in the birthplace: resolving the physician-patient conflict through informed consent, standard of care, and assumption of risk. Nebr Law Rev 1986;65:655.
31. Katz J: Informed consent: are "miracle, mystery and authority" better medicine? Conn Med 1986;50:457.
32. Semm K: Operative manual for endoscopic abdominal surgery. Chicago: Year Book Medical Publishers, 1987:20.
33. Gilhooley M: Learned intermediaries, prescription drugs and patient informed consent. St. Louis Univ Law J 1986; 30:633.
34. Rosenberg JE, Towers B: The practice of empathy as a prerequisite for informed consent. Theor Med 1986;7:181.
35. Appelbaum P, Lidz C, Meisel A: Informed consent: legal theory and clinical practice. New York: Oxford University Press, 1987.
36. Truman v Thomas, 27 Cal3d 285, 611 P2d 902, 165 Cal Rptr 308 (1980).
37. Wainess R: Physician's duty to inform patients who refuse "treatment": Truman v Thomas in perspective. Med Trial Tech Q 1986;32:444.
38. Meisel A: The "exceptions" to informed consent. Conn Med 1981;45:27.
39. Smith SR: Legal issues in trauma care. In: Richardson JD, Polk HC, Flint LM, eds. Trauma: clinical care and pathophysiology. Chicago: Year Book Medical Publishers, 1987:569.
40. Kolder VE, Gallagher J, Parsons MT: Court-ordered obstetrical interventions. N Engl J Med 1987;316:1192.
41. Cantebury v Spence, 464 F2d 772n(DC Cir), cert denied, 409 US 1064 (1972).
42. Marsh FH: Informed consent and the elderly patient. Clin Geriatr Med 1986;2:501.
43. Buchanan AE: The limits of proxy decision-making for incompetents. UCLA Law Rev 1981;29:386.
44. Holder AR: Legal issues in pediatric and adolescent medicine. New Haven, CT: Yale University Press, 1985.
45. Working Group of the Northern Region in Current Medical/Ethical Problems: Consent to treatment by parents and children. Child Care Health Dev 1986;12:5.
46. Melton G, Koocher G, Saks M, eds: Children's competence to consent. New York: Plenum Press, 1983.
47. Melton GB: Children's participation in treatment planning: Psychological and legal issues. Professional Psychology 1981;12:246.
48. American Academy of Pediatrics: Committee on Youth. A model act providing for consent of minors for health services. Pediatrics 1973;51:293.
49. Wright TE: A minor's right to consent to medical care. Howard Law J 1982;25:525.
50. Restaino JM Jr: Informed consent: should it be extended to 12-years-olds? A surgeon's view. Med Law 1987;6:91.
51. Appelbaum P, Lidz C, Meisel A: Informed consent: legal theory and clinical practice. New York: Oxford University Press, 1987.
52. Fineberg KS, et al: Obstetrics/gynecology and the law. Ann Arbor, MI: Health Administration Press, 1984.
53. Kahan JS: Medical devices reclassification: the evolution of FDA policy. Food Drug Cosmetic Law J 1987;42:288.
54. Gluck MS: Regulation of medical devices by the Food and Drug Administration. J Clin Monit 1985;1:216.
55. Killian WH: Equipment mishaps may result in lawsuits. Am Nurse 1990;22:34.
56. Agar J: Labeling of prescription devices for the Food and Drug Administration and product liability: a primer. Food Drug Cosmetic Law J 1990;45:447.
57. Keeton WP, Dobbs D, Keeton R, et al: Prosser and Keeton on the law of torts (5th ed). St. Paul, MN: West Publishing, 1984.
58. Maedgen B, McCall S: A survey of law regarding the liability of manufacturers and sellers of drug products and medical devices. St. Mary's Law J 1986;18:395.
59. Smith SR: Constitutional privacy in psychotherapy. George Washington Law Rev 1980;49:1.
60. Bruce JAC: Privacy and confidentiality of health care information. 2nd ed. Chicago: American Hospital Publishers, 1988.
61. Weisman E: Liability for medical record disclosure is real but rare. Hospitals 1990;64:28.
62. Ewald LS: Medical decision making for children: an analysis of competing interests. St. Louis Univ Law J 1982; 25:689.
63. Cole v Jordan, 161 Ga App 409, 288 SE2d 260 (1982).
64. Thornburg v American College of Obstetricians and Gynecologists, 476 US 747 (1986); Bellotti v Baird 443 US 4622 (1979).
65. Carey v Population Services, 431 US 678 (1977).
66. Wright TE: A minor's right to consent to medical care. Howard Law J 1982;25:525.
67. Ehrlich JS, Sabino JA: A minor's right to abortion—the constitutionality of parental participation in bypass hearings. N Engl Law Rev 1991;25:1185.
68. Goldberg SB: Call home: courts may interpret but not rewrite parental notice laws. ABA J 1991;77:86.
69. Moore C: The fog clears from the parental notice laws. Thurgood Marshall Law Rev 1991;16:399.
70. Morrissey J, Hofmann A, Thorpe J: Consent and confidentiality in the health care of children and adolescents: a legal guide. New York: Free Press, 1986.
71. Roe v Wade, 410 US 113 (1973).
72. Secrest SM: Minors' right to abortion. U Detroit Law Rev 1989;66:691.
73. Katz J: Experimentation with human beings. New York: Russell Sage Foundation, 1972.
74. Nuremberg Military Tribunal, The Nuremberg Code, 2: The Medical Cases 181-182 (GPO. 1947), used in United States v Karl Brandt, et al: Trials of war criminals before military tribunals under control law No 10 (Oct 1946–Apr 1949).
75. 21 CFR 50 (1990) [contains FDA regulations regarding research under the jurisdiction of the FDA]; 45 CFR 46 (1990) [regulations subject to HHS jurisdiction].
76. Glass KC, Freedman B: Legal liability for injury to research subjects. Clin Invest Med 1991;14:176.
77. Robertson J: The law of institutional review boards. UCLA Law Rev 1979;26:484.

APPENDIX 2-1: *Informed Consent*

The following is an example of a fairly complete informed consent form for an endoscopic procedure. Because it is tailored to one type of endoscopic surgery, it would not be usable, as is, for all endoscopic procedures. It does provide, however, a general approach that could be readily adapted to fit any occasion. Note particularly that the form assumes that it will be accompanied by a complete discussion(s) with the patient. The form contains several areas that the physician should complete before providing it to the patient.

Consent to Operative Laparoscopy

I understand that Dr. ____________ is recommending that I undergo laparoscopic abdominal surgery to [*describe the purposes of the laparoscopy*].

Description of the procedure. I understand that during this procedure the surgeon or surgeons first perform a diagnostic examination using the laparoscope. This requires creating one or more incisions (cuts) through the abdomen (belly) near the umbilical area (belly button). This incision (or incisions) will probably be about ½″ long per incision (if there is more than one), although the length of the cut can vary. Carbon dioxide is injected into the abdomen as part of the procedure. Other small incisions may be required to insert other instruments. I understand that the process that occurs next depends on the findings during the first part of the operation. If in the judgment of the surgeons treatment can be undertaken using the same endoscopic tube, they will use the endoscope to try to correct any problems. It is possible, however, that the surgeons may decide that it is best to perform major surgery (laparotomy), which requires a large incision in my abdomen. A hospital stay [will] [may] be required. If so, it is usually short with the laparoscopic procedure but is likely to be longer if more extensive abdominal surgery is required.

Risks. I understand that laparoscopy is major surgery. Although it is a relatively safe procedure, it does carry risks. There is a small possibility of cutting or puncturing my intestines or other organs (including reproductive organs), which may result in serious bleeding or interference with the functioning of the organs. An allergic reaction to any of the medications used is also a remote possibility. Infections may occur with any form of surgery, although these are seldom serious. I further understand that it [will] [may] be necessary that I have a general anesthetic during the surgical procedure. Although very infrequent, there may be a need for blood transfusion.

I have been informed that if it becomes necessary to perform abdominal surgery (laparotomy) there are increased risks, including additional pain after surgery and a period of hospitalization and recovery. The risk of infection is also increased. Other risks include damage to the stomach, intestines, or other organs; ruptures in the surgical wound or breathing muscles (diaphragm); burns on the skin; damage to the kidney and urinary system; blood clots in the pelvis and lungs; and allergic reactions. These reactions are rare, although there is a small risk of a serious complication causing permanent disability or death. [*Insert statement in appropriate case, regarding sterility or risk of sterility.*]

Alternatives. An alternative to the laparoscopic surgery is major abdominal surgery but that is not recommended, because it may be unnecessarily risky and painful, until after the initial endoscopic examination has been performed. [*If there are other diagnostic procedures, discuss those possibilities here.*]

I also understand that if it is determined that open abdominal surgery is necessary, it may be possible for the doctors to not perform it immediately but to wait a short time until I have discussed this matter with them further. Because of the additional difficulties and risks, I have decided against this delay. I understand that refusing this procedure may risk my health or life. Because the doctors will not know whether anything is wrong with me without this procedure, it would be risky not to undergo this surgery that they are recommending.

[*If the patient refuses the procedure, it is important to describe the risks of doing so in some detail. Also, see note below concerning research and teaching.*]

Consent. Having been informed of the above and having discussed this operation with my doctor, I consent to Dr. ____________ and such assistants as he/she may designate performing the endoscopic surgical procedures and if necessary, the abdominal surgery (laparotomy), which could include removing and studying or disposing of any tissue or organs that may be necessary or medically desirable. This consent extends to the administration of such anesthetics and medications as may be desirable. I also authorize the doctors to perform other procedures that they may determine are medically desirable or necessary during the course of this operation. I understand that the doctor cannot guarantee the success of this treatment.

I have had all of my questions answered to my satisfaction.

Signed by patient (and where appropriate, a guardian or member of the family); the physician; and at least one witness (a real witness who actually saw it signed).

Note concerning research and teaching. If anything other than a standard, commonly accepted practice is undertaken (including research), additional information *must* be given and special consent *must* be obtained. If the patient is to be used as a significant part of a teaching exercise, special consent should be obtained.

Chapter 3

Laparoscopic Surgery: An Atlas for General Surgeons, edited by
Gary C. Vitale, Joseph S. Sanfilippo, and Jacques Perissat.
J. B. Lippincott Company, Philadelphia, © 1995.

Guidelines for the Future

Gary C. Vitale
Alfred Cuschieri
Jacques Perissat

Laparoscopic surgery of the digestive tract began with laparoscopic cholecystectomy. In March 1987, Philippe Mouret, in Lyon, France, quietly and without fanfare performed a cholecystectomy laparoscopically during a gynecologic procedure. Shock and disbelief were the initial reactions when the report of the procedure was first presented at major national meetings in the United States in April 1989 (Society of American Gastrointestinal and Endoscopic Surgeons, Louisville, Kentucky) and in May 1989 (American Society for Gastrointestinal Endoscopy, Washington, DC). Could anyone at that time have predicted the revolution that has happened since that discreet beginning? The following year, the largest lecture halls at the meeting of the American College of Surgeons in San Francisco were so full that surgeons were standing in the entryways, craning their necks to get a view of the video presentations.

In retrospect, cholecystectomy was an opportune choice for the first laparoscopic procedure. It is an ablative operation that requires identification of few anatomic structures and the outcome regarding postoperative recovery and return to work is easily calculated. The explosion in laparoscopic procedures that followed was unpredictable in breadth and scope. Time must be taken for thoughtful and careful study, comparison, and evaluation of the benefits of performing a given procedure laparoscopically versus the standard open surgical approach. One point to consider is the unproved benefit of a laparoscopic approach for some procedures. Two examples of this are laparoscopic appendectomy and laparoscopic hernia repair. The laparoscopic approach in each of these procedures may increase surgical costs without clear benefit. In the case of appendectomy, recovery after laparoscopic surgery may be no faster than after open appendectomy; with hernia repair, the standard open procedure may prove to be better in terms of hernia recurrence when long-term results are in. The high cost of excessive dependence on technology and the potential adverse consequence of differences in operative technique required to accommodate the laparoscopic approach are thus important factors.

Finally, surgeons may tend to perform certain procedures more frequently because of the perceived ease of access with laparoscopy. This pressure to operate may come from the patient, who feels that the simplicity of laparoscopy is such that he or she should go ahead with an operation that may have been otherwise postponed (e.g., cholecystectomy for asymptomatic or minimally symptomatic gallstones). If the laparoscopic revolution is to move forward effectively, these issues must be addressed responsibly. This can only be achieved by a series of prospective clinical trials. The management of common duct stones is a case in point. There are several options for treating a patient with choledocholithiasis: endoscopic retrograde cholangiopancreatography (ERCP) with stone extraction (pre- or postoperatively), or laparoscopic (transcystic or transcholedochal) or open common duct exploration. All these treatment options are potentially highly successful; consequently, all the discussion in the world will not resolve the issue without clinical trials. Not only must the medical issues be addressed, but the economic issues also need to be explored in evaluating these options.

The difficulty of constructing and executing valid clinical trials to decide these issues is twofold. First, it is difficult to recruit patients to the traditional arm of a prospective study after there has been widespread acceptance of a new technique, as has occurred with laparoscopic surgery. Second, these clinical trials must be conducted by surgeons who are experienced with laparoscopic techniques for the trial to be valid. Experience varies among surgeons with many of the new techniques, particularly among academic centers in which such trials may be mounted. Those surgeons who are familiar with the new techniques may be unwilling to do half of their operations the older way, even in the interest of collecting important prospective data.

A few principles need to be adhered to as we move forward. Endoscopic surgery is not new but new applications require a relearning of basic surgical skills as they relate to laparoscopy. Proper training and credentialing should go a long way toward gaining acceptance of new, advanced laparoscopic surgical procedures. We may find controls being placed on laparoscopic approaches by third-party payers if we do not act individually and corporately as surgeons to establish good training centers and adequate credentialing procedures. The public is increasingly aware of the possibility of laparoscopic surgery being performed by those who are not adequately trained. The lack of a broadly accepted definition of adequate training is a glaring deficiency, which must be corrected. Remaining faithful to the traditional guidelines of surgical indications and therapeutics is critical while executing careful prospective studies to assist in developing new criteria and directions. With careful attention to these issues and continued commitment to technical excellence and training, these problems will be resolved.

Technical advances in certain areas are critical for the advancement of laparoscopy. Two-dimensional imaging systems are in existence. As three-dimensional systems are developed, improved, and adopted, the learning curve of the neophyte laparoscopist will also improve. Use of a two-dimensional system results in only a learned reflex or mental reconstruction that allows the surgeon to maneuver in the third dimension. The time necessary to develop these reflexes is variable. In the beginning, the surgeon is in a strange environment and again experiences the fumbling and hesitation of his or her early years as a resident. True three-dimensional imaging will certainly reduce this visual handicap and allow a more direct translation of traditional operating skills to the laparoscopic arena. With existing three-dimensional systems, there is a significant reduction of light (about two thirds), resulting from the eyewear necessary to view the image. This is true for all types of three-dimensional systems. In addition, there is no accommodation for distance from the telescope to the surgical site with these systems as a result of their fixed focal lengths.

Head-mounted displays have been touted as being capable of creating the ultimate virtual reality environment for the surgeon. With these devices, the surgeon feels as though he or she has indeed entered the peritoneal cavity because the entire field of vision is filled with the image. The disadvantage of a head-mounted display system is that the surgeon is isolated from the rest of the surgical team and the operating-room environment; the system may also reduce the intuitive reflex reactions that are necessary to conduct the overall operation. In other words, being able to see one's hands as one operates may allow certain movements to be made more smoothly or naturally. Conversely, improvements in the high-resolution image generated by today's multichip cameras will be important. The issue of orientation of the monitor to the alignment of hand, eye, and body position is being investigated. A moving ceiling-mounted monitor that automatically adjusts position when there is a change in the hand–eye axis of the surgeon has benefits that any endoscopic surgeon immediately appreciates. Similarly, robotic camera holders have been developed that can automatically zoom in and out, pan right and left, or tilt. Computer-coordinated remote-tracking systems are being developed that may allow subtle movements of the operating camera based on eye movement, as detected by tracking cameras focused on the surgeon's eyeballs. This type of tracking intelligence would greatly enhance the surgeon's ability to proceed faster in procedures such as colectomy, in which constant repositioning of the camera is necessary as the dissection progresses.

One of the main advantages of open surgery that is lost with the laparoscopic approach is tactile sensation. Pressure receptors in the fingertips allow quick confirmation of pulsation in a suspected artery or development of a tissue plane between adjacent loops of bowel. Direct cutting with cautery is more difficult without that direct touch, and careful time-consuming dissection is necessary to ensure that no vital structures are cut. Human interface technology will certainly encompass this aspect of virtual reality, transferring pressure and tactile sensory input from the operative field to remote adjacent devices that the surgeon may be able to wear, such as gloves. The surgeon would get a true "feel" of the tissue, whereas under telescopic vision, he or she directs the servo-slave device to squeeze the tissue in question. Development of these types of microsensors to detect pressure, temperature, touch, and position is not far off; indeed, they are being actively investigated for nonmedical virtual reality applications. The microtechnology required for such real-time human interfaces already exists; only time will tell how quickly it can be adapted to our surgical systems and needs.

An additional area for development is the simultaneous endoscopic and laparoscopic approach. In treating certain upper gastrointestinal, hepatobiliary, and pancreatic diseases, the use of a peroral endoscope, passed while the patient is undergoing laparoscopy, may help in the performance of a specific procedure. In the case of a perforated ulcer, endoscopes have been used to help perform an omental patch closure of the perforation. In these cases, a snare has been used to grasp the laparoscopically prepared omentum and pull it into the perforated ulcer. In common duct stone cases, a wire may be passed through the cystic duct into the duodenum. Simultaneously, a side viewing endoscope may be passed to perform a wire-guided sphincterotomy to assist in stone extraction. These examples represent a beginning to the possibility of joint endoscopic–laparoscopic work. Biliary enteric anastomosis, drainage of pancreatic pseudocysts, and laser ablation of biliopancreatic tumor obstruction may be amenable to innovative new techniques. With more surgeons becoming trained in interventional endoscopy and endoscopic retrograde cholangiopancreatography (ERCP), creative new work can be expected in this field in the next decade.

We certainly stand on an important threshold as we move into the 21st century. It may be fortuitous that laparoscopy exploded onto the general surgical scene with such great force at the beginning of this decade. The tremendous commercial competition that it engendered has tapped the inventive genius of the medical-engineering world. Gynecologists are finally getting some of the instrumentation and equipment that they sorely needed and had requested for years. Laparoscopy is not new; Palmer in the 1940s and Semm, Manhes, and Bruhat in the 1960s and 1970s deserve recognition and homage for the great centers of excellence that they developed during those years, in which 80% of the gynecologic surgery was performed laparoscopically. Urologists, orthopedists, and thoracic surgeons did not completely abandon endoscopic surgery; yet these disciplines have not seen the explosion of inventive attention that abdominal surgery has generated. Some of this may be because of the broad nature of abdominal surgery but more likely, laparoscopy was an idea whose time had truly come technologically. With the world of fiberoptics, microelectronics, and computerization all coming of age during the past decade, the timing may have been perfect for a laparoscopic revolution. Certainly the rapidity with which all of these techniques have been so universally adopted could not have been predicted.

The next important area for development may be the human–computer interface systems, which will greatly expand the sense of being able to perform laparoscopic surgery with the same tactile sense as open surgery. This will take significant investment and research but would represent a meshing of technologic advances that has unlimited potential. At least for today's surgeons, the sky is the limit for creative enterprise, so let us seize the moment and move our specialties forward in a way and on a scale that may not happen again for many generations.

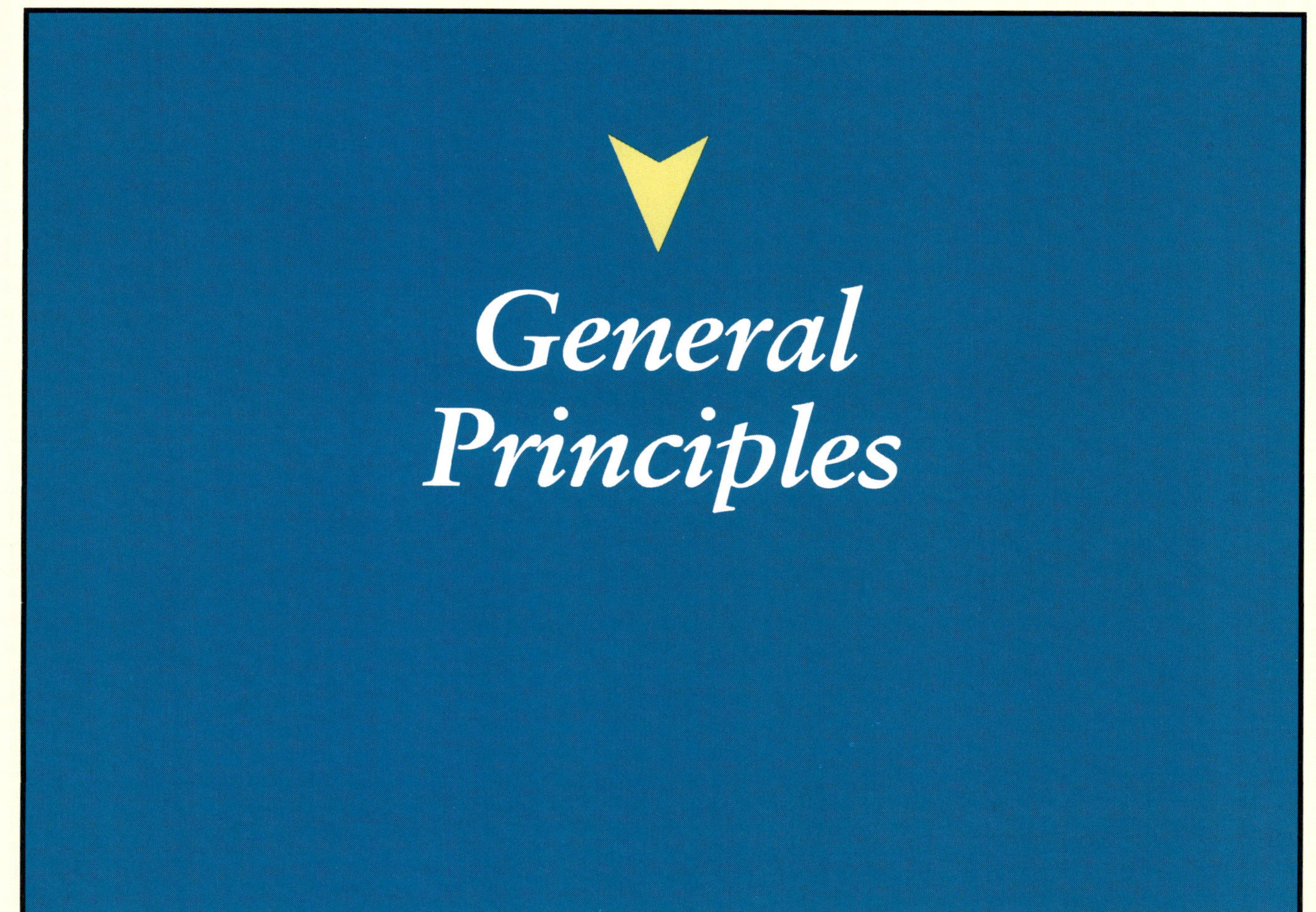

General Principles

Chapter 4

Laparoscopic Surgery: An Atlas for General Surgeons, edited by Gary C. Vitale, Joseph S. Sanfilippo, and Jacques Perissat. J. B. Lippincott Company, Philadelphia, © 1995.

Credentialing

Gary C. Vitale

Laparoscopic surgery involves the use of techniques that most practicing general surgeons do not have experience with from their residency training. This creates the problem of determining what constitutes adequate training for postresidency acquisition of these skills. Although large reported series generally document that laparoscopic cholecystectomy can be performed without increase in common duct injury as compared with historic controls, many complications including laparoscopic common duct injuries are never reported.[1–3] It is the impression of those who are managing the complications on a tertiary referral basis that the incidence of common duct injury during laparoscopic cholecystectomy was certainly high in the first 3 years after the introduction of the procedure, although it may be decreasing.[4,5]

Is it acceptable in the name of progress for patients to undergo a higher risk of complication during the early experience of surgeons learning a new technique? The potential complications in performance of complex advanced laparoscopic procedures (e.g., colon resection and Nissen fundoplication) are serious and argue for careful credentialing and verification of clinical competence.

The problem in developing national standards for credentialing is twofold. First, the educational experiences available for practicing surgeons are varied. Second, granting of clinical privileges is a local hospital-based process and the possibility of different approaches to the problem is as great as the diversity of hospitals in the United States.[6] The first step is agreement on which procedures require a special credentialing process. The second is to agree on standardized educational requirements. The third is widespread adoption of requirements for clinical privileges at the hospital level. It is this last requirement that is almost impossible to tackle in our existing medical system. It is certainly possible that third-party payers will provide the needed pressure for standardization by refusing payment to all but those who comply with a regional or national set of criteria for credentialing of laparoscopy.

The Society of American Gastrointestinal and Endoscopic Surgeons has set forth guidelines for the granting of privileges in laparoscopy that encompass all of the foregoing points. This document, prepared by the organization's credentials committee, argues for separate privileges for each new major laparoscopic procedure; defines adequate educational programs, with hands-on animal laboratory experience; and delineates the roles of preceptors and proctors in the granting and maintenance of clinical privileges at the hospital level. This document is the most comprehensive and accepted credentialing standard available at the national level. General surgeons should argue for use of this document as a standard for their hospital credentials committee as a protection to both themselves and the hospital as the indications and use of laparoscopy expand.

Credentials entitle an individual to confidence, credit, or authority. In the field of laparoscopic surgery, specific and formal guidelines are essential for the credentialing body of an institution to determine an individual's competence in the performance of these procedures, including the use of the laser. The following summarizes criteria for credentialing set forth by the Society of American Gastrointestinal and Endoscopic Surgeons:[7]

- The individual must have completed a residency in general surgery and must be board-certified or an active candidate for certification.
- The surgeon must be privileged in the performance of the procedure by open surgery for which laparoscopic privileges are being sought.

If the surgeon has completed a surgical residency that included advanced laparoscopy, the specifics of the experience should be confirmed in writing from the program director. This should include details of the individual's experience as assistant and operating surgeon and observed skill while in training.

For individualized training postresidency, the individual shall have completed a course especially designed for advanced laparoscopic surgery. Such a course should be university-sponsored or should have received the approval of an academic surgical society. It should include:

- Didactic and video material that teaches and exemplifies the principles of laparoscopic surgery, equipment, and laser use, including safety factors
- Sufficient time in a "hands-on" animal laboratory to allow demonstrations and student performance of safe techniques for tissue handling, suturing, knot tying, and stapling
- Surgeon preceptor written documentation that the individual seeking credentials has reached a satisfactory level of competence in performing the procedures in the animal model

Courses that do not have hands-on training supervised by experienced laparoscopic surgeons are not acceptable.

On completion of course work, the newly trained surgeon should first observe and then assist experienced laparoscopic surgeons in performing the procedures for which credentials are sought. The neophyte laparoscopist should then perform each procedure while being assisted by surgeons experienced in that procedure. A proctoring system should be established by the credentials committee of the institution, and a proctor should be assigned to observe the surgeon's first case of each procedure for which credentials are being sought. The proctor should be responsible to the privileging committee and not to the surgeon who is seeking credentials. The proctoring should not occur at the same session as that when the surgeon seeking credentials is assisting an experienced surgeon but should be when he or she is acting alone as the operating surgeon. The proctor should complete a standard evaluation form, rating surgical performance in several areas, including familiarity with equipment, safe access technique and tissue handling, in addition to appropriate technical performance of the operation in question.

Periodic review of performance should be required for renewal of privileges. Criteria should include frequency of performance of a given procedure, complications, tissue review, adequacy of continuing education, and experience specifically related to laparoscopy. Although most of these may already be in place as part of the quality assurance program of the institution, the delineation of these factors specifically for privileges in laparoscopic surgery is warranted given its extensive use and the difficulty of obtaining and maintaining skills. Strict adherence to standards for credentialing and renewal of privileges will improve safety and should provide a more widespread acceptance of advanced laparoscopic surgery by patients as well as the medical community at large.

References

1. Ress A, Sarr G, Nagorney D, Farnell M, Donohue J, McIlrath D: Spectrum and management of major complications of laparoscopic cholecystectomy. Am J Surg 1993;165:665.
2. Soper N, Flye M, Brunt M, et al: Diagnosis and management of biliary complications of laparoscopic cholecystectomy. Am J Surg 1993;165:663.
3. Larson G, Vitale G, Casey J, et al: Multipractice analysis of laparoscopic cholecystectomy in 1,983 patients. Am J Surg 1992;163:221.
4. Vitale G, Stephens G, Wieman T, Larson G: Use of endoscopic retrograde cholangiopancreatography in the management of biliary complications after laparoscopic cholecystectomy. Surgery 1993;114:806.
5. Ponsky J, Howerton R: Complications of laparoscopic cholecystectomy. Comp Surg 1994;13:461.
6. Dent T: Training, credentialling, and granting of clinical privileges for laparoscopic general surgery. Am J Surg 1991; 161:399.
7. Granting of privileges for laparoscopic (peritoneoscopic) general surgery. Los Angeles: Society of American Gastrointestinal Endoscopic Surgeons, 1993.

Laparoscopic Surgery: An Atlas for General Surgeons, edited by Gary C. Vitale, Joseph S. Sanfilippo, and Jacques Perissat. J. B. Lippincott Company, Philadelphia, © 1995.

Chapter 5

Photo Documentation

Joseph S. Sanfilippo
Paul D. Indman

WHAT IS DOCUMENTATION?

Documentation is simply the recording of observed phenomena. Every physician devotes a significant amount of time to graphically recording—in some form—that which he or she observes in the practice of medicine. Most often, it takes the form of written notes and diagrams but occasionally it consists of radiographs, photographs, or electronic images. In each instance, the record is meant to preserve what is seen, heard, or thought regarding a patient. The purpose is not to satisfy requirements of the record room or to protect against litigation, as it often seems, but to assist in solving a problem, arriving at a diagnosis, or recording the specifics of treatment for future reference. Therefore, every form of documentation is important to the physician as he or she attempts to solve health problems. For example, should a complication occur, review of a videotape of the procedure may help to determine the cause and prevent a similar occurrence in the future.

Most forms of traditional documentation are subjective, to a degree. They often reflect the background and prejudice of the observer as much as they do the object of observation. The written progress note or office note or the dictated operative summary is at best interpretative; in the vernacular of modern technology, they are not transportable.

Documentation thus means acquiring, transporting, and storing visual images to make them available to a multitude of secondary observers, providing them the opportunity to draw their own conclusions based on the "raw" observed material.

TYPES OF DOCUMENTATION

Written Documentation

To record surgical procedures, operative dictation is the form most widely used and that which is most familiar to surgeons. Its primary purpose is to record details of the operative procedure and observed findings for the patient's permanent record. Although this record intends to inform future readers exactly what was seen and done, for many reasons it often fails to do so. Frequently, the creation of this record is delegated to the junior member of the operating team. It may be merely a recitation of the details of the technique, with little attention given to the actual findings. Far too often, physicians dictate long after the operation, when it is impossible to accurately remember the findings or exactly what was done.

It has been suggested that the operative report be complemented by anatomic drawings that accurately identify abnormalities or lesions. Unfortunately, the wide range of artistic talent found among surgeons makes this potentially useful addition variable in accomplishment and value.

In today's litigious climate, the operative report—with or without an accompanying sketch—often assumes more importance for the medical record librarian and hospital administrators than it does for the medical care of the patient. At its best, it is only an *interpretation* of the findings and therefore never more than a subjective form of documentation.

Visual Imaging

Conversely, direct visual documentation usually is objective. As applied to operative laparoscopy, it is accomplished by any one or a combination of three technical modalities: (1) still photography, (2) cine photography, and (3) video imaging.

STILL PHOTOGRAPHY

All imaging involves the recording of an observed object on a sunlight-sensitive medium. The medium itself may be (1) sensitive to light directly (e.g., silver halide film); (2) influenced secondarily by magnetic fields that in turn are dimensioned by light (e.g., magnetic videotape); or (3) influenced by electronic signals, the value of which is determined by light (e.g., digital discs, laser discs). The degree of sensitivity of the medium to light in any documentation system depends on the type of recording equipment used.

Although all three systems (still photography, cine photography, and video imaging) are used to document laparoscopic surgery, illumination of the observed object is provided by a separate light source that is designed to work with laparoscopic recording equipment. The light source is usually the same as that used with the endoscope but most still photography systems also contain a built-in electronic flash unit.

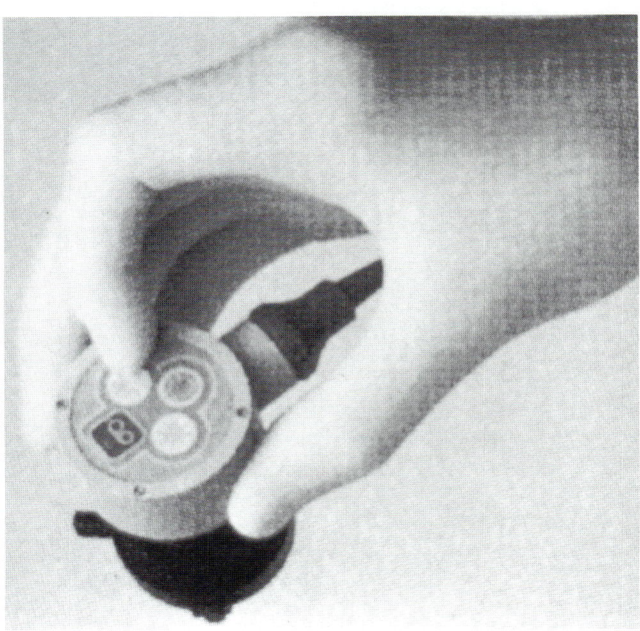

FIGURE 5-1. Microchip camera with light-gain booster capabilities. (Courtesy of Circon, Inc., Stamford, CT).

CINE PHOTOGRAPHY

The optical axis, through which light must travel to the object and return to the sensitized medium in the camera, is composed of the lens systems of both the camera and the laparoscope to which it is attached. The optical characteristics of this axis are subject to many factors that directly influence image quality. To achieve consistently high-quality visual documentation, the laparoscopic surgeon should take time to understand the interdependence of these factors as well as those basic principles that govern imaging and the lighting on which it depends.

BASICS OF VIDEO IMAGING

Modern videocameras for endoscopic use consist of a lens and one or more solid-state image sensing chips (Figs. 5-1 and 5-2). A chip converts the image into an electronic signal that can be processed and sent to a video monitor and recorder. Each chip is composed of thousands of tiny sensors (pixels), each of which corresponds to one point on the picture. High-quality cameras, designed for broadcast use, use a separate chip for each of the three light primary colors (red, green, blue). Because the chips cannot sense color, the image must be broken down into primary colors by a prism and colored filters. Most endoscopic and home video cameras use a single chip; however, high-quality cameras used in broadcasting have a separate chip for each of the three light primary colors.

The National Television Standards Committee

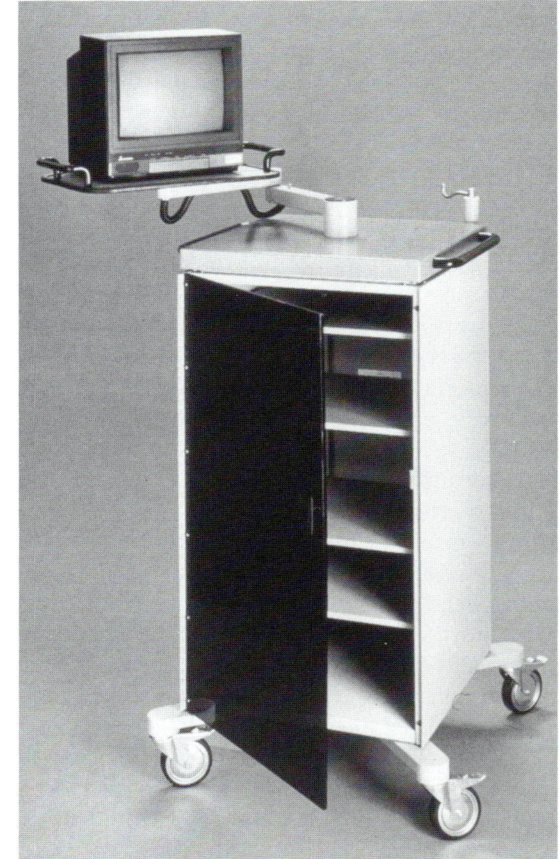

FIGURE 5-2. Monitor mounted on cabinet for video equipment.

(NTSC) video signal is the standard signal in the United States; produced by home and industrial video cameras and recorders, it only requires one cable for transmission. To understand the newer video systems, it is necessary to understand the process of creating the composite signal.

The video image in the NTSC system is composed of luminance (black and white) and chrominance (color) components. The backbone of the signal is the luminance information, to which the chrominance information is added by changing the timing or "phase" of the signal. *The process of encoding the red, green, blue signal into a composite NTSC signal causes significant degradation of the image.* One of the most noticeable resulting artifacts is called "dot crawl." This is best demonstrated by observing a pattern of color bars on the monitor. If the signal has been NTSC-encoded, the edges of the bars can be seen to consist of little squares or dots. This interferes with edge sharpness and causes colors to "bleed" into one another.

Many newer cameras provide a "Y/C" (luminance–chrominance) output. The Y/C connector actually consists of two connectors: one for luminance and one for chrominance. Many newer monitors accept a Y/C input. The resulting image is free of the dot-crawl that degrades the NTSC signal, has decreased bleeding of colors from one area to another, and is superior in quality to a composite image.

When using a Y/C system, it is essential to maintain the signal in component (Y/C) form throughout the system. The Y/C (or S) connectors must be used from the video camera to the video recorder and from the video recorder to the monitor. If the Y/C signal is converted to a composite NTSC signal at any point, the subsequent signal contains all the created artifacts, degrading the final image.

Image Quality

When performing surgery while viewing a video monitor, instead of looking directly through an endoscope, the surgeon depends on a detailed and accurate electronic image of the surgical field (Fig. 5-3). Laparoscopy also has a wider brightness range (dynamic range) because of bright reflections from shiny surfaces and from the white ovary in the female patient. It is essential to use the finest video equipment available because the video camera becomes the surgeon's eye.

Many factors affect the final quality of the picture. Resolution, commonly touted as the sole criterion by which to judge a camera, is only one measure of image quality. Resolution indicates the number of vertical lines that can be distinguished in the picture: the higher the number, the better the resolution. Single-chip cameras usually employ a ½″ chip that is capable of resolving 300 to 330 lines and occasionally up to 450 lines. Industrial and broadcast three-chip cameras commonly resolve 600 to 700 lines. A monitor capable of displaying this high resolution is needed to reproduce this detail. The increased resolution of the three-chip camera is most apparent when it is used for laparoscopy.

Every video image contains video "noise." This is the video equivalent of the "hiss" or "static" that is heard on the radio. It appears as "snow" or graininess in the picture. Video noise is greater in the red region; unfortunately, that is the color most often reproduced in endoscopy. The relative amount of noise is measured by the signal-to-noise ratio (SNR), expressed in decibels (dB);

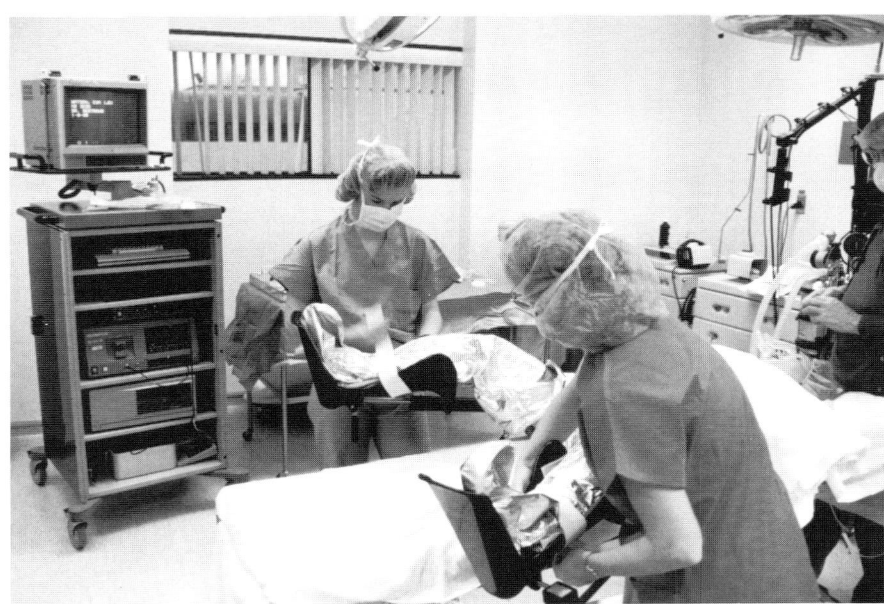

FIGURE 5-3. Room setup for laparoscopic surgery. Video monitor is located so that surgeon and assistant can both observe the intraoperative proceedings.

higher SNRs indicate less noise. The three-chip industrial and broadcast cameras have SNRs of 60 dB or greater, indicating reduced video noise. This is a major reason that images produced by these cameras are better than simple comparison of resolution figures predicts.

Some cameras offer a "low light" or increased-gain setting. It should be understood that amplifying the video signal also amplifies the noise, so the increase in sensitivity is offset by a proportional increase in noise. In selecting a camera, it is thus necessary to compare light sensitivity at a given SNR. Any camera can be made to appear more sensitive by increasing the gain but this is achieved at the expense of a decreased SNR.

Extremely bright areas can overload the camera and cause "ringing" or "blooming." This is a situation in which a bright highlight appears to spill into other areas. This problem is particularly noticeable in the numerous specular reflections from peritoneal surfaces that occur during laparoscopy.

Some cameras incorporate "edge enhancement." This may give the false appearance of increased sharpness but does not actually increase resolution. When such cameras are used for hysteroscopy or laparoscopy, video noise is significantly increased, colors may "bleed" into adjacent areas, and the overall image suffers. Adjusting the monitor may partially compensate for this but it is preferable to have the camera manufacturer adjust the unit so that color saturation is not overemphasized.

It is important to select a video system with as broad a dynamic range as possible. If the system has poor dynamic range, light-colored objects such as an ovary "white out" and lack detail, whereas dark objects or objects slightly farther away from the laparoscope are dark and lack detail. A system with a wide dynamic range may appear to have less contrast in the middle tones; this should not be mistaken for lower resolution or less detail. The ability to see detail in the highlights as well as in the shadows is essential.

Dynamic Imaging

If the ancient Chinese adage that a picture is worth a thousand words is true, a continuous series of pictures (e.g., cine or video frames) is worth infinitely more. The most useful record of any laparoscopic procedure is that which is dynamic. Whether recorded photographically (cine) or electronically (video), the "live" moving record of the procedure adds to the dimension of time, making this type of documentation more meaningful to a subsequent observer.

Electronic Imaging

It was predictable that the introduction of electronic imaging in the 1970s would impede and eventually severely restrict the future of increasingly expensive silver halide technology for dynamic imaging in medicine. Movie making was simply too much trouble to be practical for use in pelviscopic surgery. The use of increasingly smaller microprocessors in video camera design in the 1980s has produced smaller lightweight units that have good resolution and are capable of providing a wide variety of video documentation in medicine. The technology has grown so rapidly that in mid-1987, the National Library of Medicine listed in Index Medicus some 804 references on video applications in medicine.

With the capability of extreme miniaturization afforded by the microchip camera, an entirely new technical development has emerged: direct video endoscopy (see Fig. 5-1). The camera is mounted at the distal end of the endoscope and does not require a transmitting system to carry light to the microchip. Direct endoscopy was first developed for use with flexible gastrointestinal endoscopes but has been quickly adapted to rigid laparoscopes.

Continuous video monitoring offers several benefits that more than compensate for the inconvenience of having to learn to manipulate instruments while watching the monitor's screen. What is perhaps the greatest benefit has little to do with documentation but derives from allowing a procedure to be seen by all members of the operating team.

As gastrointestinal and other flexible endoscopes transmit the image through an array of flexible fibers, the image is comprised of a pattern of dots. This dot pattern, which limits the resolution of the instrument, can be eliminated by placing the camera chip at the distal end of the endoscope. In contrast, rigid telescopes (e.g., the laparoscope) use a lens system that transmits a high-resolution image, so there is less to gain by placing the chip at the distal end. A single small chip placed at the distal end should yield far less resolution than a three-chip camera placed proximally. The placement of a video camera at the proximal end of the laparoscope allows the laparoscopes to be interchanged; one does not need a separate camera for each laparoscope. Because it is not uncommon to use a 10-mm 0°, a 10-mm 30°, and a 5-mm laparoscope during a single procedure, the additional cost of a built-in camera for each laparoscope may be substantial.

A unique advantage of electronic imaging is the ability to combine simultaneous visual and audio signals on the same magnetic tape. In addition to providing an incomparable record of pelviscopic surgery, the videotape also can be used to educate the patient.

STORAGE AND ARCHIVING

The best storage place may well be within the patient's record; in the case of still photographs, at least some documentation should be placed in this record. It is es-

TABLE 5-1
Information Required on Slide, Film, or Tape

Document number
Hospital number
Date of procedure
Diagnosis
Patient name
Patient age
Operation
Key words

sential to review and edit all videotapes. An edited second-generation tape, to be shown to the patient or a colleague, is often useful later. The review should take place as soon after the procedure as is practical. If the tape is to be used for teaching purposes, the patient's permission must be obtained and all identifying information edited out. The expertise of the hospital's audiovisual department in the dubbing and editing of the videotape or film is helpful.

Color slides can be kept in plastic slide sheets (20 to a page in three-ring binders) or more conveniently, in special storage cabinets. Storage boxes are available for videotapes (VHS or beta formats). Photographic material should be kept in a dry, somewhat cool place. Ideally, a separate file cabinet for these items is placed away from direct sunlight and other sources of heat.

The identifying data on the slide, film, or tape should include information as outlined in Table 5-1.

Videodisc Recording

In the near future, archival material will be laser-recorded or laser-read optical discs. A record only 8 inches in diameter is capable of storing about 15,000 color transparencies. Each "slide" in storage is a digitalized representation of the original and from the electronic standpoint, is merely another record in a computer database. It is instantly retrievable, making it possible for someone lecturing on the East Coast to show "slides" on the West Coast without physically moving anything.

Laser-recordable optical discs of the record-once-and-read-only type are helpful (Fig. 5-4). Actual pits are burned into the optical discs by the laser during the process of recording (SONY Corporation, New York, NY). The method uses what is known as Langmuir-Blodgett (LB) thin-film technology. Langmuir-Blodgett films are extremely thin with 2.5- to 10-nm layers (10 to 40 molecules) of phthalocyanine. When applied to optical-disc recording, mixtures of organic dyes are used in the film and are made to absorb light by predictable laser-induced disordering of their structure. A laser writes information to the LB layer on the disc, creating the light-absorbing spots in the LB thin-film.

Erasure of the information is made possible by subjecting the LB layer to suitable temperature and humidity, which reverses the disordering and restores the layer to its original condition. Technology should eventually permit the precise localized erasure of selected segments of information.

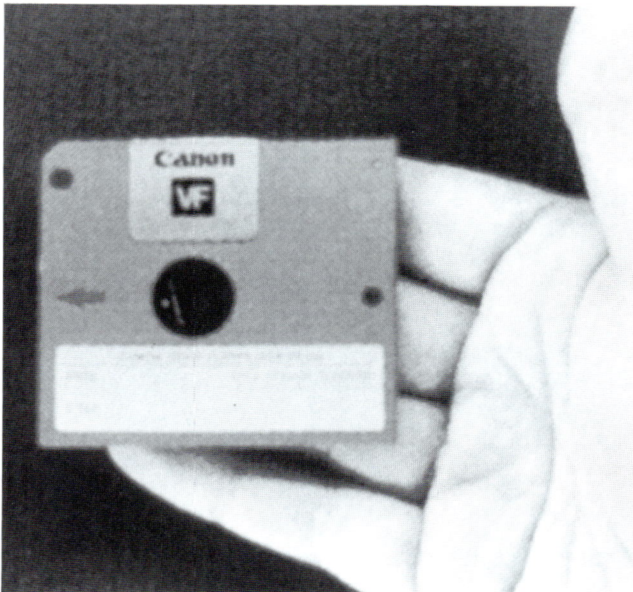

FIGURE 5-4. Laser-recordable optical discs for storage and record-once-and-read-only information.

Using the same LB thin-film technology, the SONY Corporation is developing a process to lay down multiple LB films that are sensitive to different absorbance frequencies, making it possible for a disc to hold several images, separately accessed by lasers of different colors. The capacity of the optical discs will increase sufficiently to make practical the storage of dynamic images.

Within the next 5 years, creating digital archives for virtually all visual imaging will become routine. Physical storage space will shrink to a fraction of that required by today's analogue technology and both local and remote retrieval will be almost immediate.

STERILIZATION OF DOCUMENTATION EQUIPMENT

With the exception of medical video cameras, it is not possible to sterilize those parts of the documentation system handled by the surgeon or those that must be close to the operative field. Therefore, an effort to minimize the risk of bacterial contamination of susceptible tissues is mandatory.

Newer video cameras and connecting cables are carefully sealed to protect their electronic components against moisture. Sterilization of the video camera that is used for arthroscopy is crucial because the knee joint has a relatively low level of defense against bacteria.

Whenever an instrument is removed from the abdominal cavity, it is placed with the distal (sterile) end on the surface of the instrument table, with the proximal (contaminated) end extending beyond the edge of the table.

Drapes designed for arthroscopy can be used for laparoscopy. An intermediate alternative is to have the surgeon wear double gloves, removing the outer gloves before handling any sterile instrument. Preservation of the bacterial integrity of the operative field falls far short of true barrier protection and is not recommended for pelviscopic surgery. Intraabdominal infection resulting from technique contamination is extremely rare, vindicating the common use of nonsterile documentation equipment at laparoscopy.

CONCLUSION

In an increasing number of areas of medicine—and in endoscopic surgery in particular—visual documentation has a vital role to play in both the evaluation and treatment of the patient. Acquiring skill in documentation techniques should therefore be an integral part of the training for endoscopic surgery. The tremendous advances in technology during the past decade have given the surgeon who performs endoscopic procedures an impressive array of documentation equipment to record and store findings.

The documentation objectives should be decided on, thoroughly learned, and used until they no longer satisfy the requirements of that setting. A wide range of inexpensive visual documentation technology is available, making it possible for most physicians to easily obtain and retrieve useful and objectively accurate records for an expanding variety of uses.

Suggested Readings

Jameson D, Roberts L: Interactive video: a new approach to training. Occup Health (Lond) 1987;39:88.

Lardennois B, Adnet JJ, Oismayo C, et al: The storing of medical images on videodisc lasers. Presentation of the first instructional videodisc in urology. Acta Urol Belg 1987;55:113.

Leventhal J: Visual documentation. In: Sanfilippo JS, Levine RL, eds. Operative gynecologic endoscopy. New York: Springer-Verlag, 1989:148.

Mannheim LA: Thin-film for erasable discs. Funct Photog 1987; 22:49.

Satava RM: A comparison of direct and indirect video endoscopy. Gastrointest Endosc 1987;33:69.

Wamsteker K: Documentation in laparoscopic surgery. Baillieres Clin Obstet Gynecol 1989;3:625.

Wigton RS: The new knowledge bases: CD-ROM and medicine. MD Comput 1987;4:34.

Chapter 6

Laparoscopic Surgery: An Atlas for General Surgeons, edited by Gary C. Vitale, Joseph S. Sanfilippo, and Jacques Perissat. J. B. Lippincott Company, Philadelphia, © 1995.

Instrumentation and Knot-Tying

Joseph S. Sanfilippo

INSTRUMENTATION

Preparation of Patient and Surgeon Before Surgery

Appropriate preoperative discussion with the patient and obtaining informed consent for the surgical procedure are paramount. The surgeon's knowledge of instrumentation and ability to "troubleshoot" certainly help to allay his or her anxiety and contribute to optimal patient care.

Operating Room Setup and Initial Procedures

The operating room setup includes that equipment which properly positions the patient, operative laparoscopic and video equipment, and a dedicated, well-coordinated physician and nursing team. Anesthesiologists well versed in the potential problems that are associated with laparoscopy can contribute to the success of the procedure and the management of any complications that may arise.[1] Use of Allen universal stirrups (Fig. 6-1) facilitates proper patient positioning and avoids neurologic damage.

An initial incision is made at the umbilicus. A vertical incision within the lines of turgor provides an excellent cosmetic result (Fig. 6-2). Next, a Veress needle is inserted to produce a pneumoperitoneum (Fig. 6-3). Alternative placement of the Veress needle, especially in an obese patient, largely depends on the planned procedure.

An open laparoscopic approach may be more feasible than the direct insertion of a Veress needle or trocar for the patient who has had prior abdominal surgery, especially in the area immediately beneath the incision. The Hasson cannula is specifically designed for open laparoscopy (Fig. 6-4*A* and *B*). Disposable open laparoscopic equipment is also available (see Fig. 6-4*C*). An array of new instrumentation, designed without scissors-type handles, are available (Fig. 6-5). Advances in laparoscopes include a model that permits irrigation of the laparoscope lens while in use (Fig. 6-6). A 10- to 12-mm puncture site can be reduced to 3.5 mm with the appropriate reducer (Fig. 6-7). Instrument support arms are available (Fig. 6-8) that are easily adjusted and locked in place instantly.

Insufflators

Several insufflators are available (Fig. 6-9). A basic understanding of the mechanics of high-flow insufflators is important. Generally, the operative laparoscopic insufflators are capable of delivering a 1- to 6-L/minute insufflation rate. Specific gauges indicating intraabdominal pressure and the total volume of gas delivered should be observed throughout the procedure. The end point of abdominal pressure (eg, 14 to 16 TORR) can frequently be selected on an insufflator. This setting is important to prevent compromise of venous return. Intraoperatively, O_2 saturation, end tidal CO_2, and CO_2 partial pressures in addition to cardiac status must be continuously monitored. Use of an esophageal stethoscope facilitates detection of any abnormal murmurs that can be associated with problems such as CO_2 emboli (characteristic mill-wheel murmur may be heard).

Laparoscopes, Light Sources, and Video Equipment

Generally, 10-mm laparoscopes are used, with a visual angle of 0°. This allows a "head-on" or more normal perspective for visualizing intra-abdominal structures. The laparoscope provides low-power magnification in

(text continues on page 41)

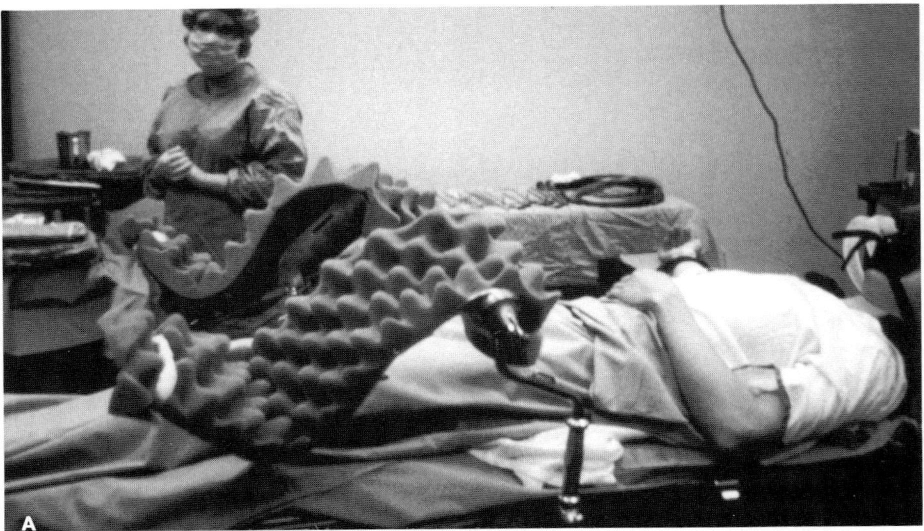

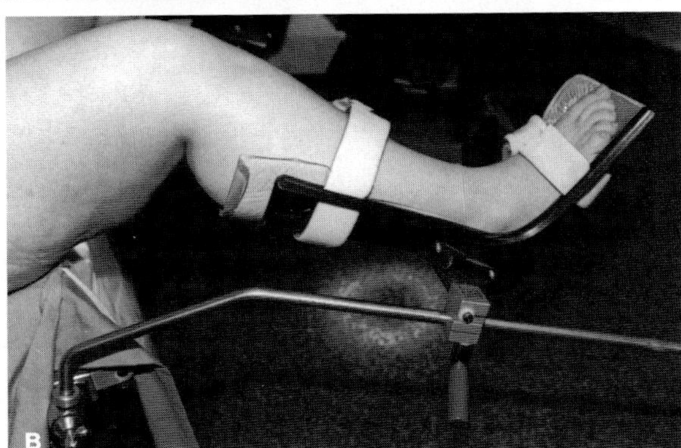

FIGURE 6-1. (**A**) Allen universal stirrups (courtesy of Allen Medical Systems, Cleveland OH). (**B**) Proper placement of foot and calf in stirrup.

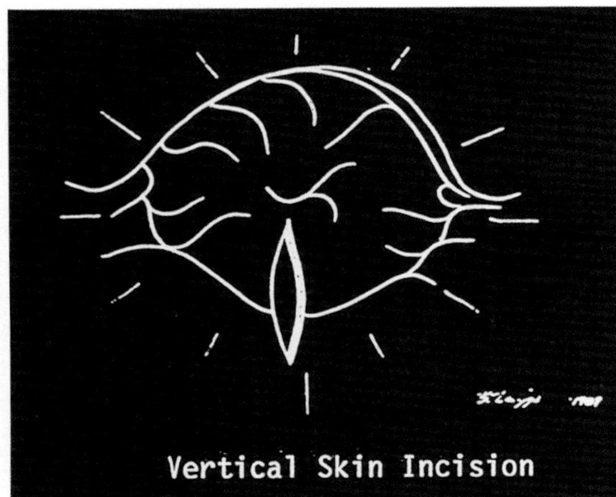

FIGURE 6-2. Vertical skin incision at umbilicus.

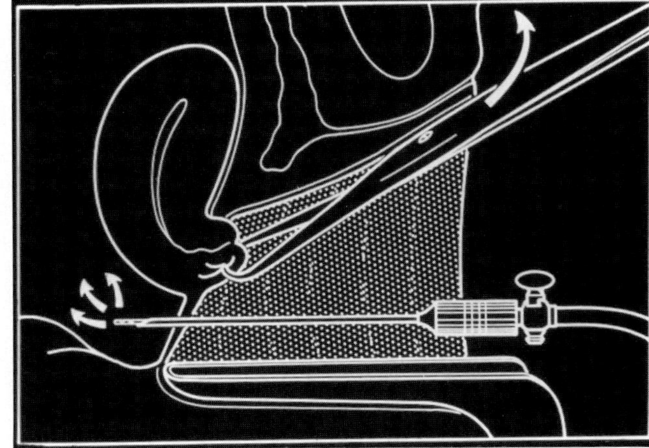

FIGURE 6-3. Veress needle insertion in cul de sac for creation of pneumoperitoneum.

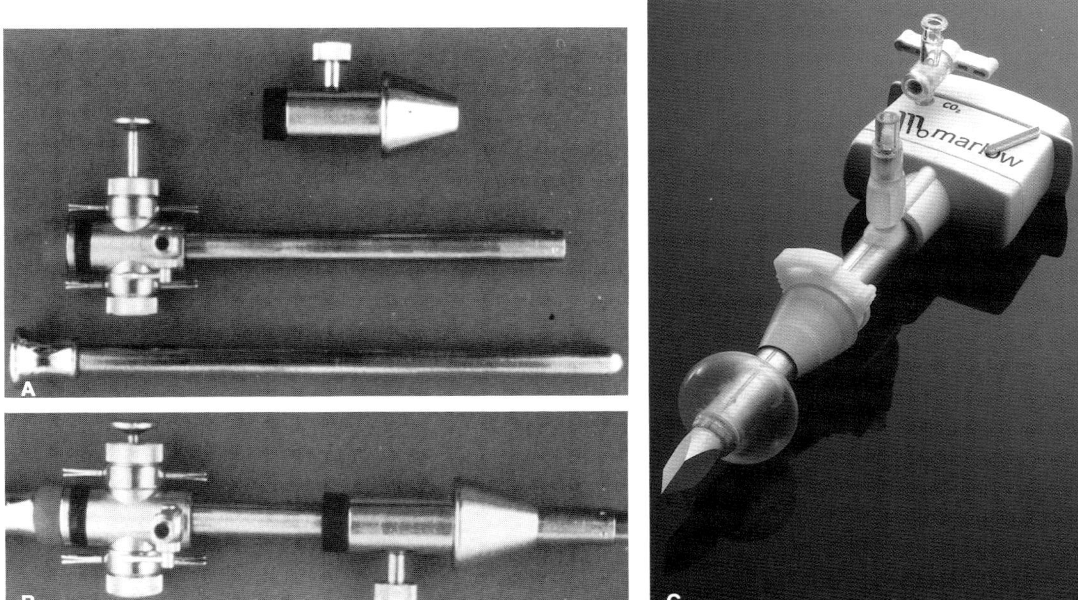

FIGURE 6-4. Hasson cannula for open laparoscopy. (**A**) Disassembled. (**B**) Assembled. (**C**) Marlow Sac 10-11 (pyramidal tip) disposable laparoscopy trocar and sleeve (courtesy of Marlow Surgical Technologies, Inc., Willoughby, OH).

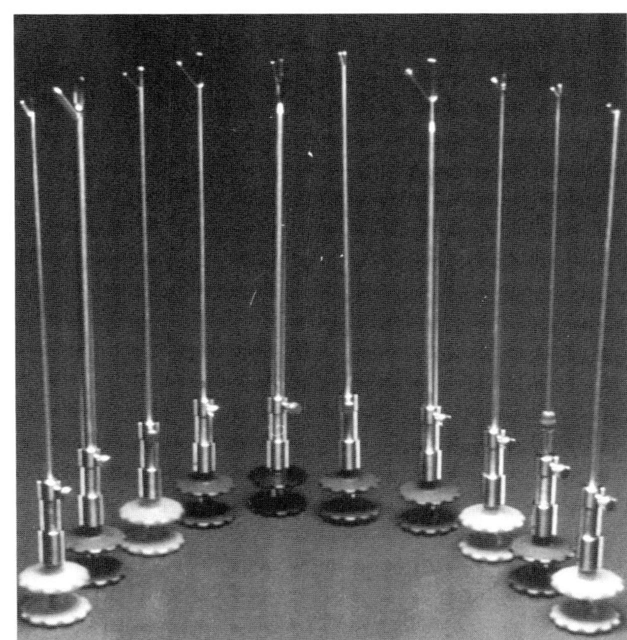

FIGURE 6-5. Alternative to a scissors-type handle, allowing placement of instrument in palm of hand. There is a movable sleeve that opens and closes the blades when the instrument is advanced or retracted. The handles are color-coded for easy identification of the type of instrument (courtesy of WISAP, Tomball, TX).

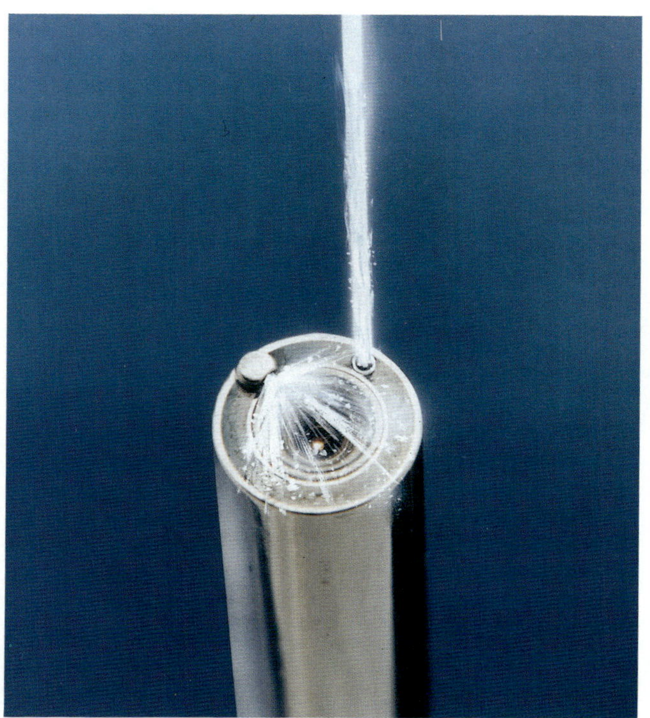

Figure 6-6. Laparoscope irrigation system for removal of blood and other debris from end of laparoscope lens (courtesy of Circon, Stamford, CT).

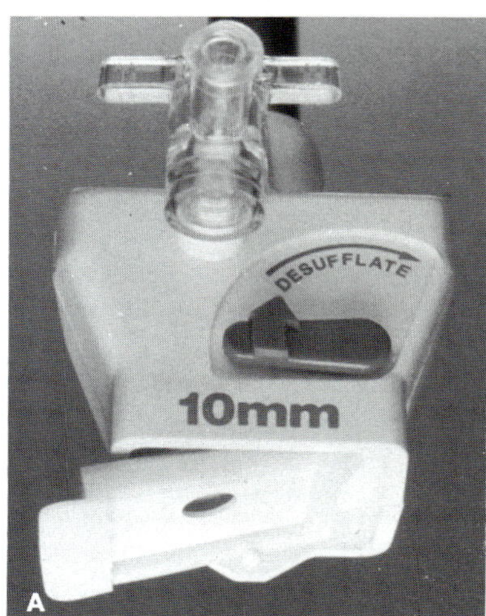

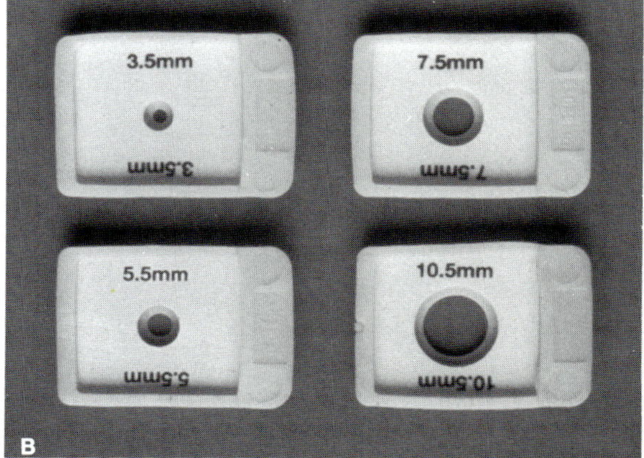

FIGURE 6-7. (A) 10-mm Disposable trocar with reducer (courtesy of US Surgical, Norwalk, CT). (B) 3.5- to 10.5-mm adapters (courtesy of US Surgical, Norwalk, CT).

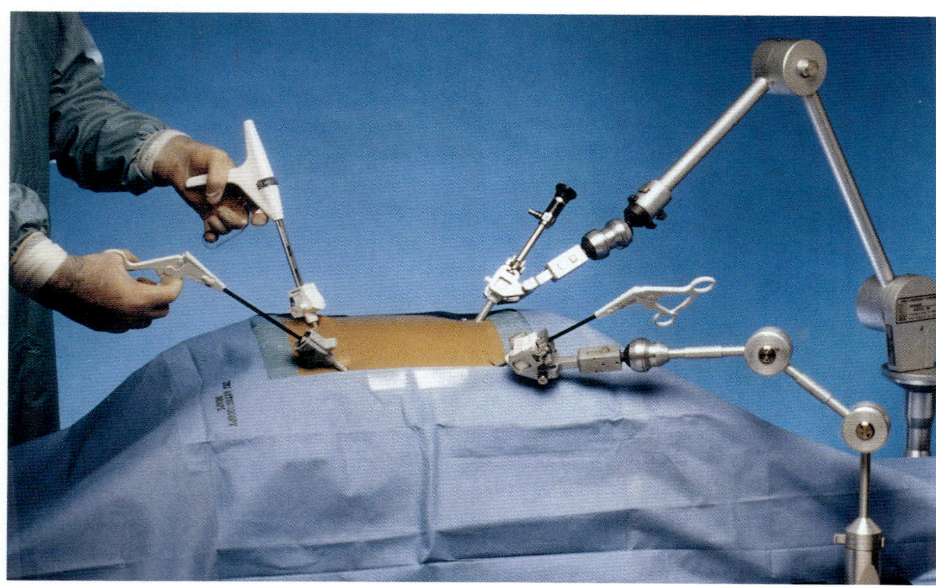

FIGURE 6-8. First Assistant and First Assistant, Jr instrument support arms (courtesy of Leonard Medical Inc., Huntingdon Valley, PA).

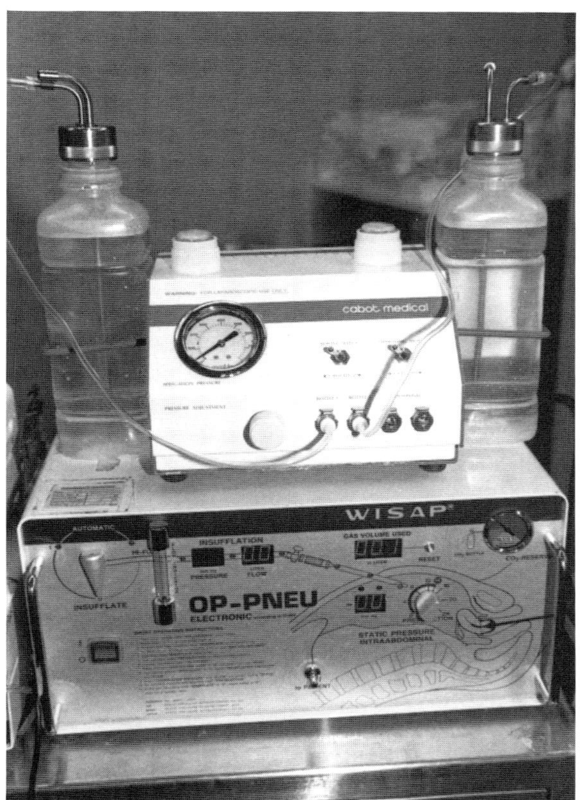

FIGURE 6-9. Electronic insufflator (Courtesy of WISAP, Tomball, TX). Suction irrigator (courtesy of Cabot Medical, Langhorne, PA).

direct proportion to distance from the object. A video monitor is highly recommended, especially for long surgical procedures; furthermore, it is helpful for the assistants to follow the procedure. Fogging of the laparoscope is often prevented by use of Ultra Stop (Richard Wolf, Vernon Hills, IL). Some surgeons use warm water or saline, perhaps kept in a thermos, to warm up the laparoscope to body temperature.

Light sources with photographic (video or still) capabilities (Fig. 6-10) and video equipment are used to record procedures (Fig. 6-11).

Suction–Irrigation Systems

Many suction–irrigation systems are available, including the Aqua-Purator (WISAP, West Germany; Fig. 6-12) and Storz system (Karl Storz, Endoscopy-America, Culver City, CA; Fig. 6-13). This instrumentation permits irrigation fluid to be instilled at a pressure up to 200 mmHg and can also be used for aspiration of serosanguinous fluid. The irrigation solution usually used is lactated Ringer's solution (ideally warmed to body temperature). These systems can also be used for aquadissection—to separate adhesions or for dissection. The handpiece for suctioning or irrigating is shown in Figure 6-14.

Basic Instrumentation

Appropriate instrumentation that is suitable for the planned procedure should be readily available (Table 6-1).

FORCEPS

There are many types of forceps or graspers (Figs. 6-15 through 6-27). They are available in 3-, 5-, and 10-mm sizes. An atraumatic grasping forceps risks little tissue damage while providing appropriate traction.

Bipolar coagulation forceps, including the Kleppinger forceps, are used for control of bleeding. The instrument can be placed through the operating channel (5 mm) of a laparoscope or through a second puncture

(text continues on page 45)

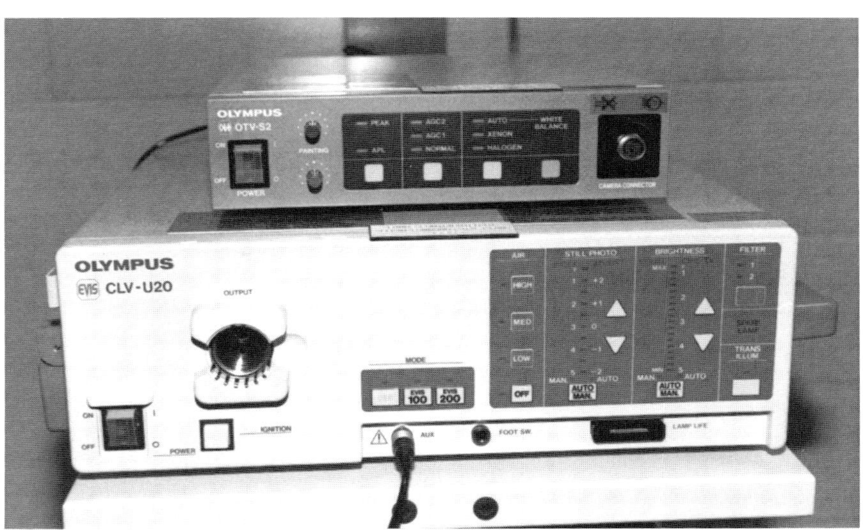

FIGURE 6-10. Light source (courtesy of Olympus, Lake Success, NY).

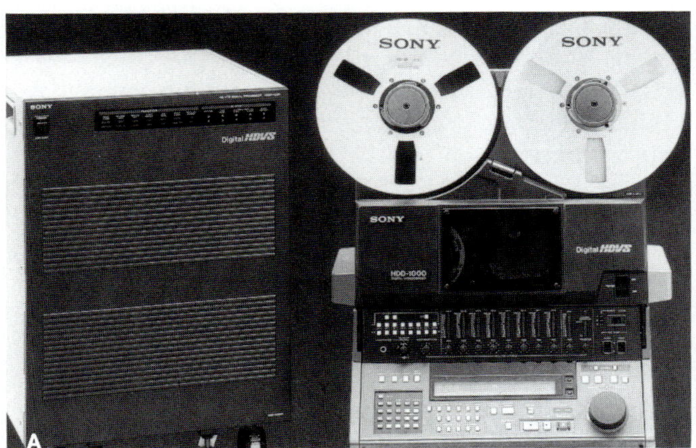
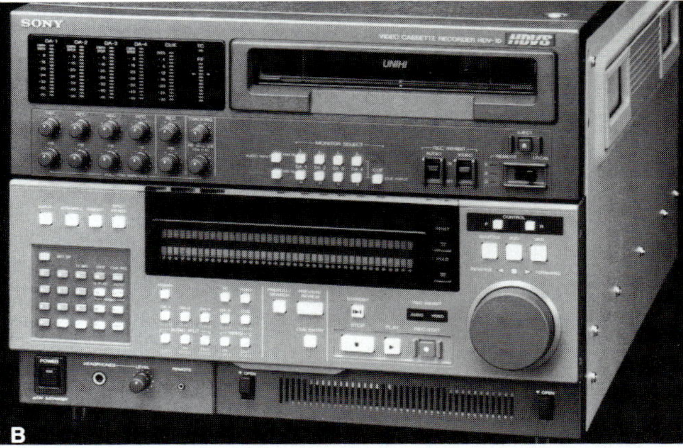

FIGURE 6-11. (**A**) SONY digital HDVS video recorder system. (**B**) SONY HDV-10 video cassette recorder. (Courtesy of SONY Medical Electronics Corp, Hackensack NJ).

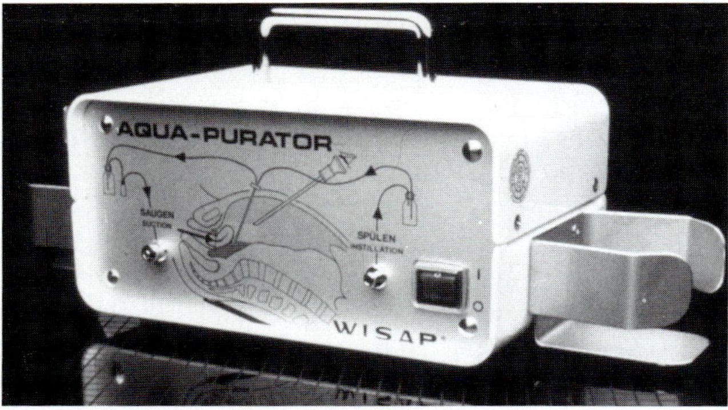

FIGURE 6-12. Aqua-Purator (courtesy of WISAP, Tomball, TX).

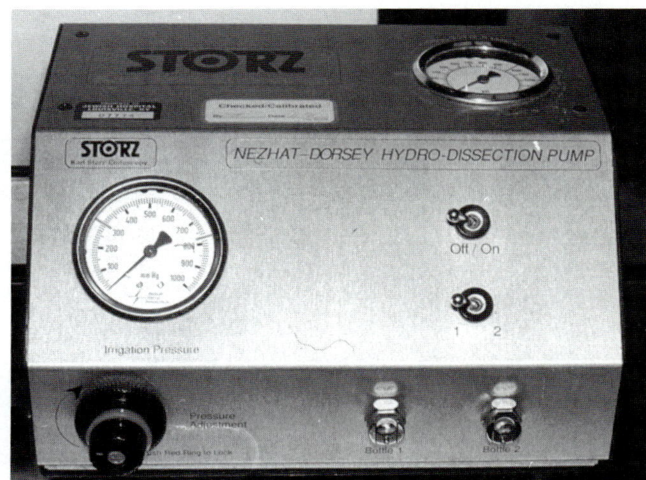

FIGURE 6-13. Nezhat-Dorsey Hydro-Dissection Pump (courtesy of Karl Storz, Endoscopy-America, Culver City, CA).

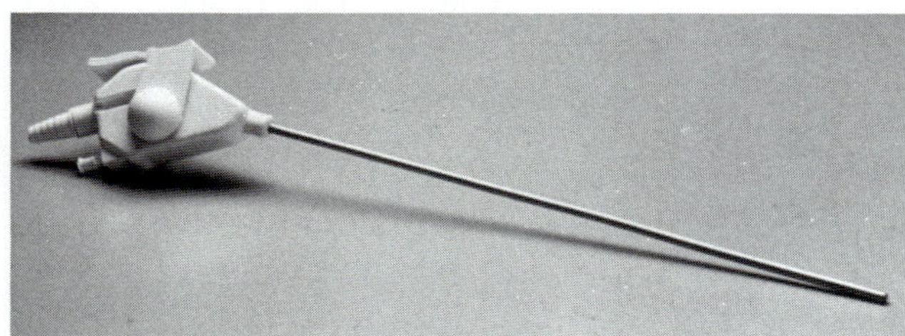

FIGURE 6-14. Corson suction irrigation applicator (courtesy of Cabot Medical, Langhorne, PA).

TABLE 6-1
Basic Instrumentation

Grasping forceps
Laparoscopic scissors
Aquadissection or suction irrigator
5 and 10 mm instrumentation
Instrumentation associated with electrosurgical systems
Bipolar
Monopolar

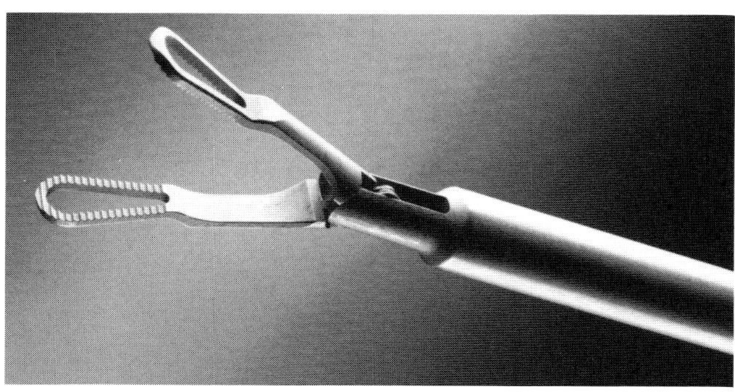

FIGURE 6-15. Ring forceps (courtesy of Marlow Surgical Technologies, Inc., Willoughby, OH).

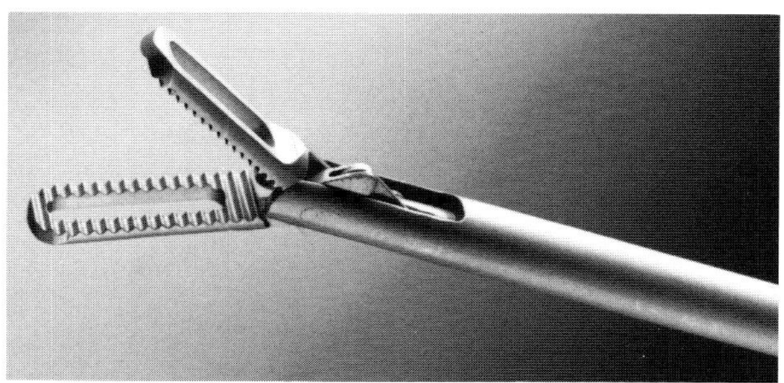

FIGURE 6-16. Paddle forceps (courtesy of Marlow Surgical Technologies, Inc., Willoughby, OH).

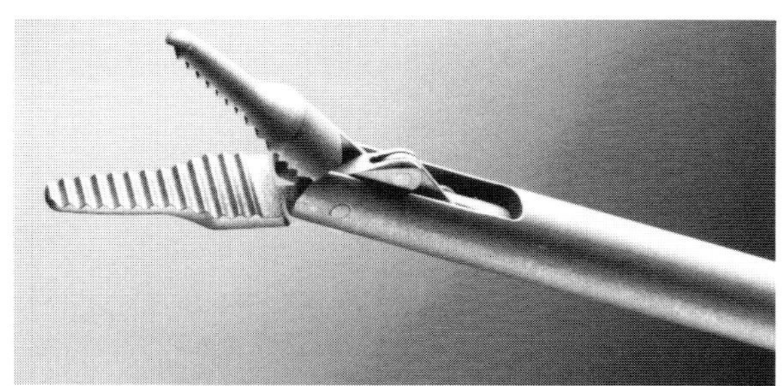

FIGURE 6-17. Dolphin nose dissector (courtesy of Marlow Surgical Technologies, Inc., Willoughby, OH).

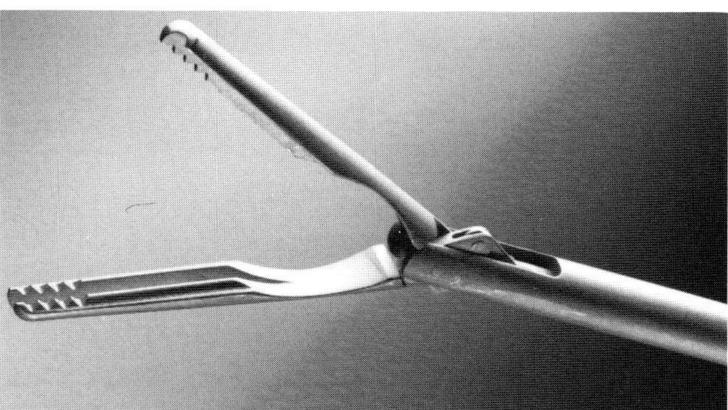

FIGURE 6-18. DeBakey forceps (courtesy of Marlow Surgical Technologies, Inc., Willoughby, OH).

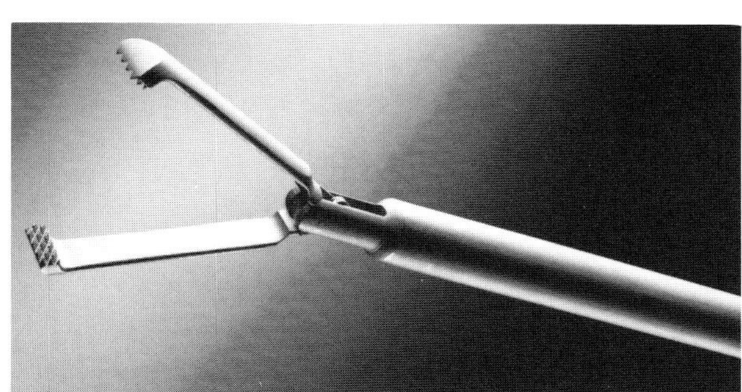

FIGURE 6-19. Allis forceps (courtesy of Marlow Surgical Technologies, Inc., Willoughby, OH).

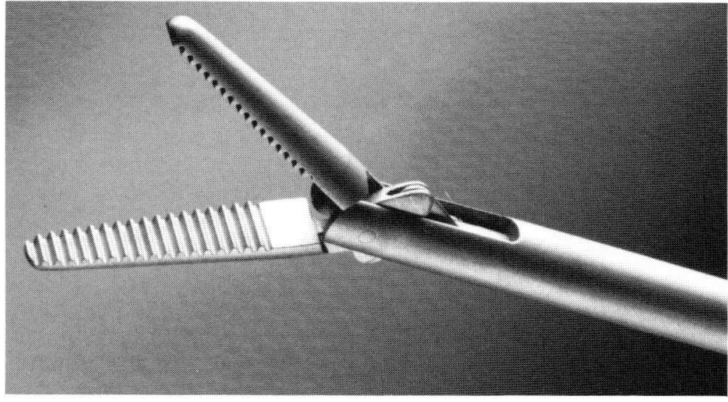

FIGURE 6-20. Pollack grasper (courtesy of Marlow Surgical Technologies, Inc., Willoughby, OH).

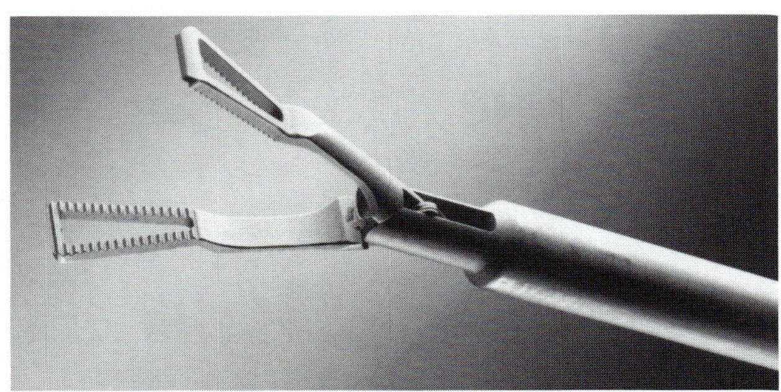

FIGURE 6-21. Pennington forceps (courtesy of Marlow Surgical Technologies, Inc., Willoughby, OH).

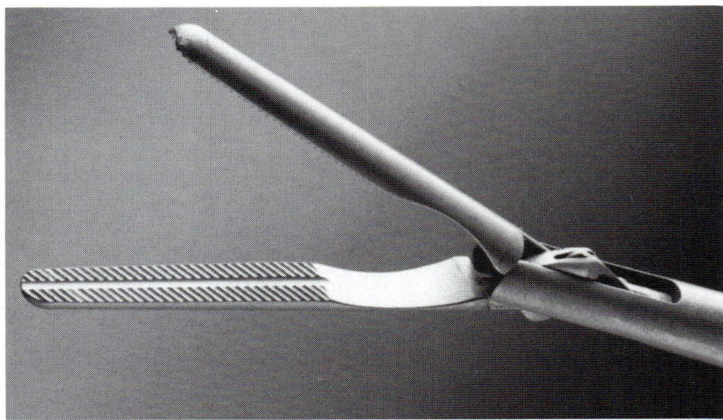

FIGURE 6-22. Glassman grasper (courtesy of Marlow Surgical Technologies, Inc., Willoughby, OH).

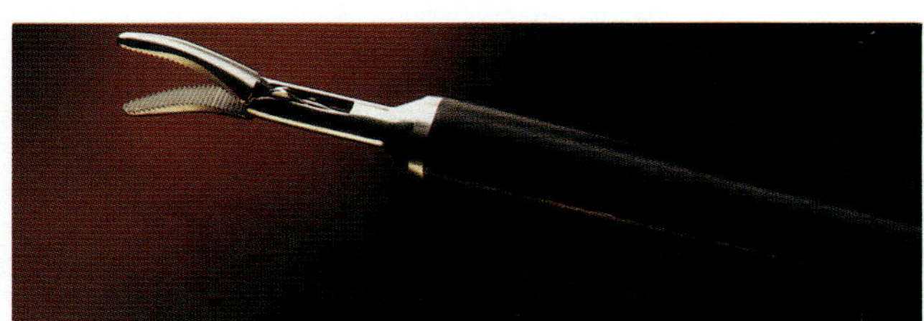

FIGURE 6-23. Maryland dissecting forceps (courtesy of Marlow Surgical Technologies, Inc., Willoughby, OH).

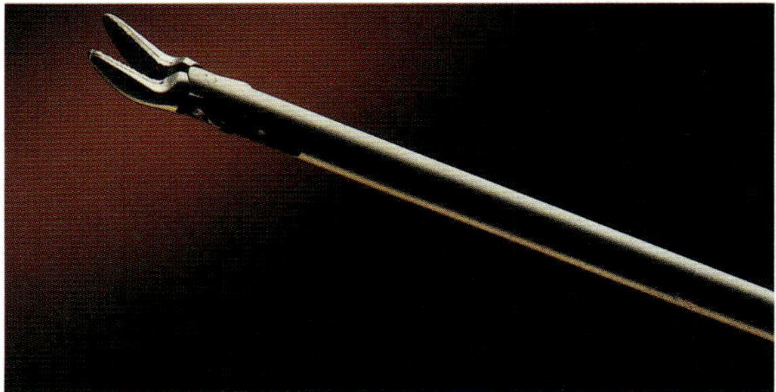

FIGURE 6-24. Reddick-Saye needle driver (courtesy of Marlow Surgical Technologies, Inc., Willoughby, OH).

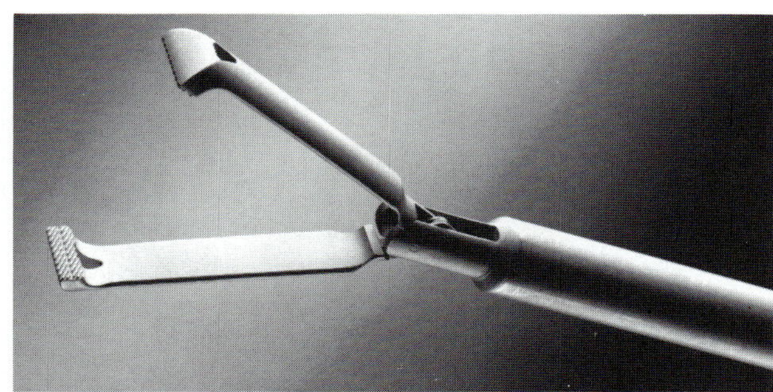

FIGURE 6-25. Duval forceps (courtesy of Marlow Surgical Technologies, Inc., Willoughby, OH).

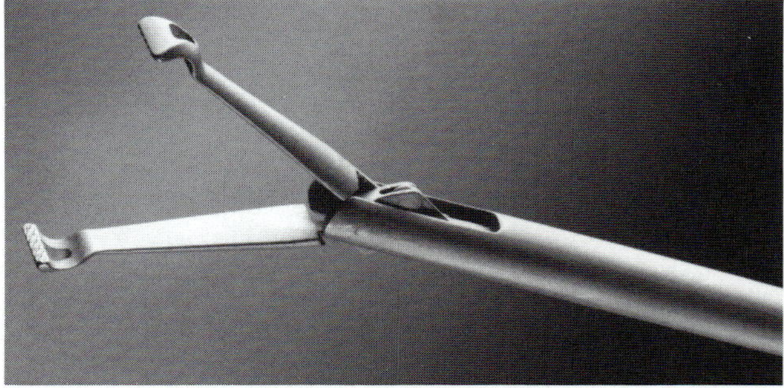

FIGURE 6-26. Babcock forceps (courtesy of Marlow Surgical Technologies, Inc., Willoughby, OH).

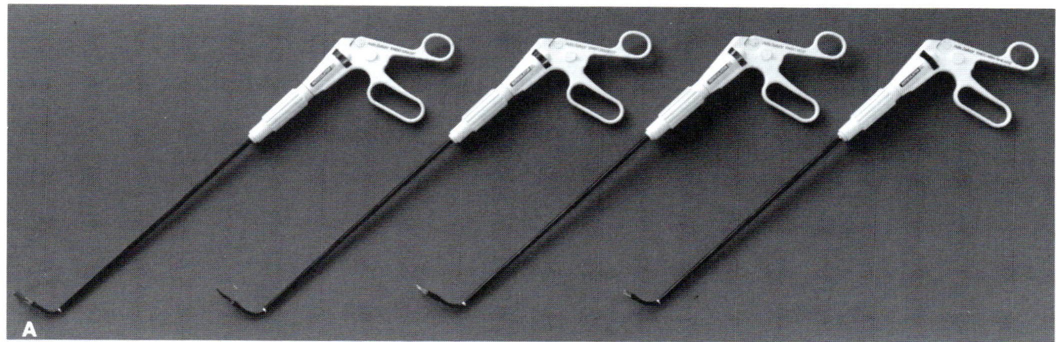

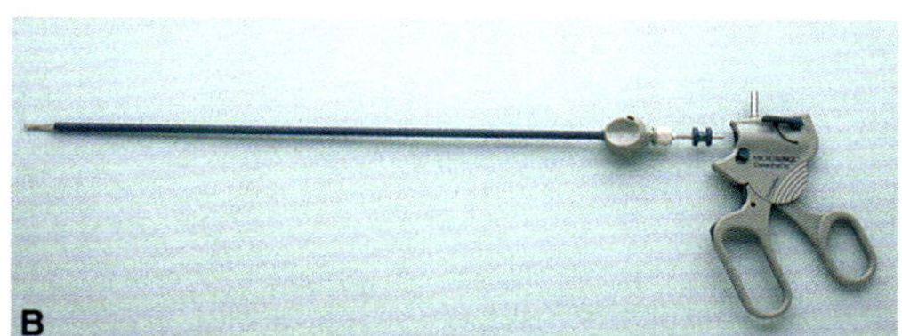

FIGURE 6-27. (A) Articulated disposable instrumentation (courtesy of US Surgical Corp., Auto Suture Co., Norwalk, CT). (B) DetachaTip, reuseable instrumentation (courtesy of Microsurge, Needham, MA).

site. Instrumentation for electrodissection includes a host of different types and application tips, as shown in Figures 6-28 through 6-30.

SCISSORS AND CLIP APPLICATORS

Many types of scissors are available, ranging in size from 3 to 10 mm. Several are presented in Figures 6-31 through 6-34. Figures 6-35 and 6-36 show examples of clip applicators.

STAPLERS

Staplers are used to achieve hemostasis. Both those with and those without an articulated head allow placement of a clip. Delivery of rows of staples with scissor-incising capabilities is also possible (Fig. 6-37).

The Endo Gauge (US Surgical Corp/Auto Suture Co., Norwalk, CT; Fig. 6-38) can be used to determine the proper size of Endo-GIA (US Surgical, Norwalk, CT) stapler to be used. Multifire cartridge applications are available (Figs. 6-39 and 6-40).

ENDOPOUCHES OR SACS

Endopouches (Ethicon, Inc., Somerville, NJ) are available to facilitate tissue removal. This type of device prevents spillage of tissue contents (Figs. 6-41 and 6-42).

KNOT-TYING

Principles of knot-tying have assumed a new and enhanced role in operative laparoscopy. The surgeon

(text continues on page 49)

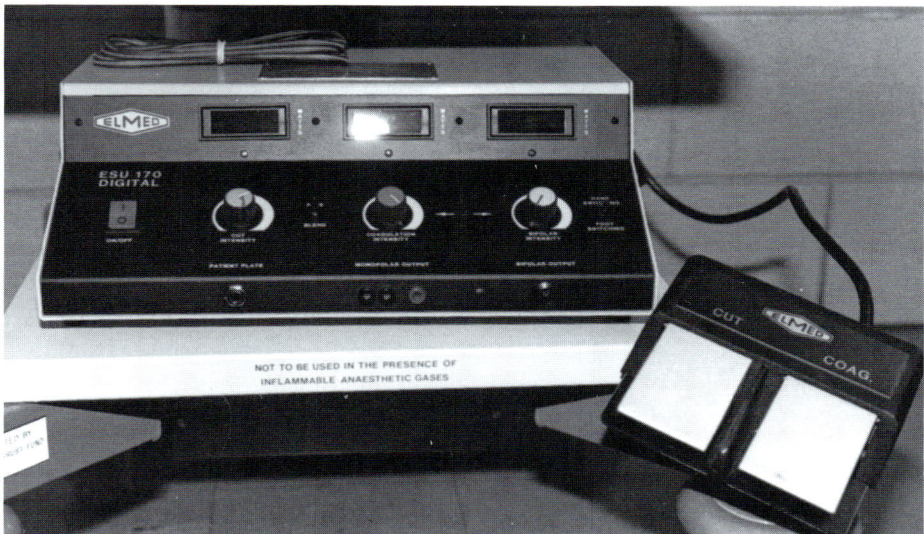

FIGURE 6-28. Electrocoagulation system with both cutting and coagulation current capabilities (courtesy of El Med, Addison, IL).

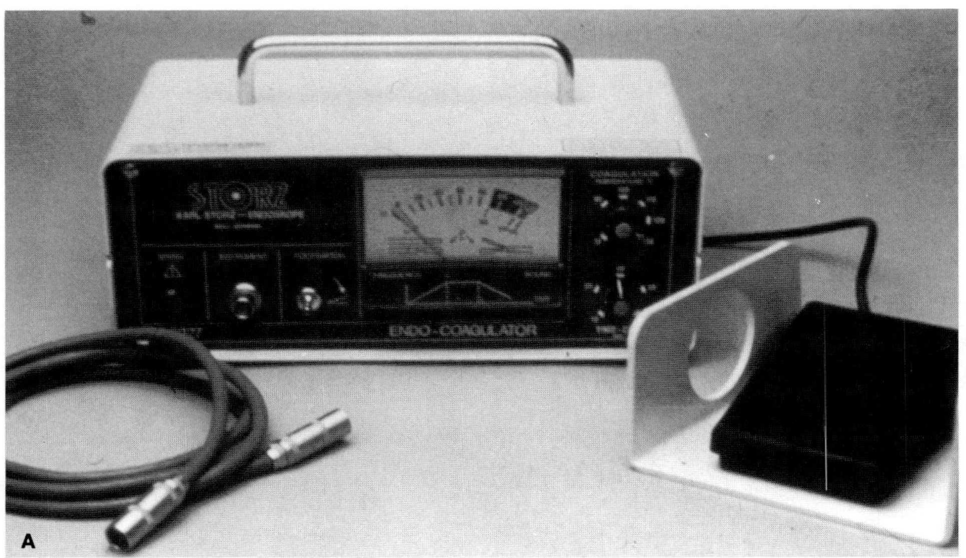

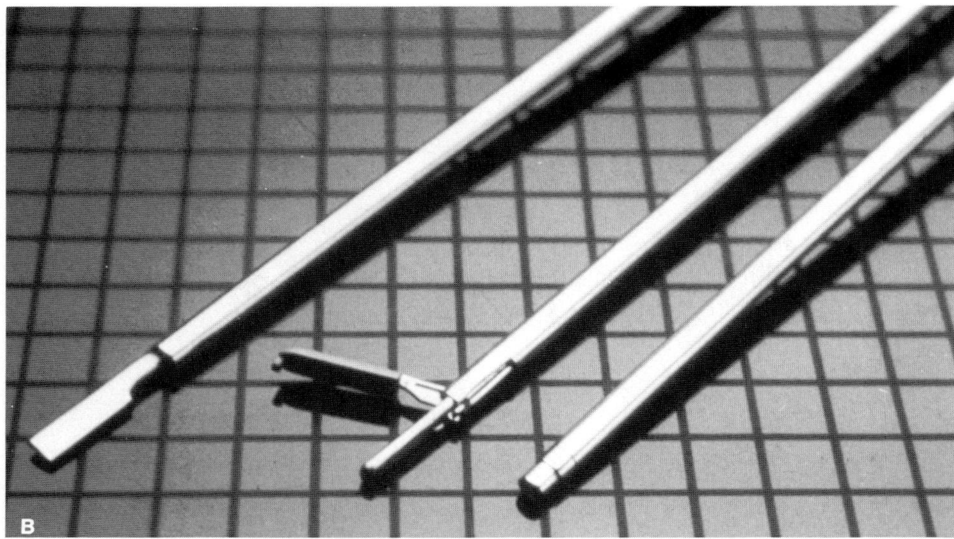

FIGURE 6-29. (**A**) Endocoagulator (courtesy of Karl Storz, Endoscopy-America, Culver City, CA). (**B**) Applicators (left-right) myoenucleator, alligator forceps and point coagulator (courtesy of WISAP, Tomball, TX).

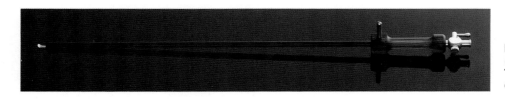

FIGURE 6-30. Spatula dissector (courtesy of Marlow Surgical Technologies, Inc., Willoughby, OH).

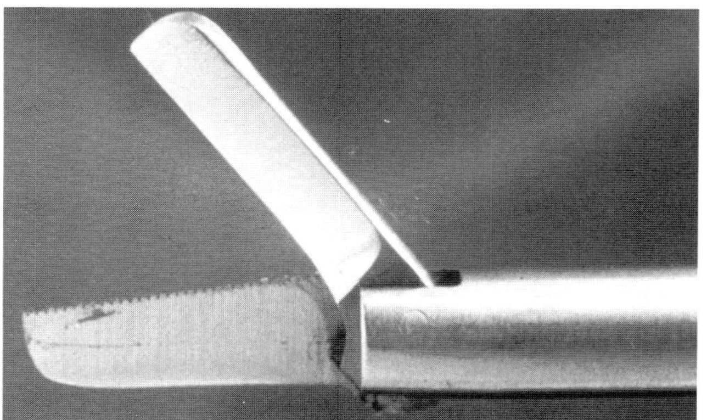

FIGURE 6-31. Hook scissors.

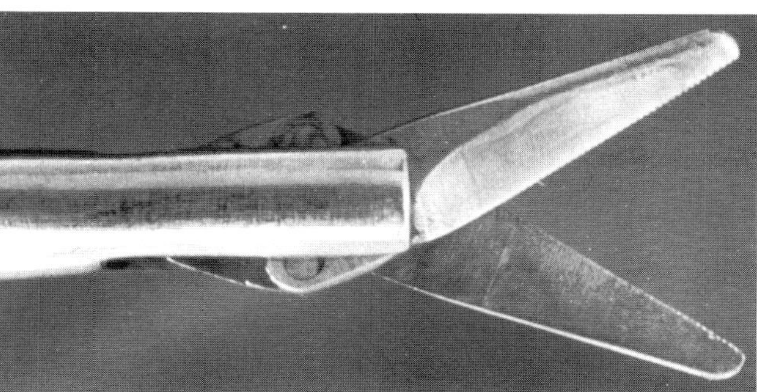

FIGURE 6-32. Straight scissors.

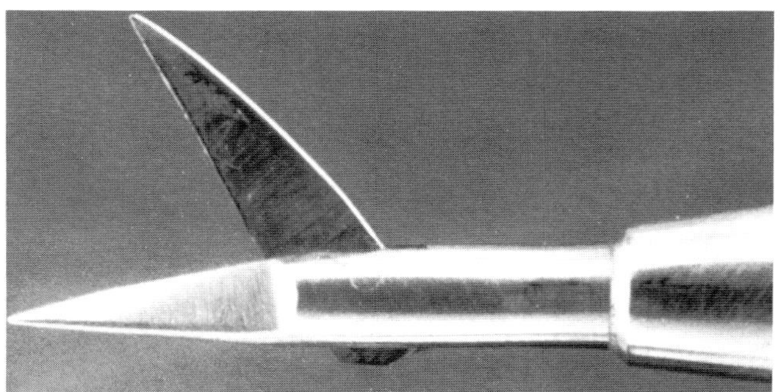

FIGURE 6-33. Microscissors.

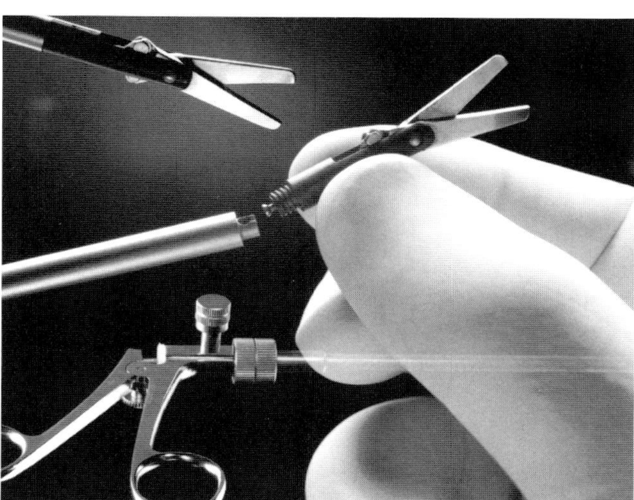

FIGURE 6-34. Disposable scissor instrumentation Nu-Tip Montage (courtesy of Marlow Surgical Technologies, Inc., Willoughby, OH).

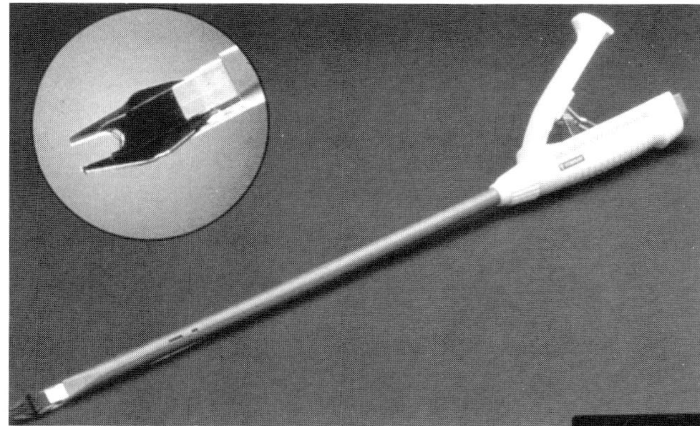

FIGURE 6-35. Auto Suture Endoclip applicator (courtesy of US Surgical Corp., Auto Suture Co., Norwalk, CT).

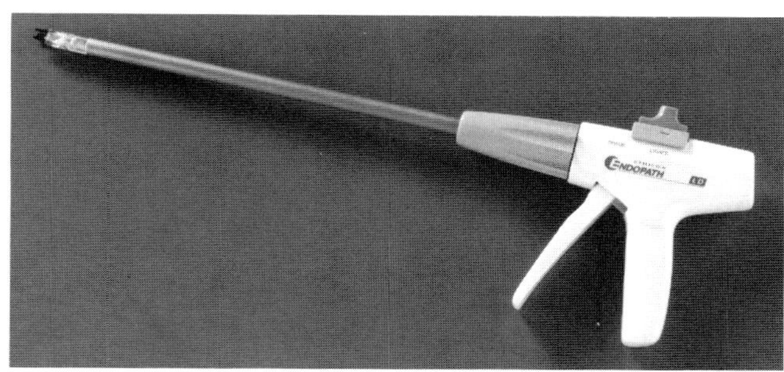

FIGURE 6-36. Endopath clip applicator with divide and ligate features (courtesy of Ethicon, Inc., Somerville, NJ).

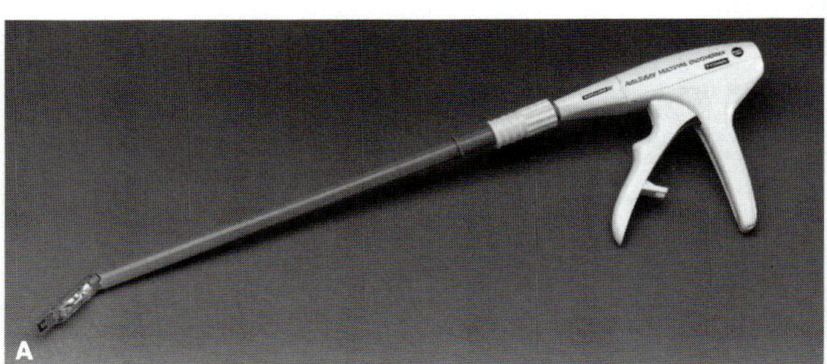

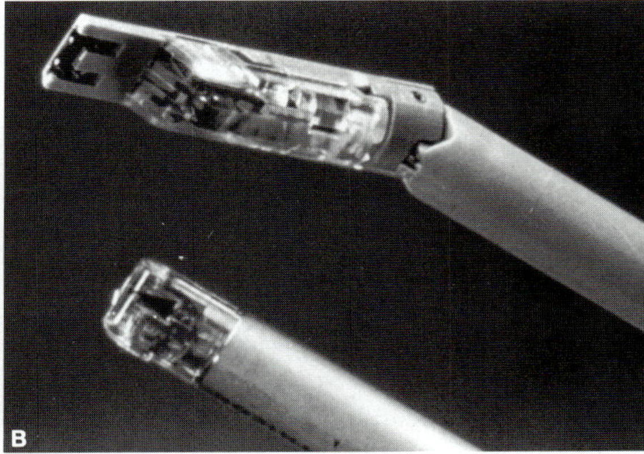

FIGURE 6-37. (**A**) Multifire Endohernia stapler with articulated head. (**B**) Articulating head for Multifire Endohernia stapler. (Courtesy of US Surgical Corp., Auto Suture Co., Norwalk, CT).

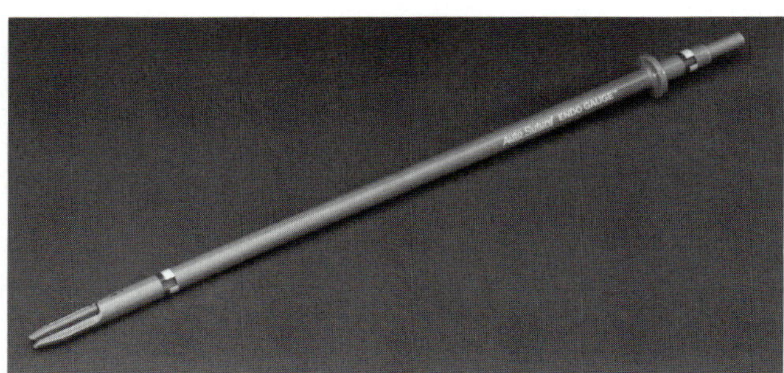

FIGURE 6-38. Use of the Endo Gauge determines the appropriate Endo-GIA stapling device to use (courtesy of US Surgical Corp., Auto Suture Co., Norwalk, CT).

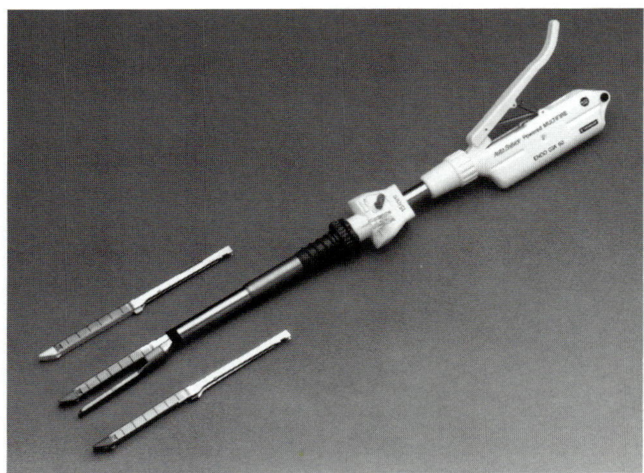

FIGURE 6-39. Endo-GIA 60 (courtesy of US Surgical Corp., Auto Suture Co., Norwalk, CT).

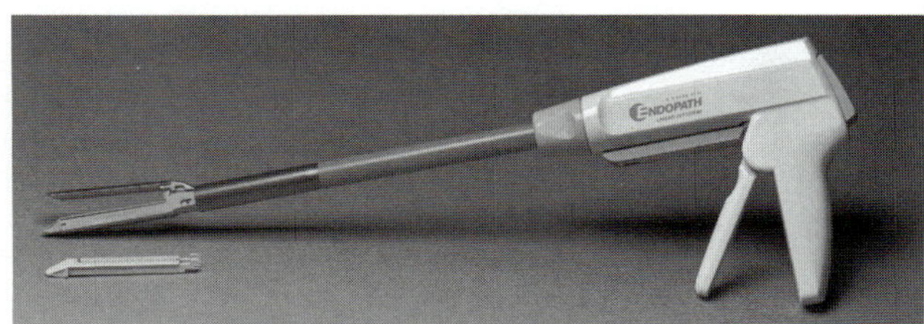

FIGURE 6-40. Endopath Stapler (courtesy of Ethicon, Inc., Somerville, NJ).

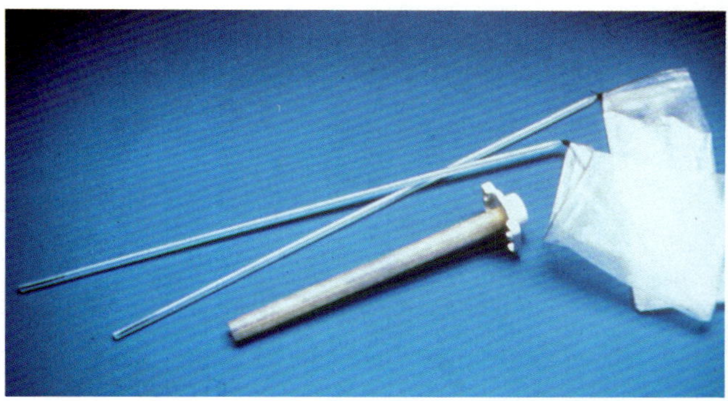

FIGURE 6-41. Endopouch Specimen Bag (courtesy of Ethicon, Inc., Somerville, NJ).

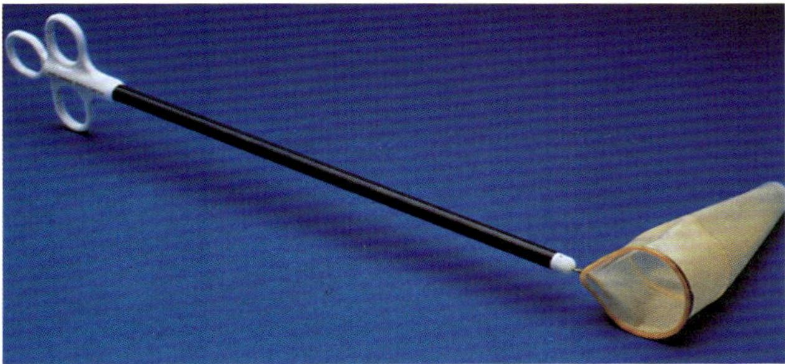

FIGURE 6-42. EndoCatch Specimen Bag (courtesy of US Surgical Corp., Auto Suture Co., Norwalk, CT).

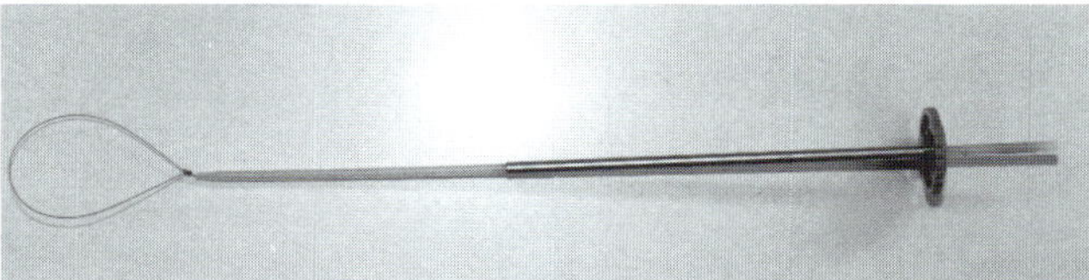

FIGURE 6-43. Endoloop back-loaded into loop applicator (e.g., 3 mm, courtesy of Ethicon, Inc., Somerville, NJ).

should be familiar with extracorporeal knot-tying techniques. It is important that the knot be placed with a smooth application because there is evidence (depending on the suture material) that shearing of the tissue as well as the integrity of the knot (i.e., tensile strength) can occur. Tensile strength of the knot has been tested.[2]

If an Endoloop (Ethicon, Inc., Somerville, NJ) ligature is to be used, it requires an applicator. Back-loading (Fig. 6-43) is necessary to properly house the Endoloop within the 3-mm applicator. This is then fitted into a 5-mm trocar sleeve; the distal end of the applicator is snapped to secure the Endoloop. Endoloop ligatures are available in PDS (polydioxan one) suture, plain and chromic gut, and coated Vicryl (polyglactin 910) suture (Ethicon, Inc., Somerville, NJ). Once the Endoloop is properly placed, scissors are used to cut the suture and the applicator is removed.

Ideally, the surgeon should be well versed in laparoscopic suture techniques, including extracorporeal knot-tying. As noted, several needle holders are available, including 3- and 5-mm sizes, as are needle holders for "curved" needles (Fig. 6-44). In addition, tissue graspers, suture introducers, and hook scissors should be readily available to accomplish the laparoscopic suturing. It is recommended that an Endotrainer be used (Fig. 6-45) to develop skill in laparoscopic suturing techniques.

Extracorporeal Knot-Tying

For extracorporeal knot-tying, the surgeon has a choice of several types of needles—straight, ski, or curved (Fig. 6-46).[3] Once the suture is properly placed, the needle is removed from the abdomen. A single-throw knot is placed outside the abdomen while the assistant prevents loss of CO_2 insufflation by placing a finger over the open port. A knot pusher (Fig. 6-47) is then used to properly secure the knot. A second throw (making a square knot) is then placed and is again tightened with the knot pusher. This is followed by a third (square) knot. A scissors is then used to cut the excess suture. An Endoknot is a pre-tied knot that facilitates laparoscopic suturing (Fig. 6-48).

One other frequently used extracorporeal knot is the Roeder loop (Fig. 6-49). When properly applied, it provides a secure hemostatic knot. A third extracorporeal knot is the fisherman's knot (Fig. 6-50). In essence, whichever knot the surgeon is most comfortable with should be used, as deemed necessary. A technique of extracorporeal knot-tying using a preplaced loop (Endoknot) is presented in Figure 6-51. Use of a Babcock grasper for placement of knots is illustrated in Figure 6-52.

Intracorporeal Knot-Tying

If the surgeon chooses, intracorporeal knot-tying can be performed (Figs. 6-53 and 6-54). To place the suture in the proper position, 3- and 5-mm needle holders are usually used. Similar to an instrument tie, two loops are placed around one of the needle holders intra-

(text continues on page 54)

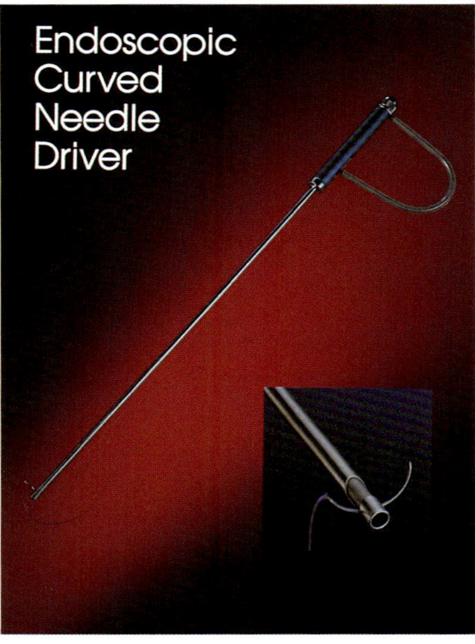

FIGURE 6-44. Curved needle holder (courtesy of Cook OB/GYN, Spencer, IN).

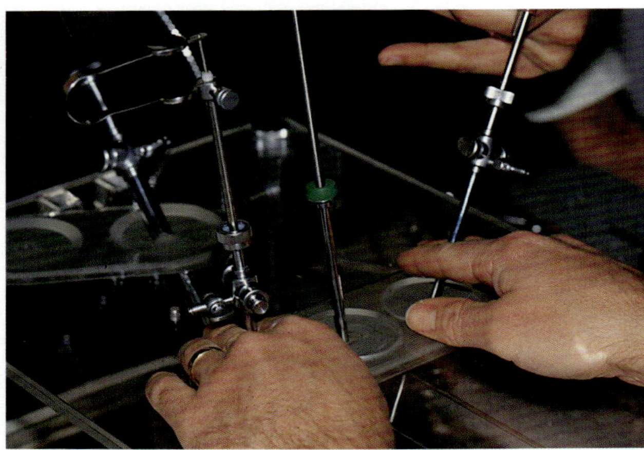

FIGURE 6-45. Ethicon Endotrainer. Develops enhanced hand–eye coordination, thus enhancing operative laparoscopic skills (courtesy of Ethicon, Inc., Somerville, NJ).

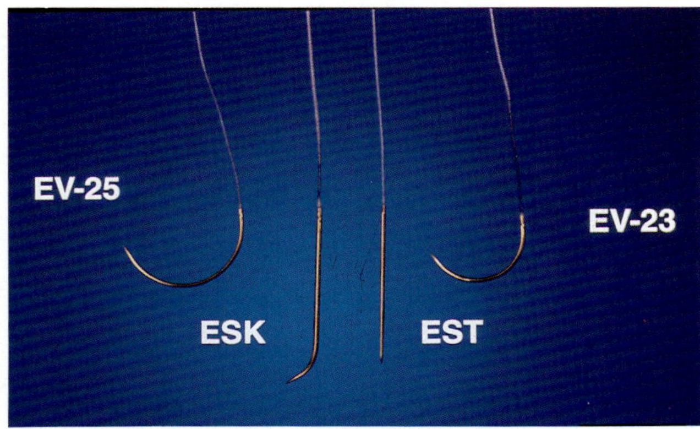

FIGURE 6-46. Array of needles available for laparoscopic suturing (courtesy of US Surgical Corp., Norwalk, CT).

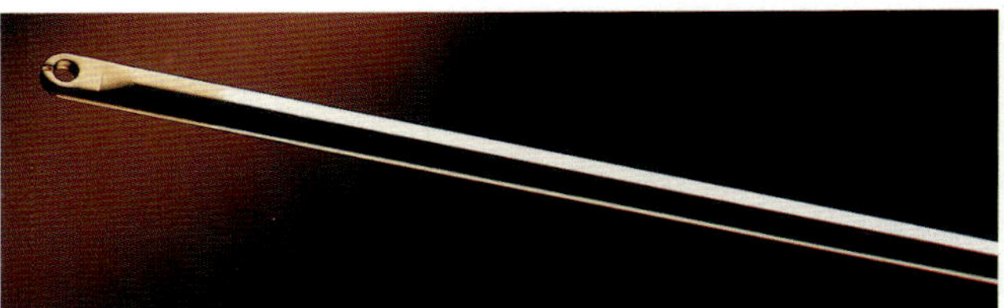

FIGURE 6-47. Clark-Reich Ligator (courtesy of Marlow Surgical Technologies, Inc., Willoughby, OH).

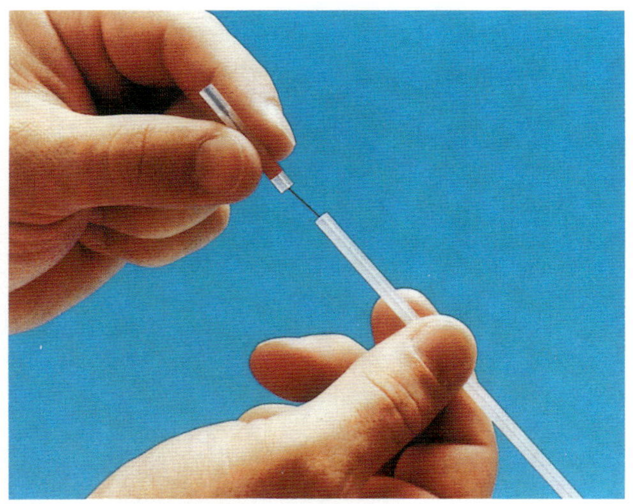

FIGURE 6-48. Snap-off end of the Endoknot shaft (at red band) allows sliding of the knot downward (courtesy of Ethicon, Inc., Somerville, NJ).

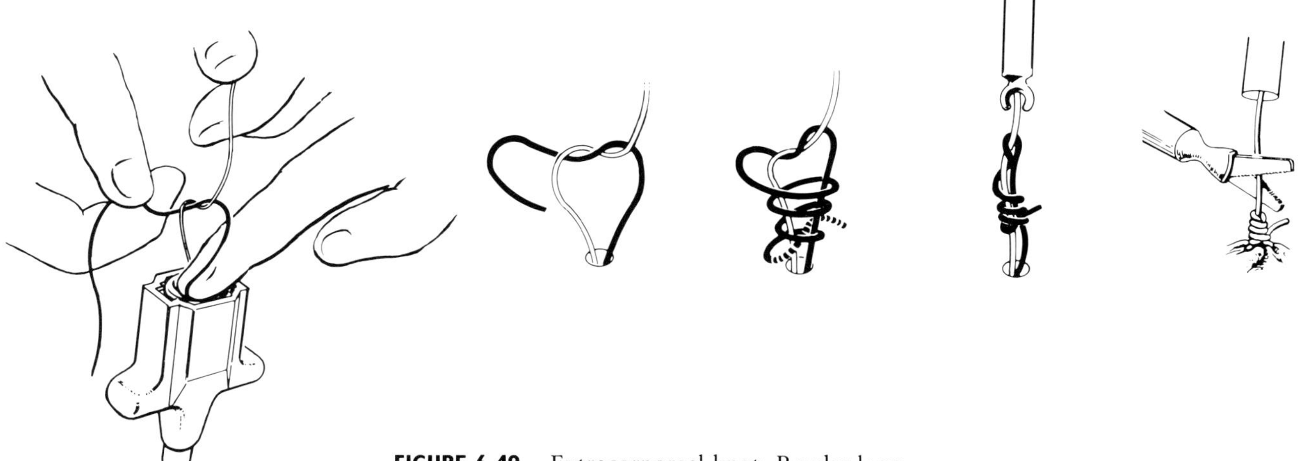

FIGURE 6-49. Extracorporeal knot; Roeder loop.

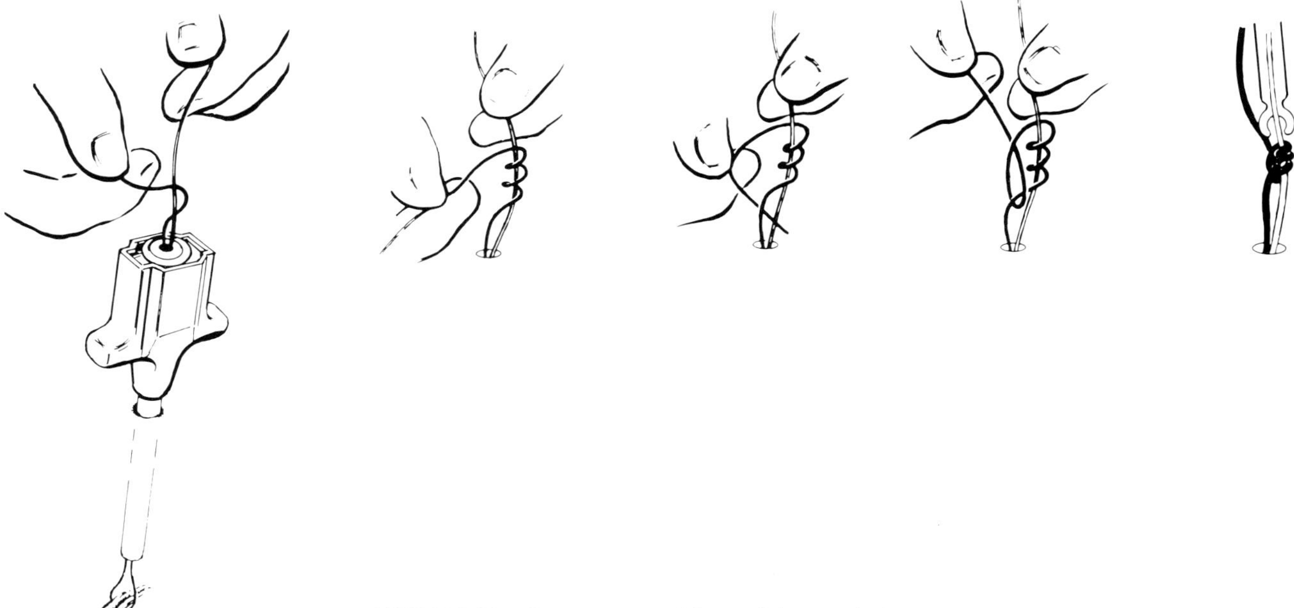

FIGURE 6-50. Extracorporeal knot; fisherman's knot.

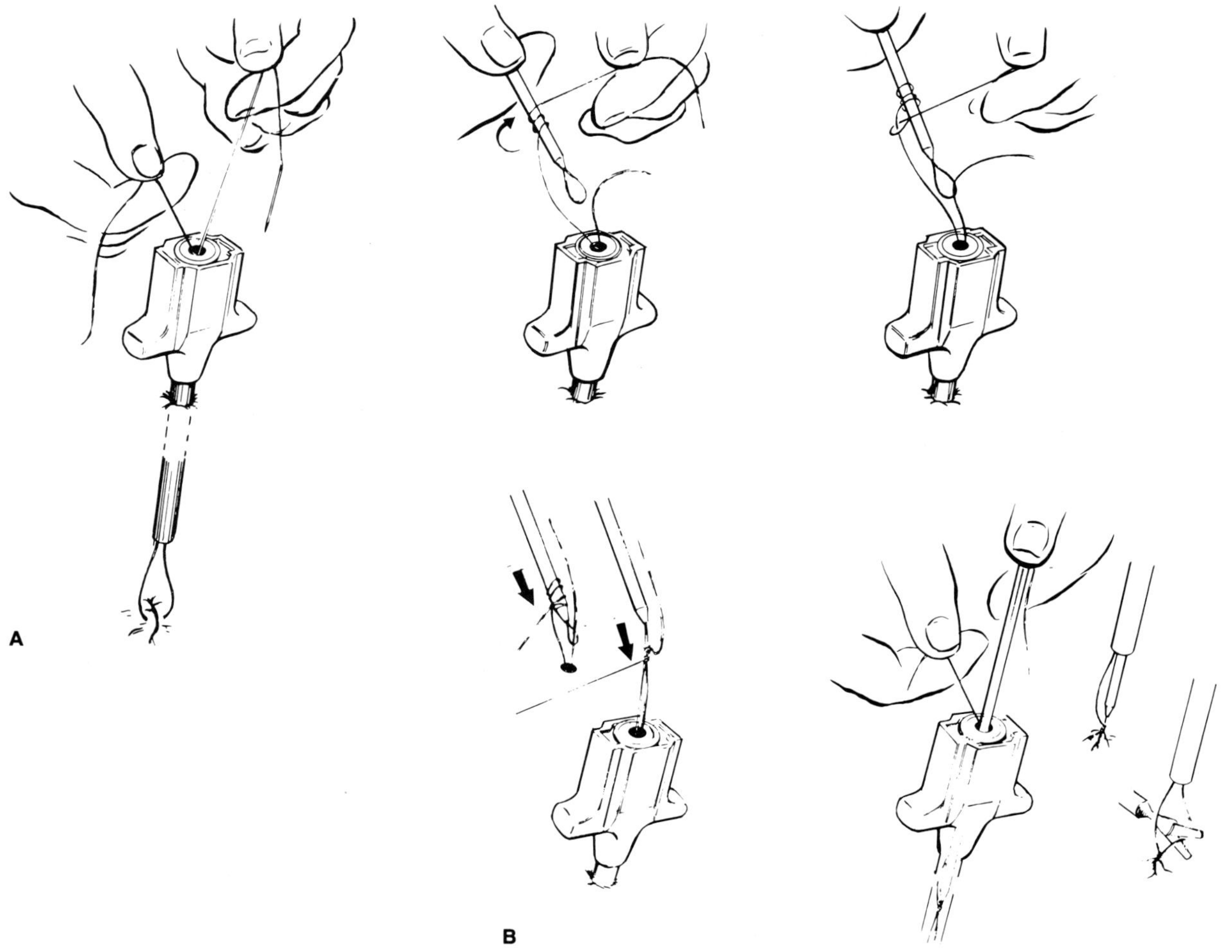

FIGURE 6-51. Extracorporeal knot tying with use of an Endoknot.

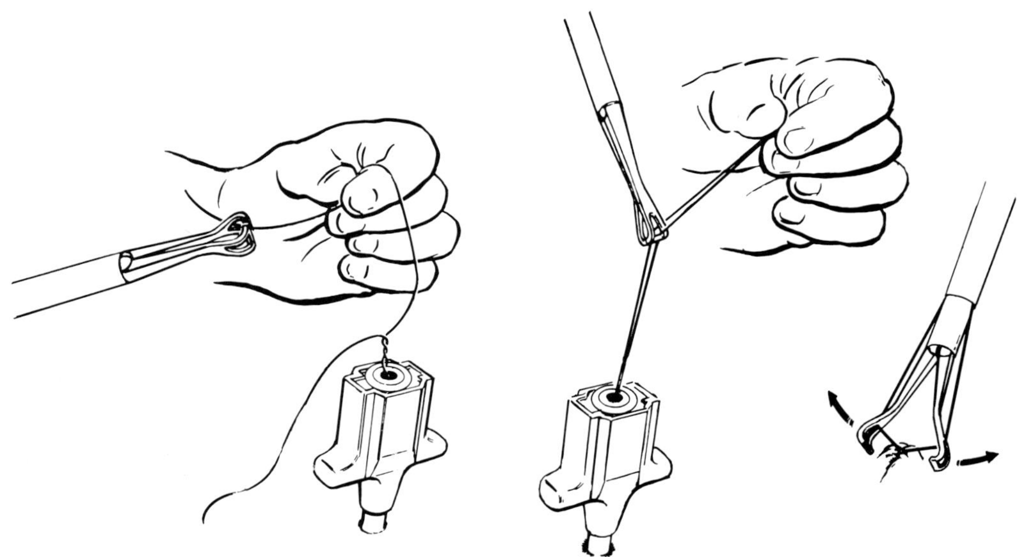

FIGURE 6-52. Use of a Babcock grasper for extracorporeal knot-tying.

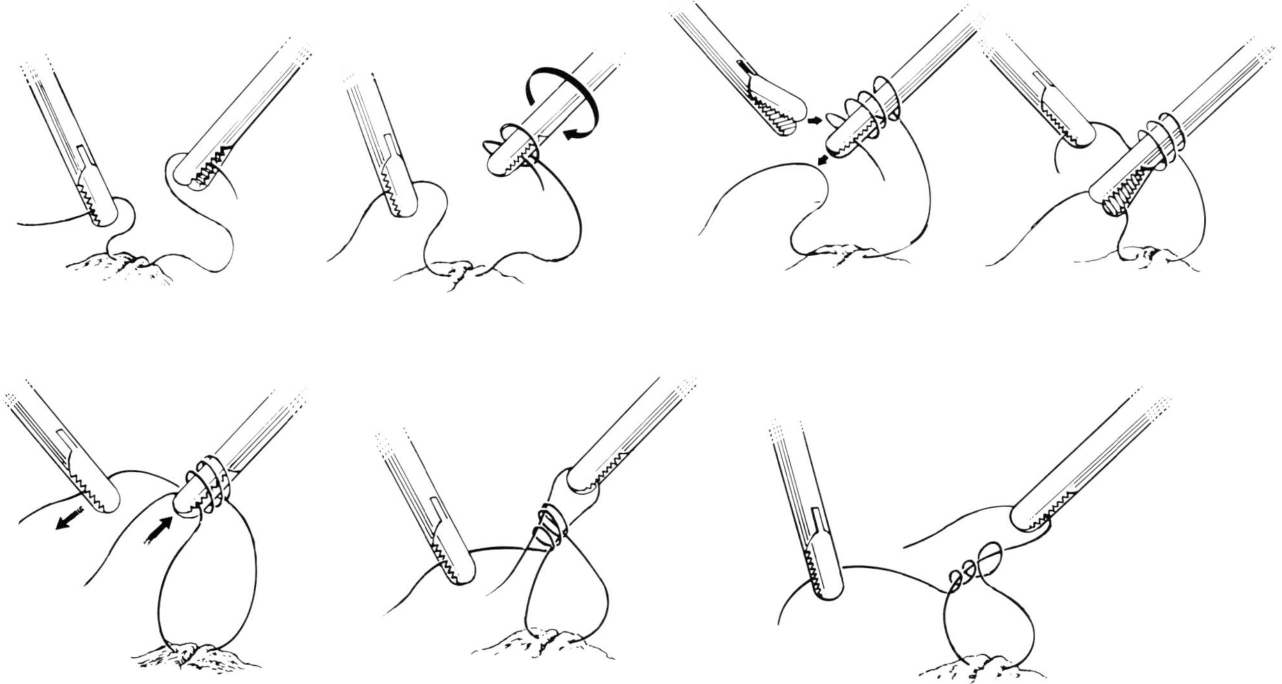

FIGURE 6-53. Intracorporeal twist.

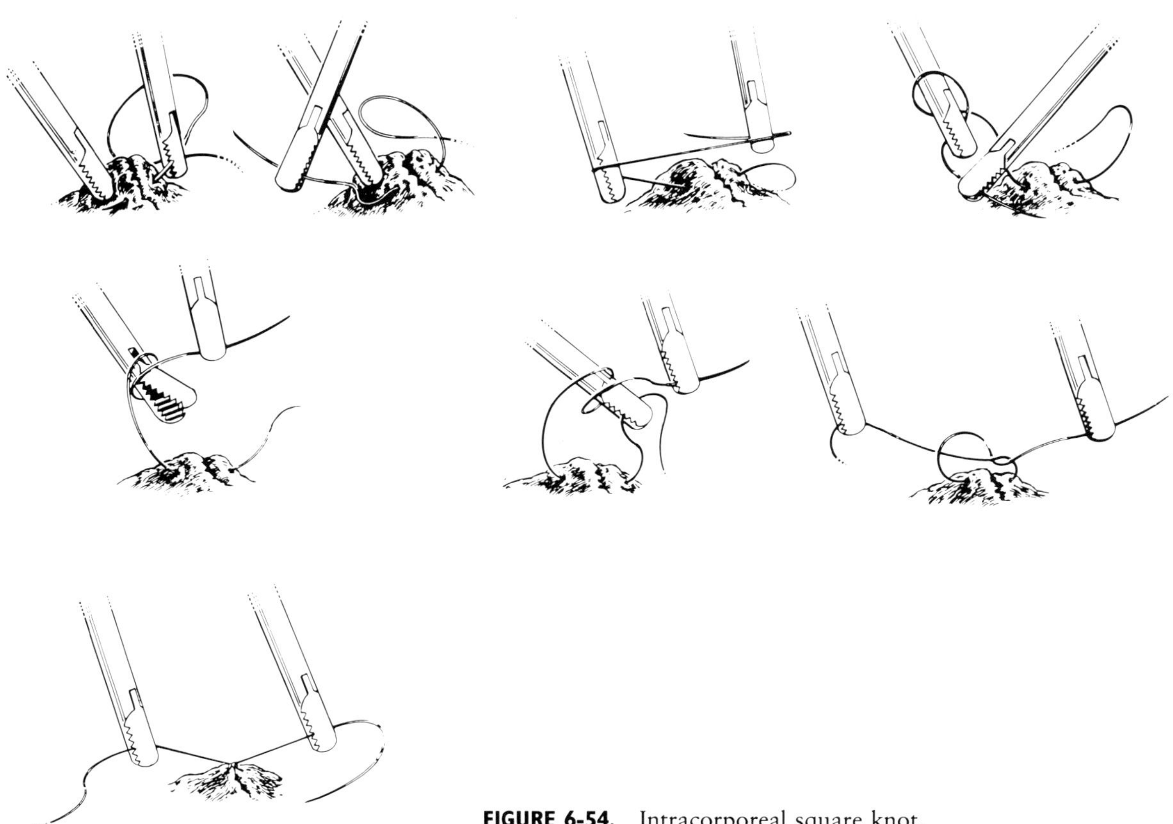

FIGURE 6-54. Intracorporeal square knot.

abdominally (after the needle has been removed from the abdomen), and a single-throw surgeon's knot is then placed. It is helpful to minimize the amount of "journeying" (movement with loop around instrument) once the loops are placed (i.e., have the needle holder with the loops in the immediate vicinity of the opposite [free] suture end). It is also helpful to keep the jaw of the needle holder that has the loop or loops slightly open to prevent loss of the loops.

SUMMARY

A large array of instrumentation is available for operative laparoscopic procedures. Knowledge of indications for specific instrumentation is important for successful completion of the surgical task. Acquiring skills of laparoscopic knot-tying adds a new dimension to operative laparoscopy.

References

1. Mackety JC: Operative room personnel. In: Sanfilippo JS, Levine RL, eds. Operative gynecologic endoscopy. New York: Springer-Verlag, 1989:179.
2. Hay DL, Levine RL, von Fraunhofer JA, Masterson BJ: Chromic gut pelviscopic loop ligature. Effect of the number of pulls on the tensile strength. J Reprod Med 1990;35:260.
3. Reich H, Clarke HC, Sekel L: A simple method for ligating with straight and curved needles in operative laparoscopy. Obstet Gynecol 1992;79:143.

Laparoscopic Surgery: An Atlas for General Surgeons, edited by Gary C. Vitale, Joseph S. Sanfilippo, and Jacques Perissat. J. B. Lippincott Company, Philadelphia, © 1995.

Chapter 7

Anesthesia for Laparoscopic General Surgery

Linda F. Lucas
Eleanor F. Asher
Julia A. Schroeder
Benjamin M. Rigor

Laparoscopic techniques are gaining wide acceptance for surgical diagnosis and treatment. General, regional, and local anesthesia have all been used effectively for laparoscopic procedures. The suitability of each depends on the type of procedure, the physiologic status of the patient, and the preferences of the surgeon and patient. Physiologic changes that occur during laparoscopy must be considered in the choice of appropriate anesthetic for each procedure.

RESPIRATORY AND CARDIAC EFFECTS OF POSITIONING AND PNEUMOPERITONEUM

Effects of Positioning

For cholecystectomy and appendectomy, the patient is placed supine or in the lithotomy or modified lithotomy position. With the former, the patient is placed in an extreme reverse Trendelenburg's position to allow the colon and the omentum to be displaced inferiorly. With the latter the patient is placed in the supine or modified lithotomy position, with the addition of a moderate Trendelenburg's tilt.

The lithotomy position alone may decrease tidal volume by as much as 13% in the anesthetized patient. When combined with a Trendelenburg's position of 20°, tidal volume is decreased by 15%.[1,2] Pulmonary compliance is also reduced, especially in obese patients.[3,4] Diaphragmatic excursion is limited and pulmonary blood flow is increased with the lithotomy and Trendelenburg's positions, resulting in decreases in vital capacity and functional residual capacity (Table 7-1).[5–8] Distribution of airflow within the lungs is also altered (Fig. 7-1).[9]

Such changes in pulmonary function may predispose the patient to postoperative atelectasis and pneumonia. Patients undergoing laparoscopic cholecystectomy, however, appear to have fewer pulmonary complications than those who undergo open procedures. We attribute this to the use of the reverse Trendelenburg's position during laparoscopy, which allows increased physiologic air flow to basilar lung segments. It also reduces pain and improves ambulation in the early postoperative period. In most cases, the clinical problems associated with respiratory changes produced by positioning for laparoscopy can be prevented with the use of general anesthesia and controlled ventilation to restore normal lung volumes.

Using the reverse Trendelenburg's position during laparoscopic cholecystectomy may reduce ventilatory abnormalities but—conversely—may increase circulatory compromise and hypotension (Fig. 7-2). Adequate hydration preoperatively should prevent (or minimize) hypotension due to blood pooling in the lower extremities. Any intraoperative changes in positioning should be made slowly to compensate for intravascular volume shifts that may contribute to hypotension. This is especially important because both regional and general anesthesia compromise the body's compensatory mechanisms for cardiovascular adjustments to positional change (Tables 7-2 and 7-3).

Effects of Pneumoperitoneum

In addition to the changes produced by positioning, pneumoperitoneum also produces changes in pulmonary and circulatory mechanics. Total respiratory compliance and diaphragmatic movement are reduced.[10,11] Increases in airway pressure and intrathoracic pressure

TABLE 7-1
Effect of Position on Lung Volume

Position	Vital Capacity (% Decrease from Standing)
Recumbent	10
Gallbladder rest	13
Head down	15
Trendelenburg's	15
Lithotomy	18

Modified from Collins V: Principles of anesthesiology. 2nd ed. Philadelphia: Lea & Febiger, 1976:153.

also occur at intraperitoneal pressures above 20 mmHg. In spontaneously breathing patients' respiratory rate increases, causing an increase in minute ventilation despite reduced tidal volumes.[10–13] Vital capacity is reduced but remains sufficient for tidal volumes to increase in healthy nonobese patients if necessary.

Although at least five different gases or combinations of gases have been used for pneumoperitoneum, carbon dioxide (CO_2) is used most commonly. Carbon dioxide is rapidly absorbed and excreted and does not support combustion. It is the most soluble in blood of all the agents used for pneumoperitoneum and is safer than oxygen and nitrous oxide (N_2O) in preventing air embolism.[12,14] Absorption of CO_2 into the blood contributes to hypercarbia. The arterial CO_2 tension is raised about 8 mmHg in patients undergoing gynecologic laparoscopic procedures with CO_2 pneumoperitoneum when compared with patients with N_2O insufflation.[15] Patients breathing spontaneously with halothane–N_2O–oxygen anesthesia compensate by increasing their respiratory rate by as much as 75% to 100%.[10] Minute ventilation is increased despite a reduction in tidal volume.[10,12,13] Respiratory and metabolic acidosis may result.[10,16,17] Hypoxia may follow, with values as low as a PaO_2 of 46 to 64 mmHg when the inspired oxygen concentration is less than 40%.[16] Hypercarbia and acidosis are not seen in patients when N_2O is used.[15] Although experienced anesthesiologists may prefer to maintain general anesthesia with a mask and spontaneous ventilation for short cases, it is generally recommended that respiratory and acid–base homeostasis be maintained with mild hyperventilation and adequate muscle relaxation by administration of a general anesthetic and use of endotracheal intubation.[17,18]

When it occurs, hypercarbia contributes to hyperten-

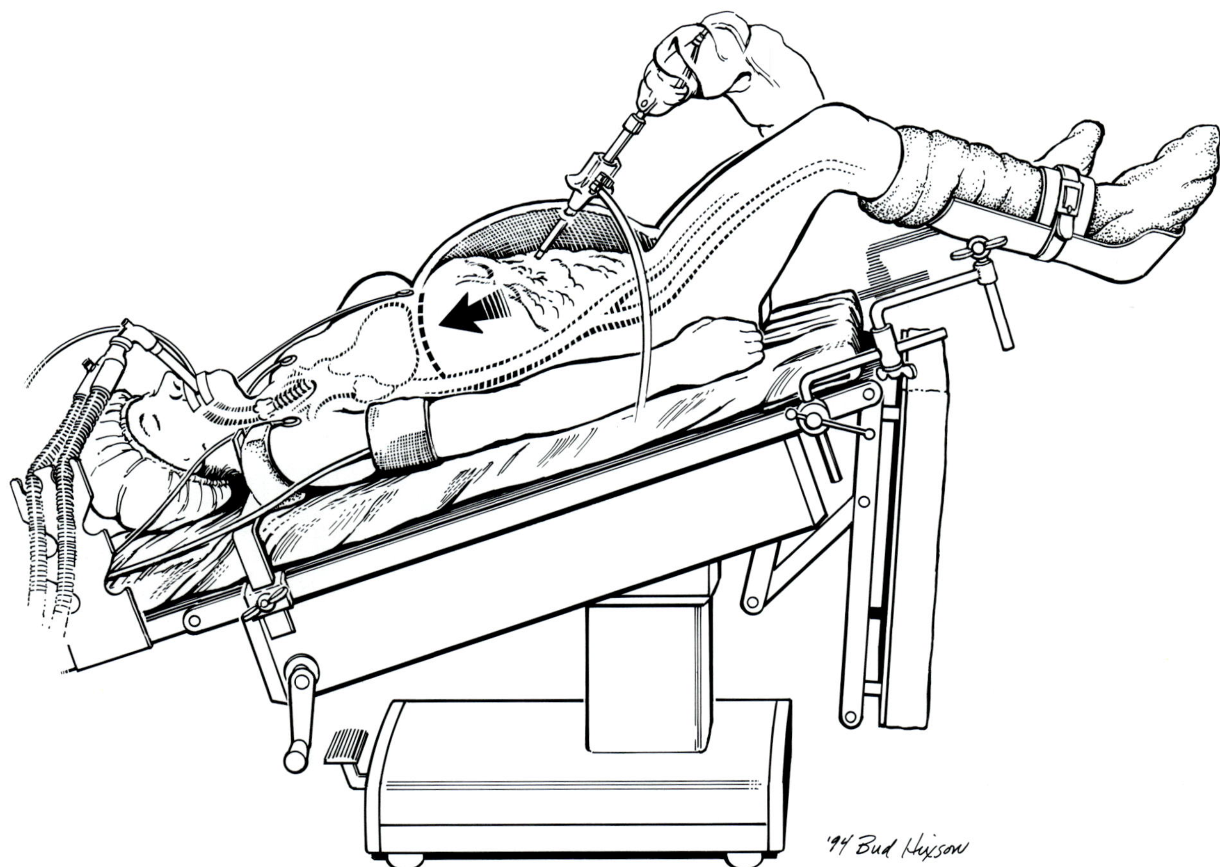

FIGURE 7-1. Trendelenburg and lithotomy positions limit diaphragmatic excursion and increase pulmonary blood flow.

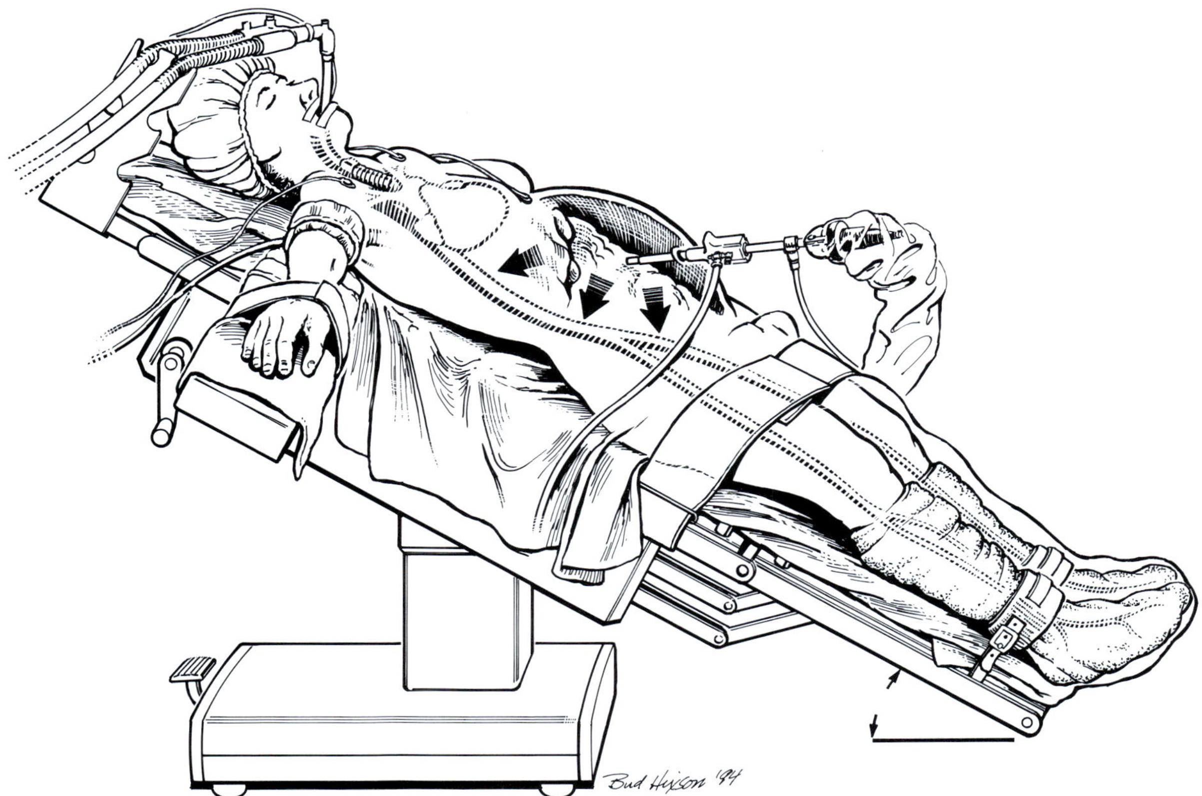

FIGURE 7-2. Reverse Trendelenburg position reduces ventilatory abnormalities but may increase circulatory compromise and hypotension.

sion, tachycardia, and cardiac arrhythmias and to vasodilation and myocardial depression. Sympathetic responses to pneumoperitoneum and hypercarbia, however, counter these responses by increasing plasma catecholamines that produce vasoconstriction, elevate central venous pressure, and increase cardiac chronotropy, inotropy, and arrhythmias (Fig. 7-3).[19,20] Additionally, halothane general anesthesia contributes to cardiac conduction abnormalities and arrhythmias. Plasma concentrations of cortisol, prolactin, and glucose also increase significantly in response to the stress of peritoneal distention.[21]

TABLE 7-2
Head-Up Position (Erect) Cardiocirculatory Changes

CARDIAC	
Cardiac rate	Increased
Cardiac volume	Decreased
Stroke volume	Decreased
A-V oxygen	Increased
Cardiac output	Unchanged or decreased
CIRCULATORY	
Systolic pressure	Decreased
Diastolic pressure	Increased
Venous pressure	Decreased
CAUSES	
Hydrostatic blood displacement	
Physiologic edema	
Changes in leg volume	

Modified from Collins V: Principles of anesthesiology. 2nd ed. Philadelphia: Lea & Febiger, 1976:152.

TABLE 7-3
Head-Down Position (45°) Cardiocirculatory Changes

CARDIAC	
Cardiac rate	Slowed (reflex)
Cardiac volume	Increased
Superior vena cava	Doubled
Stroke volume	Increased
A-V oxygen	Decreased
Cardiac output	Unchanged or increased
CIRCULATORY	
Systolic pressure	Slightly increased
Diastolic pressure	Slightly decreased
Venous pressure	Decreased
Cerebral venous pressure	Increased
Cerebral blood flow	Decreased

Modified from Collins V: Principles of anesthesiology. 2nd ed. Philadelphia: Lea & Febiger, 1976:152.

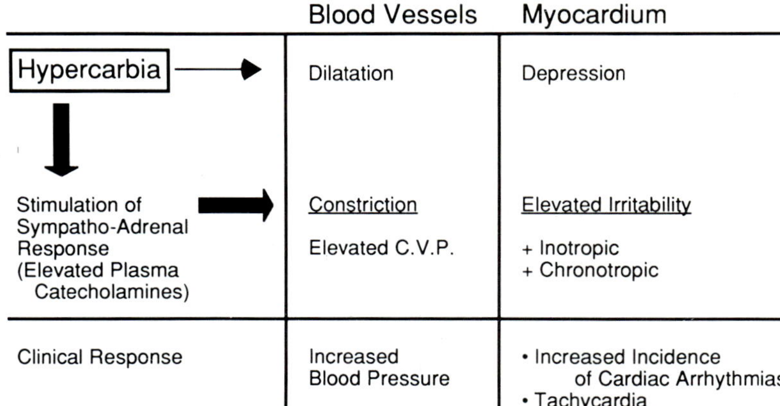

Effects of Hypercarbia Related to Anesthesia for Laparoscopy
Blood Vessels
Myocardium
Hypercarbia
Dilatation
Depression
Stimulation of Sympatho-Adrenal Response (Elevated Plasma Catecholamines)
Constriction
Elevated C.V.P.
Elevated Irritability
+ Inotropic
+ Chronotropic
Clinical Response
Increased Blood Pressure
• Increased Incidence of Cardiac Arrhythmias
• Tachycardia

FIGURE 7-3. Cardiovascular response to hypercarbia. (Modified and reprinted with permission from Peterson EP: Anesthesia for laparoscopy. Fertil Steril 1971;22:696.)

Cardiac arrhythmias (most commonly sinus tachycardia), ventricular arrhythmias, and asystole have been attributed to hypercarbia. Arrhythmias most often occur, however, during the preinsufflation period and may be the result of light anesthesia.[22] More commonly, we have noticed bradycardia resulting from peritoneal distention and stimulation. The administration of atropine, either as a premedicant or with the occurrence of bradycardia and hypotension, effectively antagonizes these vagal reflexes.

Stroke volume and cardiac output are depressed up to 60% during insufflation of the peritoneum.[23] Cardiac index and stroke index may be reduced by an average of 42%.[24] Some studies, however, show no hemodynamic change when intra-abdominal pressures reach 20 to 25 mmHg.[11,25–27] At pressures of 30 mmHg or greater, decreases in systolic pressure, pulse pressure, and cardiac output (due to impedance of venous return to the heart from compression of the inferior vena cava) produce arterial hypotension, with a rise in central venous pressure.[16,28] An even greater degree of cardiovascular depression has been demonstrated in anesthetized hypovolemic animals after pneumoperitoneum, as compared with awake normovolemic controls.[26] It is important to maintain proper hydration in patients undergoing laparoscopy because hypovolemic patients have a poor tolerance for further reductions in cardiac output. This is especially true with procedures such as cholecystectomy, wherein the reverse Trendelenburg's position results in vascular pooling in the lower extremities (see Fig. 7-2).

Hypotension may also be the result of hypoxia, particularly in patients administered general anesthesia with a low inspired oxygen concentration or in patients with preexisting pulmonary disease. General anesthesia for laparoscopy should include administration of at least 35% oxygen. The use of an oxygen analyzer and continuous pulse oximetry should prevent unrecognized hypoxemia.

ANESTHETIC TECHNIQUES APPROPRIATE FOR LAPAROSCOPY

General Anesthesia

Although regional anesthesia has been successfully used for laparoscopy, most procedures are performed under general anesthesia. Most investigations of anesthesia for laparoscopy have been conducted during gynecologic procedures. The anesthesia requirements for most intra-abdominal procedures, including cholecystectomy and appendectomy, should not differ significantly from those for gynecologic laparoscopic procedures (Fig. 7-4).

Advantages of general anesthesia include rapid onset, amnesia, complete analgesia, good muscle relaxation, and a quiet surgical field. General anesthesia is most appropriate for long procedures and patients with adhesions from previous intra-abdominal surgery or pathology. It is also appropriate for critically ill patients who may require resuscitative efforts. Respiratory and acid–base homeostasis is best maintained with general anesthesia, endotracheal intubation, and controlled ventilation, particularly in obese or older patients who may have preexisting impairment of pulmonary compliance, decreased vital capacity, and decreased functional residual capacity.[4,29]

The anxious patient may also benefit from general anesthesia. Those who are unable to cooperate, such as those with a language barrier, mental retardation, or hearing impairment may also benefit. Some surgeons, as a result of their training or experience, prefer to have the patient asleep. In this way, the surgeon may avoid the distraction of communicating with an awake patient or of causing the patient any discomfort during the procedure.

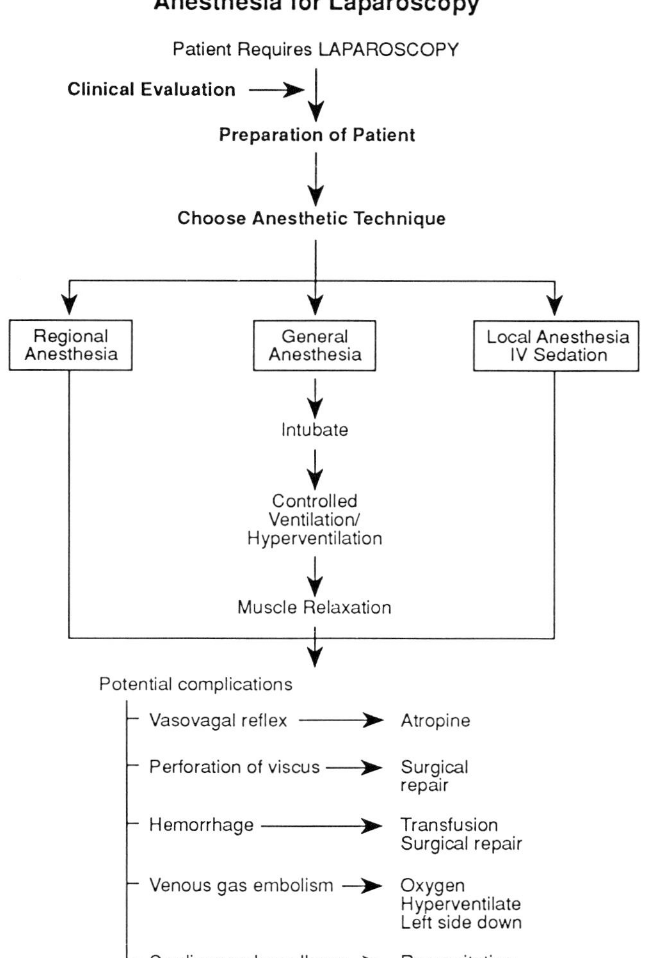

FIGURE 7-4. Anesthetic considerations in laparoscopy. (Reprinted with permission from Bready LL: Laparoscopy. In: Bready LL, Smith RE, eds. Decision making in anesthesiology. Philadelphia: BC Decker, 1987:119.)

General anesthesia is appropriate for the experienced and the novice laparoscopist. It is preferable for inexperienced personnel until equipment and viscera can be handled gently and smoothly. In training institutions, techniques and anatomic structures can more easily be demonstrated with the patient asleep. Regional and local anesthetic techniques are often more time-consuming and less reliable than those for general anesthesia; therefore, they are more likely to delay a busy operating room schedule. Many surgeons and anesthesiologists consider general anesthesia to be safer than regional or local anesthesia for procedures using lasers because it provides an immobile surgical field. General anesthesia also allows immediate laparotomy should major complications or unexpected findings occur.

Disadvantages of general anesthesia include an increased incidence of major and minor complications. Mask ventilation before intubation may cause gastric distention, contributing to nausea, vomiting, and an increased risk of aspiration. Controlled ventilation may result in increased airway pressures, causing barotrauma and pneumothorax, especially in emphysematous or other patients with poor pulmonary compliance. Sore throat, myalgia, hoarseness, nausea, and vomiting are frequent postoperative complaints.[30,31] These sequelae usually resolve in 24 to 48 hours. In a report of patients for minor outpatient gynecologic laparoscopic procedures, however, as many as 57% were unable to return to their usual activities for 48 hours after the surgery.[32,33] Postoperative morbidity appears to be highest in female patients, patients undergoing procedures lasting more than 20 minutes, intubated patients, and those who have not had general anesthesia previously.[34] In patients undergoing laparoscopic cholecystectomy, older patients and those with adhesions from previous surgery suffered more morbidity than other patients, often delaying discharge.[35]

Anesthesia is most frequently induced with a rapid-acting intravenous barbiturate solution or other induction agents, including etomidate, propofol, and short-acting narcotics. These agents allow rapid awakening and recovery. Etomidate and methohexital are associated with a high incidence of minor adverse side effects, including pain on injection and myoclonus.[36] Etomidate transiently depresses adrenocortical function.[37] Propofol is being used extensively for general anesthesia and for conscious sedation for outpatient procedures, including gynecologic laparoscopy, because it allows extremely rapid recovery with minimal adverse effects.[38]

A Foley catheter and a nasogastric tube are placed before trocar insertion to decompress the bladder and the stomach. The nasogastric tube is initially suctioned and then left open for gravity drainage, with intermittent suctioning to relieve gastric distention from gas diffused into the stomach from the pneumoperitoneum.

Maintenance of anesthesia may be accomplished with inhalational or intravenous anesthetic agents. Halothane, enflurane, and isoflurane, often in combination with N_2O, have been used for laparoscopy. Halothane is not recommended for laparoscopic procedures because it may predispose patients to life-threatening ventricular arrhythmias, especially in the presence of hypercarbia or acidosis.[10,11,13] Enflurane has been recommended for outpatient procedures because it may allow more rapid recovery than halothane and has fewer side effects than isoflurane. A newer study, however, concludes that there is no significant difference in recovery from enflurane and isoflurane (Table 7-4).[39] Isoflurane may also decrease the risk of arrhythmias induced by hypercarbia.[40] The administration of N_2O as it relates to postoperative nausea and vomiting has been studied, but it remains unclear whether it is a causative factor.[41,42]

Propofol is a new intravenous anesthetic agent that can be administered for maintenance of anesthesia as

TABLE 7-4
Morbidity After the Use of Halothane, Enflurane, or Isoflurane for Outpatient Gynecologic Surgery

	Incidence (%)		
Postoperative Symptoms	*Halothane*	*Enflurane*	*Isoflurane*
Sore throat	68	64	64
Pain (analgesic)	52	68	54
Malaise	28	44	44
Cough	16	40	44*
Dizziness	16	28	52*
Drowsiness	16	36	40
Myalgia	16	28	20
Smell of anesthetic	28	12	40*
Headache	20	12	44*
Nausea	8	12	32*
Vomiting	4	4	12

* *Significantly different from halothane or enflurane groups,* $p < .05$.

Reprinted with permission from White PF: Outpatient anesthesia. In: Miller RD, ed. Anesthesia. 3rd ed, vol 2. New York: Churchill Livingstone, 1990:2039.

well as its induction. Although it is expensive, its use almost eliminates postoperative adverse effects. In combination with short-acting narcotics such as alfentanil, propofol is particularly suitable for outpatient procedures.[43] Potent short-acting narcotics such as fentanyl, sufentanil, and alfentanil are also effective for anesthetic induction and maintenance when used in conjunction with an inhalational agent, oxygen, and a muscle relaxant.[44,45] These narcotics provide potent analgesia, are rapidly eliminated or easily reversed, and maintain cardiovascular stability, even in critically ill patients. Although outpatients who have received a balanced anesthetic with these narcotics appear to develop a higher incidence of early postoperative complications including nausea, vomiting, and respiratory depression, the incidence of complications following discharge does not differ significantly from patients administered inhalational anesthetics.[44] Outpatients for laparoscopic procedures, including cholecystectomy, have a high incidence of postoperative anesthetic adverse effects, regardless of the anesthetic employed.[34,45]

Intravenous muscle relaxants are used during maintenance of general anesthesia to relax the chest and abdominal wall musculature, to improve chest wall compliance, and to improve operating conditions. Succinylcholine is a depolarizing muscle relaxant used to facilitate intubation and may be continuously infused to provide muscle relaxation for diagnostic and other short procedures. There are, however, major and minor complications associated with the use of succinylcholine, including arrhythmias, hyperkalemia, myoglobinemia, malignant hyperthermia, sore throat, myalgia, prolonged apnea, and weakness in patients with plasma pseudocholinesterase deficiencies. Nondepolarizing muscle relaxants, including pancuronium, atracurium, and vecuronium, can be administered without these complications.[45–47] Atracurium and vecuronium are intermediate-duration agents with a length of action appropriate for diagnostic procedures, appendectomy, and cholecystectomy. Pancuronium is suitable for cholecystectomy and other procedures when they take longer than 1 hour to complete.

Regional Anesthesia

Although general anesthesia is used for most laparoscopic procedures, major regional anesthesia has been administered successfully for cholecystectomy and has been recommended for appendectomy.[48–50] Regional and local anesthetics have been widely accepted for pelviscopic surgery.[51–53] As anesthesiologists continue to gain experience in this area, regional anesthesia techniques may advance accordingly, providing suitable anesthesia for many general surgical laparoscopic procedures.

Advantages of regional and local anesthesia include an awake patient capable of giving information, which may lead to early detection and treatment of complications. Many of the major and minor complications associated with general anesthesia can be avoided with the administration of regional or local anesthesia, often decreasing recovery time. Fewer pharmacologic agents may be used, limiting allergic or other adverse pharmacologic reactions. Spinal anesthesia provides excellent muscle relaxation, an immobile surgical field, decreased intestinal peristalsis, and bowel shrinkage to improve operating conditions. The adverse effects of pneumoperitoneum and the length of most procedures, however, limit the safety and effectiveness of regional anesthesia for most general surgical procedures.

TABLE 7-5
Preoperative Work-Up in the Laparoscopic Patient

Investigation/Procedure	*Usage by Surgeons (%)*
Liver function tests	100
Gallbladder ultrasound examination	100
Oral cholecystography	20
Intravenous cholangiography	75
Group and save	95
Crossmatch	0
Prophylactic antibiotics	95

Reprinted with permission from Cuschieri A, Dubois F, Mouiel J, et al: The European experience with laparoscopic cholecystectomy. Am J Surg 1991;161:385.

Local Anesthesia

Local anesthesia provides rapid recovery and cost-effectiveness. Combined with sedation, it has gained acceptance for outpatient laparoscopic procedures in many specialties.[27,54,55] In general surgery, use of local anesthesia has been limited to diagnostic and occasional short therapeutic procedures. Percutaneous laparoscopic cholecystectomy has been performed successfully with local anesthesia in a patient unable to tolerate other anesthetic modalities.[56]

Preoperative Preparation of the Patient and Premedication

Preparation of the patient, including history, physical examination, and laboratory tests, is not significantly different from that of the patient undergoing a comparable open procedure (Table 7-5), especially because unforeseen circumstances may make it necessary to change to an open procedure. Depending upon the procedure, patients are generally typed and screened for blood products before surgery in case of hemorrhage. Anesthetic procedures, with their risks and benefits, are discussed with the patient preoperatively. Patients scheduled for outpatient procedures such as cholecystectomy benefit from more extensive counseling concerning recovery and discharge than do those who are admitted after surgery.[35]

Goals of premedication include amnesia, analgesia, anxiolysis, and the reduction of nausea, vomiting, and total anesthetic requirements. Benzodiazepines have become the most commonly used preoperative pharmacologic agents because of their anxiolytic, amnestic, and sedative properties.[57] Fentanyl and alfentanil (short-duration narcotics) and nalbuphine and butorphanol (combined narcotic agonist–antagonists) are often used in combination with small doses of benzodiazepines (such as midazolam or diazepam) to provide sedation and analgesia.

Antihistamines (e.g. hydroxyzine); butyrophenones (e.g., droperidol); and phenothiazines (including prochlorperazine and promethazine) may also be administered preoperatively, intraoperatively, or postoperatively for sedative and antiemetic effects. Transdermal scopolamine may be administered preoperatively to control postoperative nausea and vomiting.

Patients undergoing laparoscopy are at increased risk for vomiting and aspiration pneumonitis due to the increased intra-abdominal and intragastric pressures created by the pneumoperitoneum. Premedication with H_2-antihistamine receptor antagonists—including cimetidine, ranitidine, famotidine, or a nonparticulate antacid such as sodium citrate or Alka-Seltzer effervescent antacid—should be considered in all patients for laparoscopy to decrease gastric acidity.[58–61] Metoclopramide is also useful to reduce the incidence of pneumonitis if aspiration occurs because it reduces gastric volume and may decrease postoperative nausea and vomiting.[62,63]

Monitoring and Safety Considerations

Sophisticated monitoring techniques have improved the safety of anesthesia for all procedures, including laparoscopy. Electrocardiography, continuous temperature and noninvasive blood pressure monitoring, in-line oxygen concentration monitoring, capnography, and pulse oximetry should be used for all patients. Routine laboratory analysis (including hemoglobin or hematocrit, electrolyte, and blood gas assays; radiographs; and 12-lead electrocardiograms) should also be readily available.

Complications may occur as the result of laparoscopic procedures, including hemorrhage, injury to viscera, subcutaneous emphysema, and pneumothorax.[64] Laparoscopy should only be performed where equipment is immediately available for general anesthesia, emergency laparotomy, and resuscitation.

TABLE 7-6
Reasons for Admission of Patients Who Have Had Outpatient Laparoscopic Cholecystectomy

Reason	*(%)*
Patient preference	23.9
Age	17.3
Urinary retention	10.8
Distance of home from hospital	10.8
Acute cholecystitis	10.8
Ileus	8.6
Nausea	8.6
Pain	4.3
Pulmonary complications	2.1
Bleeding	2.1

Modified from Reddick EJ, Olsen DO: Outpatient laparoscopic laser cholecystectomy. Am J Surg 1990;160:485.

TABLE 7-7
Postoperative Characteristics of Patient Undergoing Laparoscopic Surgery

Characteristic	*IV*	*IM*	*PO*	*None*	
Narcotic requirement (n = 96)	2	30	71	25	
	DOS	POD 1	POD 2	POD 3	POD 4
Hospital stay (n = 93)	3	80	7	3	
Regular diet (n = 95)	6	77	9	2	1
Return to full activity*	12.8 ± 6.8 days (range 3–34)				

IV = intravenous morphine; IM = intramuscular meperidine; PO = oral oxycodone; DOS = day of surgery; POD = postoperative day.

**Mean ± standard deviation.*

Reprinted with permission from Peter JH, Elliso EC, Innes JT, et al: Safety and efficacy of laparoscopic cholecystectomy. A prospective analysis of 100 initial patients. Am J Surg 1991;213:7.

Recovery

Advances in laparoscopic surgery allow a more rapid recovery than do comparable open procedures. Patients are remarkably mobile and pain-free after surgery. At least 50% of cholecystectomy patients may be discharged the day of surgery.[35,48] For these patients, the adverse effects of anesthesia may be the limiting factor to early discharge. Other patients are usually ready for discharge on the first postoperative day.[35,36,50,65–70]

Factors unrelated to anesthesia also affect recovery and time of discharge. Young patients and those without previous upper abdominal surgery are most suitable for undergoing laparoscopic cholecystectomy as an outpatient procedure. Patients older than 70 years of age and those with acute inflammatory gallbladder disease are more likely to require hospitalization. Other reported reasons for postoperative hospital admission in uncomplicated cases include patient preference, urinary retention, ileus, nausea, pain, postoperative bleeding, and distance to home from the hospital (Table 7-6).[35]

Postanesthetic care for inpatients who have undergone laparoscopy does not differ significantly from the care of patients who have undergone nonlaparoscopic procedures for similar conditions. Although patients for laparoscopic appendectomy and cholecystectomy have more postoperative nausea and vomiting than diagnostic laparoscopy patients, they have greatly increased mobility and decreased pain medication requirements when compared with patients undergoing comparable open procedures.[66–68]

SUMMARY

An understanding of the physiologic effects of positioning and pneumoperitoneum is essential to the safe administration of anesthesia for laparoscopy. Hypercarbia, acidosis, aspiration, arrhythmias, and cardiovascular instability may occur as the result of patient positioning and increased intraperitoneal pressure. Although general, regional, and local anesthesia have all been used successfully, general anesthesia with endotracheal intubation and controlled ventilation is usually administered because of the need for pneumoperitoneum at high pressures for prolonged periods of time.

Technologic advances in surgical equipment and technique, patient monitoring, and pharmacologic agents have improved the safety and contributed to the rapid recovery of patients undergoing laparoscopic surgery. Many patients can safely undergo laparoscopic cholecystectomy, and those undergoing laparoscopic appendectomy may be discharged within 24 hours after surgery, with good mobility and little pain (Table 7-7). With the emphasis on rapid recovery, outpatient surgery, and cost-effectiveness, it is increasingly important to use short-duration inhalational and intravenous anesthetics that produce minimal postoperative adverse effects.

References

1. Jones JR, Jacoby J: The effect of surgical positions on respirations. Surg Forum 1954;5:686.
2. Henschel AB, Wyant GM, Dobkin AB, Henschel EO: Posture as it concerns the anesthesiologist: a preliminary study. Anesth Analg 1957;36:69.
3. Sharp JT: The effect of body position change on lung compliance in normal subjects and in patients with congestive heart failure. J Clin Invest 1959;38:659.
4. Waltemath CL, Bergman NA: Respiratory compliance in obese patients. Anesthesiology 1974;41:84.
5. Wood-Smith FF, Horne GM, Nunn JF: Effect of posture on ventilation of patients anaesthetized with halothane. Anaesthesia 1961;16:340.
6. Swain J: The case for abandoning the Trendelenburg position in pelvic surgery. Med J Aust 1960;47:536.
7. Martin JT: Positioning in anesthesia and surgery. Philadelphia: WB Saunders, 1978:142.
8. Case EH, Stiles JA: The effect of various surgical positions on vital capacity. Anesthesiology 1946;7:29.
9. Altschule MD, Zamcheck N: Significance of changes in subdivisions of the lung volume in the Trendelenburg position. Surg Gynecol Obstet 1942;74:1061.
10. Lewis DG, Ryder W, Burn N, Wheldon JT, Tacchi D: Laparoscopy—an investigation during spontaneous ventilation with halothane. Br J Anaesth 1972;44:685.
11. Hodgson C, McClelland RMA, Newton JR: Some effects of

the peritoneal insufflation of carbon dioxide at laparoscopy. Anaesthesia 1970;25:382.

12. Scott DB: Some effects of peritoneal insufflation of carbon dioxide at laparoscopy. Anaesthesia 1970;25:590.
13. Desmond J, Gordon RA: Ventilation in patients anaesthesized for laparoscopy. Can Anaesth Soc J 1970;17:378.
14. Graff TD, Arbegast NR, Phillips OC, Harris LC, Frazier TM: Gas embolism: a comparative study of air and carbon dioxide as embolic agents in the systemic venous system. Am J Obstet Gynecol 1959;78:259.
15. Alexander GD, Noe FE, Brown EM: Anesthesia for pelvic laparoscopy. Anesth Analg 1969;48:14.
16. Motew M, Ivankovich AD, Bieniarz J, et al: Cardiovascular effects and acid–base and blood gas changes during laparoscopy. Am J Obstet Gynecol 1973;115:1002.
17. Seed RF, Shakespeare TF, Muldoon MJ: Carbon dioxide homeostasis during anaesthesia for laparoscopy. Anaesthesia 1970;25:223.
18. Magno R, Medegard A, Bengtsson R, Tronstad S-E: Acid–base balance during laparoscopy. Acta Obstet Gynecol Scand 1979;58:81.
19. Price HC: Effects of carbon dioxide on the cardiovascular system. Anesthesiology 1960;21:652.
20. Peterson EP: Anesthesia for laparoscopy. Fertil Steril 1971; 22:695.
21. Cooper GM, Scoggins AM: Laparoscopy—a stressful procedure. Anaesthesia 1982;37:266.
22. Harris MNE, Plantevin OM, Crowther A: Cardiac arrhythmias during anaesthesia for laparoscopy. Br J Anaesth 1984;56:1213.
23. McKenzie R, Wadhwa RK, Bedger RC: Noninvasive measurement of cardiac output during laparoscopy. J Reprod Med 1980;24:247.
24. Johannsen G, Andersen M, Juhl B: The effect of general anaesthesia on the haemodynamic events during laparoscopy with CO_2-insufflation. Acta Anaesthesiol Scand 1989; 33:132.
25. Smith I, Benzie RJ, Gordon NLM, Kelman GR, Swapp GH: Cardiovascular effects of peritoneal insufflation of carbon dioxide for laparoscopy. Br Med J 1971;3:410.
26. Ivankovich AD, Miletich DJ, Albrecht RF, Heyman HJ, Bonnet RF: Cardiovascular effects of intraperitoneal insufflation with carbon dioxide and nitrous oxide in the dog. Anesthesiology 1975;42:281.
27. Diamant M, Benumof JL, Saidman LJ: Hemodynamics of increased intra-abdominal pressure. Anesthesiology 1978; 48:23.
28. Lee CM: Acute hypotension during laparoscopy. A case report. Anesth Analg 1975;54:142.
29. Couture J, Picken J, Trop D, et al: Airway closure in normal, obese, and anesthetized supine subjects. Fed Proc 1970;29:269. Abstract 131.
30. Metter SE, Kitz DS, Young ML, Baldeck AM, Apfelbaum IL, Lecky JH: Nausea and vomiting after outpatient laparoscopy: incidence, impact on recovery room stay and cost. Anesth Analg 1987;66:S116.
31. White P: Outpatient anesthesia. In: Miller RD, ed. Anesthesia. 3rd ed., vol 2. New York: Churchill Livingstone, 1990:2025.
32. Brindle GF, Soliman MG: Anaesthetic complications in surgical out-patients. Can Anaesth Soc J 1975:22:613.
33. Collins KM, Docherty PW, Plantevin OM: Postoperative morbidity following gynaecological outpatient laparoscopy. A reappraisal of the service. Anaesthesia 1984; 39:819.
34. Fahy A, Marshall M: Postanaesthetic morbidity in outpatients. Br J Anaesth 1969;41:433.
35. Reddick EJ, Olsen DO: Outpatient laparoscopic laser cholecystectomy. Am J Surg 1990;160:485.
36. Miller BM, Hendry JGB, Lees NW: Etomidate and methohexitone. A comparative clinical study in out-patient anaesthesia. Anaesthesia 1978;33:450.
37. Wagner RL, White PF: Etomidate inhibits adrenocortical function in surgical patients. Anesthesiology 1984;61:647.
38. DeGrood RM, Harbers JBM, van Egmond J, Crul JF: Anaesthesia for laparoscopy. A comparison of five techniques including propofol, etomidate, thiopentone and isoflurane. Anaesthesia 1987;42:815.
39. Tracey JA, Holland AJC, Unger L: Morbidity in minor gynaecological surgery: a comparison of halothane, enflurane and isoflurane. Br J Anaesth 1982;54:1213.
40. Kenefick JP, Leader A, Maltby JR, Taylor PJ: Laparoscopy: blood-gas values and minor sequelae associated with three techniques based on isoflurane. Br J Anaesth 1987; 59:189.
41. Lonie DS, Harper NJ: Nitrous oxide anaesthesia and vomiting. The effect of nitrous oxide anaesthesia on the incidence of vomiting following gynaecological laparoscopy. Anaesthesia 1986;41:703.
42. Hovorka J, Korttila K, Erkola O: Nitrous oxide does not increase nausea and vomiting following gynaecological laparoscopy. Can J Anaesth 1989;36:145.
43. Weightman WM, Zacharias M: Comparison of propofol and thiopentone anaesthesia (with special reference to recovery characteristics). Anaesth Intensive Care 1987; 15:389.
44. Karp KB: Anesthetic recovery after ambulatory laparoscopy: a comparison of isoflurane and alfentanil infusion. J Am Assoc Nurse Anesthetists 1990;58:83.
45. Raeder JC, Hole A: Out-patient laparoscopy in general anaesthesia with alfentanil and atracurium. A comparison with fentanyl and pancuronium. Acta Anaesthesiol Scand 1986;30:30.
46. Greville AC, Clements EAF: Anaesthesia for laparoscopic cholecystectomy using the Nd:Yag laser. The implications for a district general hospital. Anaesthesia 1990;45:944.
47. Bailey DM, Nicholas AD: Comparison of atracurium and vecuronium during anaesthesia for laparoscopy. Br J Anaesth 1988;61:557.
48. Zucker KA, Bailey RW, Gadacz TR, Imbembo AL: Laparoscopic guided cholecystectomy. Am J Surg 1991;161:36.
49. Gadacz TR, Talamini MA, Lillemoe KD, Yeo CJ: Laparoscopic cholecystectomy. Surg Clin North Am 1990; 70:1249.
50. Leahy PF: Technique of laparoscopic appendicectomy. Br J Surg 1989;76:616.
51. Aribarg A: Epidural analgesia for laparoscopy. J Obstet Gynaecol Br Commonw 1973;80:567.
52. Bridenbaugh LD, Soderstrom RM: Lumbar epidural block anesthesia for outpatient laparoscopy. J Reprod Med 1979; 23:85.
53. Mulroy M, Bridenbaugh LD: Regional anesthesia techniques for outpatient surgery. In: Wood SW, ed. Ambulatory anesthesia care. Boston: Little Brown, 1982:71.
54. Penfield AJ: Gynecologic surgery under local anesthesia. Baltimore: Urban & Schwarzenberg, 1986:21.
55. Wheeless CR Jr: Anesthesia for diagnostic and operative laparoscopy. Fertil Steril 1971;22:690.
56. Auguste L: Laparoscopy-guided percutaneous cholecystostomy. Gastrointest Endosc 1990;36:58.
57. Lichtor JL: Psychological preparation and preoperative medication. In: Miller RD, ed. Anesthesia. 3rd ed., vol 1. New York: Churchill Livingstone, 1990:895.
58. Richardson CT: Effect of H2-receptor antagonists on gas-

tric acid secretion and serum gastrin concentration: a review. Gastroenterology 1978;74:366.

59. Berardi RR, Tankanow RM, Nostrant TT: Comparison of famotidine with cimetidine and ranitidine. Clin Pharm 1988;7:271.

60. Eyler SW, Cullen BF, Murphy ME, Welch WD: Antacid aspiration in rabbits: a comparison of Mylanta and Bicitra. Anesth Analg 1982;61:288.

61. Chen CR, Toung TJK, Haupt HM, et al: Evaluation of the efficacy of Alka-Seltzer effervescent in gastric acid neutralization. Anesth Analg 1984;63:325.

62. Rao TLK, Madhavareddy S, Chinthagada M, El-Etr AA: Metoclopramide and cimetidine to reduce gastric fluid pH and volume. Anesth Analg 1984;63:1014.

63. Cohen SE, Woods WA, Wyner J: Antiemetic efficacy of droperidol and metoclopramide. Anesthesiology 1984; 60:67.

64. Marco AP, Yeo CJ, Rock P: Anesthesia for a patient undergoing laparoscopic cholecystectomy. Anesthesiology 1990;73:1268.

65. Miller TA: Laparoscopic cholecystectomy: passing fancy or legitimate treatment option? Gastroenterology 1990; 99:1527.

66. Peters JH, Ellison EC, Innes JT, et al: Safety and efficacy of laparoscopic cholecystectomy. A prospective analysis of 100 initial patients. Ann Surg 1991;213:3.

67. Griffith DP, Rubio PA, Gleeson MJ: Percutaneous endoscopic treatment of cholelithiasis. Surg Endosc 1990; 4:141.

68. Browne DS: Laparoscopic-guided appendicectomy. A study of 100 consecutive cases. Aust NZ J Obstet Gynaecol 1990;30:231.

69. Gangal HT, Gangal MH: Laparoscopic appendicectomy. Endoscopy 1987;19:127.

70. Berci G, Sackier JM: The Los Angeles experience with laparoscopic cholecystectomy. Am J Surg 1991;161:382.

Chapter 8

Laparoscopic Surgery: An Atlas for General Surgeons, edited by
Gary C. Vitale, Joseph S. Sanfilippo, and Jacques Perissat.
J. B. Lippincott Company, Philadelphia, © 1995.

Tissue Effects of Lasers and Electrosurgery

Dan C. Martin

Although lasers and pelviscopic techniques appear to be the driving forces behind the revolution of laparoscopic surgical procedures, their long-term role has yet to be determined.[1–3] Lasers and electrosurgery can be used to produce excellent surgical results.[4] When corrected for a power density of about 60,000 W/cm^2, both have similar tissue effects. The tissue effects at lower power densities are more variable. This variation has been collated for the carbon dioxide (CO_2) laser (Fig. 8-1).[5–8]

Much of the developmental work in electrosurgery was completed more than 60 years ago and that in lasers more than 20 years ago.[9–12] Several summaries of electrosurgery and lasers emphasize use and safety.[13–17] The objective of this chapter is to present the essential concepts of the principles of electrosurgery and lasers.

ENERGY CONVERSION

Tissue is cut or coagulated by converting or distributing energy. The primary method is conversion of either electric energy or laser energy into heat. The secondary effect is thermal conduction of this heat into the lateral tissue. When absorption occurs at high power densities with little penetration, the power density (PD) is based on the formula:

$$PD = 0.86 \times \frac{\text{power}}{\pi \times \text{radius}^2}.$$

When there is deeper penetration, however, a cylindrical, parabolic, or other distribution formula is required. This would take the form of:

$$PD = F_d \times \frac{\text{power}}{\pi \times \text{radius}^2 \times \text{penetration}},$$

where F_d is a correction for the noncylindrical distribution of the penetration.[5,18]

Tissue and cellular change occurs with progressive heating. Heating tissue to 60°C uncoils the helix and results in welding as the tissue cools; however, 65°C coagulates the protein and tissue necrosis occurs.[15]

As the power density of laser or electrosurgical units exceeds the threshold of vaporization, water explodes into vapor and a crater is produced. This crater can be called an incision. The heat at the base of a vaporization crater depends on the water content. It stays at 100°C as long as the tissue is predominantly water. Fat heats to about 200°C, dry tissue is hotter, and carbon sublimates at 3652°C (Table 8-1).[5]

High-power densities produce rapid heating and vaporization; low-power density is more useful for coagulation and hemostasis. The distinction between low- and high power density depends on the purpose of the operation and the experience of the operator.

When the power density of lasers or electrosurgery exceeds a threshold of vaporization, water-containing tissue sublimates at higher temperatures and may reach 3652°C.[3,5]

Lasers are named for the molecules used to generate the beam. Carbon dioxide, argon, and helium neon (HeNe) lasers use gas-containing tubes, whereas potassium-titanyl-phosphate (KTP) and the neodymium: yttrium-aluminum-garnet (Nd:YAG) lasers are generated by using modified YAG crystals within the resonator chamber. The laser beam is monochromatic, coherent, and collimated. Although these characteristics are constant for a given type of laser, the color (wavelength), penetration, absorption, scatter, and extinction coefficients vary from one laser to another (Table 8-2). The color can vary from ultraviolet (excimer); to visible (argon, HeNe, KTP); to infrared (CO_2, Nd:YAG). In addition, lasers such as the tunable free-electron laser can vary the color.[15,19]

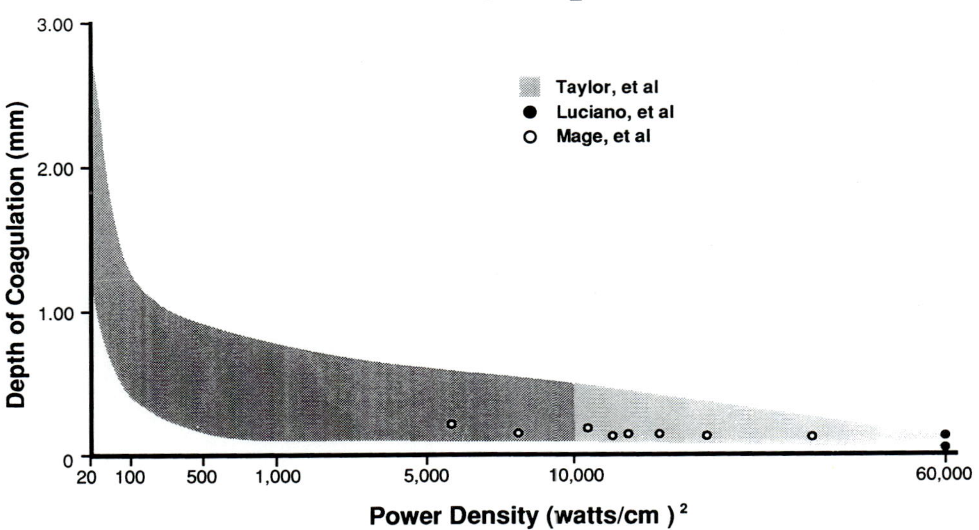

FIGURE 8-1. The depth of coagulation (tissue necrosis) decreases with increasing power density.[6–8] (Reproduced with permission of Martin DC: Tissue effects of lasers. Semin Reprod Endocrinol 1991;9[2]:132.)

POWER DENSITY

The tissue effects of laser and electrosurgery depend on many parameters. The penetration and power density of lasers appear to be the major contributors to the speed of action and the amount of deep thermal damage. In electrosurgery, the power density and waveform appear to have the same effects. The minimal penetration of the CO_2 laser and the rapid cutting of the undamped electrosurgical waveform create clean incisions and limit coagulation and hemostasis. The deep penetration and slow cutting speed of fiber lasers and the increased heat of the damped (coagulating) electrosurgical waveform create more thermal damage and increase hemostasis.

High-power density is created by spot lasers, small fiber diameters, and small electrodes for electrosurgical units. Low-power densities can be created with a defocused mode, large fiber contact areas, or broad electrosurgical tips.

TABLE 8-1
Effect of Tissue Heating

Temperature	*Effect*
42.5°C	Death of malignant cells
44.0°C	Death of normal cells
60.0°C	Collagen helix uncoils
65.0°C	Coagulation of protein
100.0°C	Vaporization of water
3652.0°C	Sublimation of carbon

Reproduced with permission of Martin DC: Tissue effects of lasers. Semin Reprod Endocrinol 1991;9(2):128.

COAGULATION

Although coagulation is used here as a basic term, its tissue effect is more complex and includes conversion of electric energy to thermal energy, conduction of thermal energy (cautery), fulguration of tissue, tissue heating, tissue necrosis, uncoiling of collagen helix, coagulation of protein, desiccation of water, and carbonization of dry tissue.[5,15] There is no general attempt to distinguish between electrosurgical coagulation, thermal coagulation, and cautery. Thermal coagulation, however, is a cautery unit, which causes tissue effects by direct transfer of heat. In contrast, electrosurgical units convert electric energy into heat and produce secondary cautery as the heat conducts into the surrounding tissue. Similarly, laser converts light energy into heat; there is primary coagulation or vaporization from the absorption of this heat and secondary cauterization as this heat source conducts into the lateral tissue.

CARBON DIOXIDE LASER

The CO_2 laser power density is controlled by a lens system, which is used to focus the beam to a small spot. In the vicinity of the spot, power densities are generally adequate for vaporization but, if the laser is pulled back and allowed to defocus, surface coagulation can be accomplished (Fig. 8-2). The depth of penetration of a defocused low-power density CO_2 laser beam is minimal; there is limited use for this technique.[2]

The CO_2 laser is most commonly spoken of as a "what you see is what you get" laser. The thermal necro-

TABLE 8-2
General Laser Characteristics

Name	Color	Wavelength (nm)	Extinction Coefficient	
			Water (cm)	Tissue (mm)
CO_2	Infrared	10,600	0.001	0.02
Argon	Blue-green	488–515	4000	0.5
KTP	Green	532	*	*
Nd:YAG	Infrared	1064	10	1.25

**Approximately equal to argon laser.*
Reproduced with permission of Martin DC: Tissue effects of lasers. Semin Reprod Endocrinol 1991;9(2):128.

sis is generally limited to 0.04 to 0.5 mm. The CO_2 laser beam is used in a "no touch" technique. The tissue effect is determined by the settings on the panel, the lens system, and the alignment of the beam. Surgeons can operate from a distance and watch the entire area of vaporization. There is no mechanical tissue resistance. Decreased smoke and cleaner cuts occur when traction is placed on tissue.

One problem with the use of low-power density CO_2 laser is carbonization, which creates what has been called a "charcoal briquette."[2] This briquette decreases tissue recognition and can interfere with diagnosis at subsequent second look laparoscopy.[20,21]

ARGON AND POTASSIUM-TITANYL-PHOSPHATE LASERS

Argon and KTP lasers are generally transmitted along fiberoptic systems. Both are absorbed by hemoglobin but pass through water and the vitreous of the eye. The argon laser has been used for retina surgery because it can coagulate areas of the retina without damaging the interior chambers. Using small fibers (0.3 and 0.6 mm), high-power densities can be created. These produce general effects similar to those of the CO_2 laser but with a slight increase in hemostatic capabilities because of the increased beam penetration.[2,5]

Surgeons who desire to use a touch technique or have experienced problems with CO_2 laser alignment may find fibers more acceptable. This requires control of both the power setting and the manual pressure because pressure on the fiber can cause a deeper cut than intended, similar to cuts made with a monopolar electrosurgical unit.[22–24] Fibers also produce a blind spot on the back side of the fiber.

As opposed to CO_2 lasers, which are focused, the fiber laser has its greatest power density as it exits from a fiber (Fig. 8-3). The power density decreases rapidly and may lose as much as 98% of the power density at 1 cm from the fiber tip.[25] Although vaporization is accomplished in the immediate vicinity of the fiber, the spread of energy results in zones of coagulation and heating as the fiber is withdrawn.

NEODYMIUM: YTTRIUM-ALUMINUM-GARNET LASER

The Nd:YAG laser is most valuable when used to coagulate highly vascular areas. This includes gastrointestinal hemorrhage and endometrial ablation.[26–28] When small sapphire tips or extruded rods are used, however, its power can be concentrated and used for vaporization, producing more predictable tissue damage than the noncontact mode, with effects similar to those of the CO_2

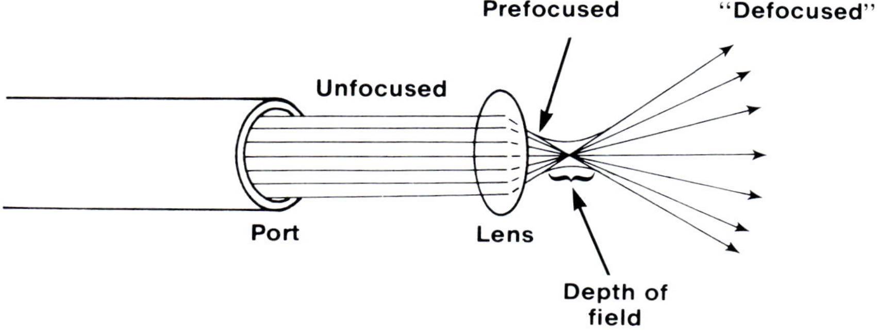

FIGURE 8-2. Focusing of the laser beam with a lens. Although this is generally used with a CO_2 laser, it may be used with other lasers. (Reproduced with permission of Martin DC: Tubal microsurgery. In: Martin DC, Absten GT, Levinson CJ, Photopulos GJ, eds. Intra-abdominal laser surgery. Memphis: Resurge Press, 1986; 123.)

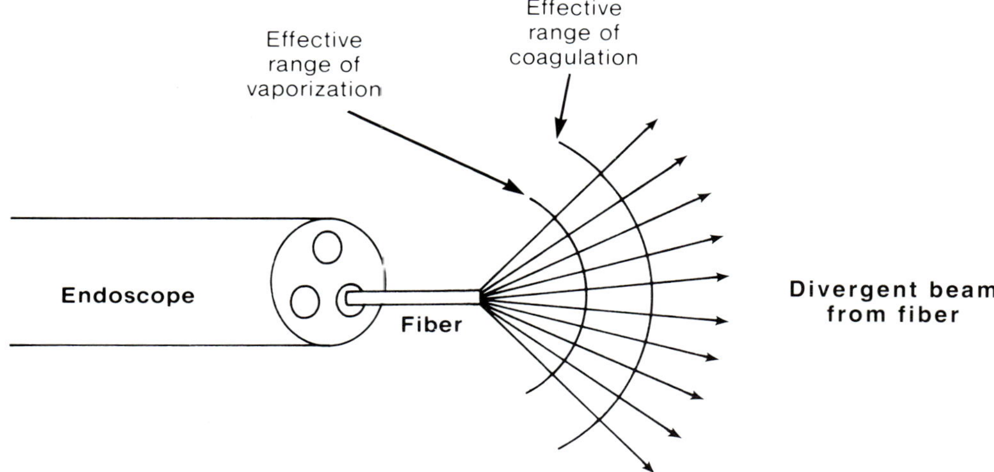

FIGURE 8-3. Fiber-directed laser beams diverge rapidly from the end of the fiber. With a high enough power density, the initial zone is vaporization. At a distance from this is coagulation; past this point, there is only heating. (Reproduced with permission of Martin DC. Tubal microsurgery. In: Martin DC, Absten GT, Levinson CJ, Photopulos GJ, eds. Intra-abdominal laser surgery. Memphis: Resurge Press, 1986;123)

laser.[8,29,30] A large component of the conversion of laser energy appears to occur in the tip, so that the tip serves as a combination of laser guide and thermal probe.[31]

MONOPOLAR ELECTROSURGERY

Electrosurgical units are generally monopolar or bipolar and produce damped waves, undamped waves, or blended waves. Monopolar systems return the active current to the generator through a patient-return electrode (ground plate). The surface area of a patient-return electrode is typically 120 cm^2. The surgical operative site tissue has the same electrical potential as the patient-return electrodes. This potential depends on the output characteristics of the electrosurgical generator and may be grounded or isolated from ground.

Monopolar current is undamped (cutting) or damped (coagulating) (Fig. 8-4).[32] Although called cutting and coagulating modes, respectively, at low-power densities both can coagulate and at high-power densities both can vaporize (cut). The difference is in the level of tissue penetration at a given power density. These terms are most relevant for monopolar electrosurgery and may be misleading when applied to bipolar electrosurgery. Undamped (vaporizing) current produces tissue effects similar to the CO_2 laser.[7]

Damped waves are good for superficial coagulation, using monopolar electrosurgery. Undamped waves are better for monopolar cutting and for deep bipolar electrosurgery. Undamped waves are best used with monopolar cutting current and for deep bipolar coagulation, such as in tubal sterilization or in the bipolar coagulation of large vessels.[13] When using a monopolar electrosurgi-

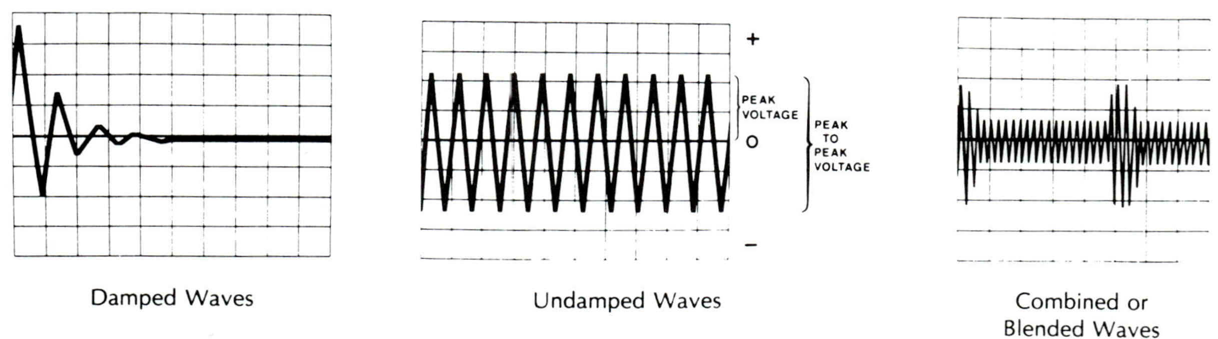

FIGURE 8-4. Frequency patterns of electrosurgical current used in surgery. (Reproduced with permission of Reich H, Vancaillie TG, Soderstrom RM: Electrical techniques. In: Martin DC, ed. Manual of endoscopy. Santa Fe Springs: American Association of Gynecologic Laparoscopists, 1990:105)

cal knife, the current does the cutting in many situations.[9,23] Excess pressure on the tip can cause unintended deep cuts, and it can produce a blind spot similar to that of the fiber laser.

BIPOLAR ELECTROSURGERY

Bipolar units have both the positive (active) and negative (patient-return) electrodes assembled on the same surgical instrument. Bipolar electrosurgery is useful for hemostatic coagulation by desiccating (dehydrating) the tissue. Although not used as cutting instruments, bipolar units use undamped current to achieve deep penetration of the energy. Small bipolar forceps can be used to limit the spread of unintended thermal damage.

SAFETY

Although a comprehensive review of safety aspects is beyond the scope of this chapter, researchers are encouraged to expand their level of knowledge by reading safety manuals or specific textbooks.[33–39]

Backstops

Backstops can either be intentional or unintentional. Surgeons have performed electrosurgery, using the tissue as its own backstop, with a high degree of safety.[23] Occasionally, deep burns have occurred, with significant tissue damage to ureters, bowel, and nerves. These burns have occurred with both electrosurgery and lasers. The techniques used in electrosurgery and lasers should be controlled to avoid inadvertent deep penetration and damage.[16,17] Avoiding distal targets with the CO_2 laser involves the use of fluid media or a backstop to stop laser penetration.

Pulmonary Hazards

Excess smoke from CO_2 lasers has been associated with bronchitis and pneumonitis. These acute responses suggest that chronic exposure to this smoke may be as dangerous as cigarette smoke.[36,40] This is in agreement with the observation that laser smoke is similar to cigarette and other particulate smoke and that vaporization of 1 gm of tissue produces mutagenicity equal to three to six cigarettes.[40] The smoke from electrosurgical units has equal or greater mutagenic potential than that from lasers.[36,40]

Although it seems reasonable to use filtration masks, the only, but impractical, mask that has been effective in laboratory testing is the North respirator (North Safety Equipment, Cranston, RI), an individually fitted, full-face mask with filter cartridges.[41] When high filtration surgical masks are efficient enough to stop the particles, the air is drawn around the edge of the mask and escapes the filter.

Electrosurgical Bowel Burn

Breaks in the insulation of monopolar electrosurgical equipment can cause damage to organs within 1/8 inch of the break, based on an anticipated maximum of 5000V peak and 100W output in a CO_2 environment.[42] These breaks can be too small to be identified on routine examination but can be detected with dynamic systems such as the Electroshield (EM1 Electroscope, Inc.). Capacitive coupling to a nongrounded metal trocar can transfer up to 40% of the energy and spark within 1/8 inch of the trocar (Fig. 8-5).[42,43] Although causing skin burns has been the greatest concern when the trocar is pulled out of the abdomen during long procedures, bowel burns can also occur if the trocar is insulated from the skin. In addition, using the abdominal wall as the ground for the trocar to avoid bowel burns may result in low-power

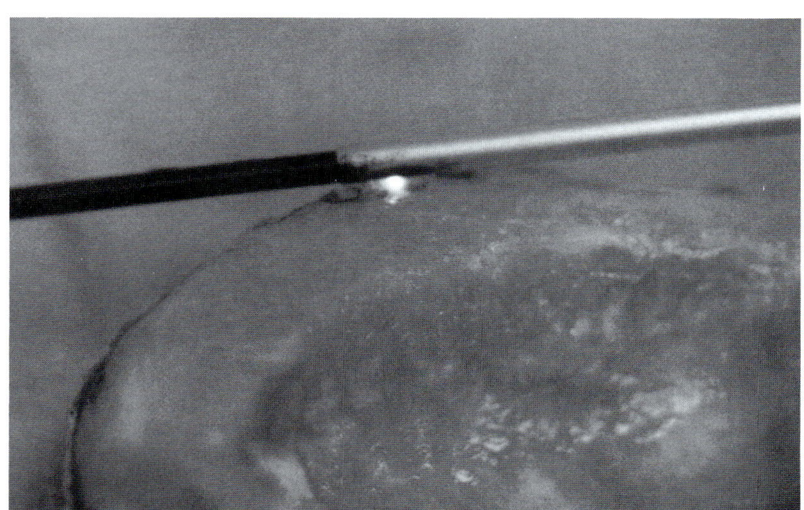

FIGURE 8-5. Sparks can occur to grounded tissue that is within 1/8 inch of an active electrode. This picture demonstrates sparking from an active electrode, produced by capacitive coupling. A monopolar electrosurgical instrument is placed through a metal trocar. The active element of the instrument is not in contact with a grounded target. The active element is insulated from the metal trocar by the normal insulation, which has been checked and is intact. When the unit is activated, up to 40% of the energy is coupled into the metal trocar and sparks and flows directly into a grounded target. The target in this picture is cantaloupe but sparks also occur to bowel and intra-abdominal organs.

density burns of the skin and abdominal wall. Avoiding prolonged activation of the electrosurgical unit helps to decrease the chance of low-power density burn of the abdominal wall.

Conversely, bowel damage (originally reported to have caused two deaths from overwhelming sepsis secondary to profound peritonitis)[44] may be caused by a needle or a trocar.[14,44,45] Moreover, the massive damage of the bowel[46] may result from direct application of electrosurgery to the bowels, similar to the misapplication of tubal rings to the sigmoid colon and appendix (King TM, personal communication, 1986).

Ureteral Injury

Grainger and coworkers summarized 13 cases of ureteral damage from bipolar electrosurgery, monopolar electrosurgery, and trocar injury.[47] This damage occurs with all equipment but appears to be rare. Caution is required in the proximity of the ureter and other delicate structures.

Tubal Damage

When lasers are used in tubal surgery, thermal damage can produce tubal occlusion. Low power density (less than 4000 W/cm^2) has been associated with tubal stenosis at the anastomotic site. In addition, a brushing technique that is used to remove adhesions from the mesosalpinx has been associated with subsequent necrosis and loss of the mesosalpinx per se (Fig. 8-6).[5]

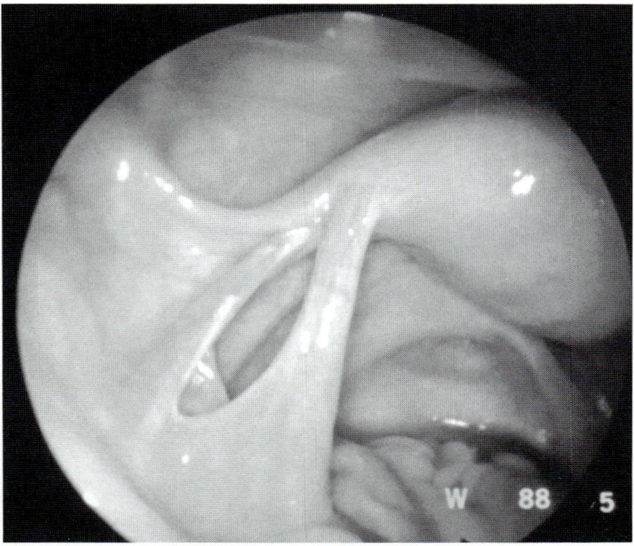

FIGURE 8-6. This defect in the mesosalpinx was associated with cornual occlusion after low-power density preparation of the tube for cornual anastomosis. Note the lack of adhesions despite the thermal necrosis. (Reproduced with permission of Martin DC: Tissue effects of lasers. Semin Reprod Endocrinol 1991;9[2]:133.)

ANIMAL MODELS

Incisions made with either a sharp knife or the Shaw scalpel cause less initial damage than incisions made with electrosurgery or lasers. Although lasers create a wider scar than the electrosurgical unit in skin incisions, the same degree of damage has been noted when either was used at high speed.[48–50] The zone of thermal necrosis appears to be related to the power density and the speed of the incision. The narrow zone of thermal damage noted with high-power density laser has also been noted with high-power density electrosurgery.[4,6,7] Healing was slower in skin incisions but not in abdominal wall incisions when incisions made with laser and electrosurgical units were compared with those made with a scalpel.[51] Minimal residual damage occurred in peritoneal incisions made with the laser, when compared with incisions made with the electrosurgical unit.[52]

Incisions made by lasers heal more slowly than those made by electrosurgical units.[12,49,53] There appears to be a decreased resistance to bacterial infection when lasers are used.[48,49]

Pulsing lasers decrease thermal spread and thermal necrosis, when compared with continuous output lasers.[8,54,55] This technique is used to maintain high instantaneous peak power densities while producing low average power densities. It decreases the thermal damage by using a high, peak, power density but increases control by using a low, average, power density, produced by mechanical pulsing, superpulse, or ultrapulse. Thus, this combination of high peak power and low average power density produces a clean incision while maintaining a slow speed. A zone of coagulation of 100 to 500 μm appears to offer the best combination of hemostasis in a clean incision.[8] This is generally produced with power densities in excess of 4500 W/cm^2 with the laser.[5] At 60,000 W/cm^2, cleaner incisions with the laser and electrosurgery are noted, whereas the thermal damage for these is limited to 40 to 160 μm.[7] Hemostasis at these high power densities is generally adequate for most procedures but lower power densities may be required in highly vascular areas. The deep penetration and low-power density of the Nd:YAG laser appear to be advisable with hepatic surgery.[51,56]

CLINICAL USE

Cholecystectomy

Laparoscopic cholecystectomy can lead to a marked reduction in morbidity for one of the most commonly performed operations in general surgery. Voyles and coworkers report 350 consecutive patients with no mortality, no reoperations, and no ductal injury.[57] There are many published reports of cholecystectomy completed with the use of laser but in this report, the authors changed to electrosurgery and performed their last 280 procedures with electrosurgery exclusively. This group points out that the use of the laser increased the total patient costs and the total time for the procedures.[58] They concluded that promotion of the laser for this procedure may limit its availability in hospitals with progressively limited budgets, without contributing to patient care.

Complications are related to experience. The incidence of bowel duct injuries was 2.2% in a surgeon's first 13 procedures and 0.1% thereafter.[59]

Appendectomy

High-power density electrosurgery or lasers may be useful in dissection and in developing planes for the excision of large tissue. Deeper coagulation or mechanical occlusion is generally required for hemostasis when cutting across large vessels, however. Large vessels can be coagulated with bipolar or thermal coagulators, harmonic scalpel or occluded with ties, sutures, clips, or staples.[32]

LOOPS, SUTURES, CLIPS, AND STAPLES

Any discussion of operative laparoscopy requires the mention of mechanical devices. The development of suture ligation and loops by Clarke and the adaptation of Roeder loops (WISAP Instruments, Inc.) by Semm preceded the ongoing development of absorbable clips (Ethicon-Endosurgery, Cincinnati, OH) and Endo-GIA (United States Surgical Corporation, Norwalk, CT) stapling devices.[60,61] More recently, the harmonic scalpel has been introduced. These mechanical devices increase a surgeon's ability to use lasers or electrosurgery or may replace lasers and electrosurgery in specific instances.

COST

Although one study showed that operative laparoscopy decreased costs by $1,007 to $1,581 when used instead of laparotomy, lasers and disposable equipment may negate these savings.[62] An increase of $1,271 was noted when laser and disposable equipment were used for cholecystectomy.[58] This is similar to the $579 increase noted for the overall costs when laparoscopic surgery was compared with laparotomy for cholecystectomy (Blue Cross/Blue Shield of South Carolina).[63] Laparoscopic techniques have the potential for decreasing costs but further analysis is required to determine if this potential is realistic. Furthermore, the use of electrosurgical techniques and nondisposable equipment appears to decrease costs, compared with the use of laser and disposable equipment.[58]

Although high-power density lasers and electrosurgery are more predictable for certain applications, this predictability is not always an indication for their use. Large vessels may require increased thermal necrosis or mechanical techniques for hemostasis. In contrast, coagulation for hemostasis may result in inadvertent detrimental thermal effect. There is ongoing debate regarding the merits of touch and no-touch surgical techniques. Continued study is paramount in determining the most useful and most effective equipment for the specific clinical circumstance.

References

1. Martin DC: Infertility surgery using the carbon dioxide laser. Clin Gyn Briefs 1983;4:1.
2. Martin DC, Diamond MP: Operative laparoscopy: comparison of lasers with other techniques. Curr Probl Obstet Gynecol Fertil 1986;9:563.
3. Martin DC: Therapeutic laparoscopy. In: Martin DC, ed. Laparoscopic appearance of endometriosis. 2nd ed., vol I. Memphis: Resurge Press, 1990:21.
4. Filmar S, Jetha N, McComb P, Gomel V: A comparative histologic study on the healing process after tissue transection. I. Carbon dioxide laser and electromicrosurgery. Am J Obstet Gynecol 1989;160:1062.
5. Martin DC: Tissue effects of lasers. Semin Reprod Endocrinol 1991;9(2):127.
6. Mage G, Pouly JL, Bruhat MA: Laser microsurgery of the oviducts. In: Baggish MS, ed. Basic and advanced laser surgery in gynecology. Norwalk, CT: Appleton-Century-Crofts, 1985:299.
7. Luciano AA, Whitman G, Maier DB, Randolph J, Maenza R: A comparison of thermal injury, healing patterns, and postoperative adhesion formation following CO_2 laser and electromicrosurgery. Fertil Steril 1987;48:1025.
8. Taylor MV, Martin DC, Poston W, Dean PJ, Vander Zwaag R: Effect of power density and carbonization on residual tissue coagulation using the continuous wave carbon dioxide laser. Colposcopy & Gynecologic Laser Surgery 1986;2:169.
9. Cushing H: Electro-surgery as aid to removal of intracranial tumors. Surg Gynecol Obstet 1928;47:751.
10. Kelly HA, Ward GE, eds: Electrosurgery. Philadelphia: WB Saunders, 1932.
11. Ketcham AS, Hoye RC, Riggle GC: A surgeon's appraisal of the laser. Surg Clin North Am 1967;47:1249.
12. Fox JL: The use of laser radiation as a surgical "light knife." J Surg Res 1969;9:199.
13. Reich H, Vancaillie TG, Soderstrom RM: Electrical techniques. In: Martin DC, ed. Manual of endoscopy. Santa Fe Springs: American Association of Gynecologic Laparoscopists, 1990:105.
14. Levy BS, Soderstrom RM: Electrical techniques in sterilization. In: Martin DC, ed. Manual of endoscopy. Santa Fe Springs: American Association of Gynecologic Laparoscopists, 1990:57.
15. Harris DM, Werkhaven JA: Biophysics and applications of medical lasers. Arch Otolaryngol Head Neck Surg 1989;3:91.
16. Martin DC: Laser physics and practice. In: Hunt RB, ed.

Atlas of female infertility surgery. Chicago: Year Book Medical Publishers, 1986:103.

17. Martin DC, Diamond MP, Yussman MA: Laser laparoscopy for infertility surgery. In: Sanfilippo JS, Levine RL, eds. Operative gynecologic endoscopy. New York: Springer-Verlag, 1989:211.

18. Burington RS: Handbook of mathematical tables and formulas, 3rd ed. Sandusky, OH: Handbook Publishers, 1958:14.

19. Crowgey SR: Laser physics, applications and safety. In: Hezhat C, ed. Videolaseroscopy course syllabus. Atlanta: Northside Hospital, 1990:1.

20. Martin DC, Absten GT, Levinson CJ, Photopulos GJ, eds: Intra-abdominal laser surgery. Memphis: Resurge Press, 1986:28.

21. Martin DC: Laparoscopic appearance of endometriosis. 2nd ed. Memphis: Resurge Press, 1990:49.

22. Patton GW: A concept of gynecologic microsurgery. In: Behrman SJ, Kistner RW, Patton GW, eds. Progress in infertility. Boston: Little, Brown, 1988:107.

23. Anderson RM, Romfh RF: Electrocautery. In: Technique in the use of surgical tools. Norwalk, CT: Appleton & Lange, 1980:141.

24. Stangel JJ: Electrosurgery. In: Stangel JJ, ed. Infertility surgery. Norwalk, CT: Appleton & Lange, 1990:110.

25. Keye WR, McArthur GR: Laser laparoscopy: argon. In: Keye WR, ed. Laser surgery in gynecology and obstetrics. 2nd ed. Chicago: Year Book Medical Publishers, 1990:208.

26. Swain CP: Endoscopic Nd: YAG laser control of gastrointestinal bleeding. In: Joffe SN, ed. Neodymium-YAG laser in medicine and surgery. New York: Elsevier, 1983:15.

27. Lomano JM: Laparoscopic ablation of endometriosis with the YAG laser. Lasers Surg Med 1983;3:179. Abstract.

28. Kojima E, Yanagibori A, Yuda K, Hirakawa S: Nd:YAG laser endoscopy. J Reprod Med 1988;33:907.

29. Joffe SN, Foster J, Schroder T, Brackett K: Splenic resection with the contact Nd:YAG laser system. J Pediatr Surg 1988;23:829.

30. Schroder T, Brackett K, Joffe SN: An experimental study of the effects of electrocautery and various lasers on gastrointestinal tissue. Surgery 1987;101:691.

31. Shirk GJ: Use of the Nd:YAG laser with sapphire scalpels. In: McLaughlin DS, ed. Lasers in gynecology. Philadelphia: JB Lippincott, 1991:290.

32. Soderstrom RM, Levy BS, Engle T: Reducing bipolar sterilization failures. Obstet Gynecol 1989;74:60.

33. Levinson CJ, Wattiez A: Complications and safety of laparoscopy. In: Martin DC, ed. Manual of endoscopy. Santa Fe Springs: American Association of Gynecologic Laparoscopists, 1990:35.

34. Corson SL, Soderstrom RM, Levy BS: Emergencies and laparoscopy. In: Martin DC, ed. Manual of endoscopy. Santa Fe Springs: American Association of Gynecologic Laparoscopists, 1990:47.

35. Soderstrom RM, Levy BS: Medical and legal aspects of laparoscopy. In: Martin DC, ed. Manual of endoscopy. Santa Fe Springs: American Association of Gynecologic Laparoscopists, 1990:53.

36. Martin DC: Laser safety. In: Keye WR, ed. Laser surgery in gynecology and obstetrics. 2nd ed. Chicago: Year Book Medical Publishers, 1990:35.

37. Rockwell J, ed: Laser safety training manual. 6th ed. Cincinnati: Rockwell Associates, 1983.

38. American national standard for the safe use of lasers (ANSI Z136.1-1986). New York: American National Standards Institute, 1986.

39. American national standards for the safe use of lasers in health care facilities (ANSI Z136.3-1988). New York: American National Standards Institute, 1988.

40. Tomita Y, Mihashi S, Nagata K, et al: Mutagenicity of smoke condensates induced by CO_2 laser irradiation and electrocauterization. Mutat Res 1981;89:145.

41. Akale D, Streifel A, Ahrens R: A method for limiting laser plume during bronchoscopic and laryngoscopic surgery. In: Rockwell Laser Industries. Proceedings of technical papers, international laser safety conference. Cincinnati, OH, November 29, 1990, Section 6:39.

42. Gallagher TJ, Pearmain AJ: High voltage measurements testing and design. New York: John Wiley & Sons, 1983:44.

43. Pearce JA: Electrosurgery. New York: John Wiley & Sons, 1986:60.

44. Deaths following female sterilization with unipolar electrocoagulating devices. MMWR 1981;30:49.

45. Levy BS, Soderstrom RM, Dail DH: Bowel injuries during laparoscopy. Gross anatomy and histology. J Reprod Med 1985;30:168.

46. Wheeless CR: Thermal gastrointestinal injuries. In: Phillips JM, ed. Laparoscopy. Baltimore: Williams & Wilkins, 1977:231.

47. Grainger DA, Soderstrom RM, Schiff SF, Glickman MG, DeCherney AH, Diamond MP: Ureteral injuries at laparoscopy: insights into diagnosis, management, and prevention. Obstet Gynecol 1990;75:839.

48. Masterson BJ, Nealon N, Sowas D: Tissue effects of lasers on wound healing. Lasers Surg Med 1983;3:153. Abstract.

49. Madden JE, Edlich RF, Custer JR, Panek PH, Thul J, Wangensteen OH: Studies in the management of the contaminated wound. IV. Resistance to infection of surgical wounds made by knife, electrosurgery and laser. Am J Surg 1970;119:222.

50. Nishimura M, Tanino R, Miyasaka M, et al: Comparative study of CO_2 laser scalpel with electroscalpel. In: Atsumi K, Nimsakul N, eds. Laser-Tokyo '81. The 4th Congress of the International Society for Laser Surgery. Tokyo: The Japan Society for Laser Surgery 1981;21.

51. Hall RR, Beach AD, Hill DW: Partial hepatectomy using a carbon-dioxide laser. Br J Surg 1973;60:141.

52. Bellina JH, Hemmings R, Voros JI, Ross LF: Carbon dioxide laser and electrosurgical wound study with an animal model: a comparison of tissue damage and healing patterns in peritoneal tissue. Am J Obstet Gynecol 1984; 148:327.

53. Hall RR: The healing of tissues incised by a carbon-dioxide laser. Br J Surg 1971;58:222.

54. Ohshiro T, Itoh E, Kato Y: Multi- and one-shot laser therapy: which is better in clinical use? In: Atsumi K, Nimsakul N, eds. Laser-Tokyo '81. The 4th Congress of the International Society for Laser Surgery. Tokyo: The Japan Society for Laser Surgery, 1981:3.

55. Yamamoto T, Fukomoto I, Saito M: Dynamic characteristics of the light reflected from the living tissue under laser irradiation. In: Atsumi K, Nimsakul N, eds. Laser-Tokyo '81. The 4th Congress of the International Society for Laser Surgery. Tokyo: The Japan Society for Laser Surgery, 1981:2,8.

56. Joffe SN, Brackett KA, Sankar MY, Daikuzono N: Resection of the liver with the Nd:YAG laser. Surg Gynecol Obstet 1986;163:437.

57. Voyles CR, Meena AL, Petro AB, Haick AJ, Koury AM: Electrocautery is superior to laser for laparoscopic cholecystectomy. Editorial. Am J Surg 1990;160:457.

58. Voyles CR, Petro AB, Meena AL, Haick AJ, Koury AM: A practical approach to laparoscopic cholecystectomy. Am J Surg 1991;161:365.

59. Southern Surgeons Club: A prospective analysis of 1518 laparoscopic cholecystectomies. N Engl J Med 1991; 324:1073.

60. Clarke HC: Laparoscopy: new instruments for suturing and ligation. Fertil Steril 1972;23:274.

61. Semm K: Historical review: from diagnostic laparoscopy to operative pelviscopy. In: Semm K, Friedrich ER, eds. Operative manual for endoscopic abdominal surgery. Chicago: Year Book Medical Publishers, 1987:5.

62. Levine RL: Economic impact of pelviscopic surgery. J Reprod Med 1985;30:655.

63. Jordan AM: Hospital charges for laparoscopic and open cholecystectomy. (Letters) JAMA 1991;266:3425.

Chapter 9

Laparoscopic Surgery: An Atlas for General Surgeons, edited by Gary C. Vitale, Joseph S. Sanfilippo, and Jacques Perissat. J. B. Lippincott Company, Philadelphia, © 1995.

Operative Laparoscopy in the Pediatric Patient

Joseph S. Sanfilippo
Thom E. Lobe

The addition of operative laparoscopy to the armamentarium of the gynecologist and general surgeon for the surgical treatment of pediatric and adolescent patients clearly represents the "neophyte" of technologic advances. When one realizes that operative laparoscopy has been performed successfully in pre-term infants, neonates, and young children, one becomes aware that surgical horizons appear to be on a continuum of exploration and unprecedented achievement. Carbon dioxide (CO_2) insufflation is attributed to Zollikofer and we have Veress to thank for the insufflation needle.[1] The first English textbook is attributed to Steptoe.[2]

Better instrumentation has made endoscopic operative intervention available to children. Gans is given major credit for convincing pediatric surgeons that laparoscopy has a major role in the management of diseases in children.[3–5] In the mid- to late 1970s—shortly after the availability of pediatric-sized Hopkins rod lens "telescopies"—Gans traveled to Stuttgart, Germany, to the Stortz research and development department and with them designed the first laparoscope suitable for use in infants and small children. Since then, the refinement of lightweight video cameras and the development of better endoscopic instrumentation, including endoscopic surgical staplers and devices for delivering various forms of thermal energy (e.g., laser and monopolar and bipolar electrosurgical tools), have facilitated endoscopic advanced operative procedures.

In any discussion of laparoscopy, two issues surface: (1) which procedures can be performed laparoscopically and how to perform them, and (2) which procedures can be performed closed more efficaciously than by the conventional operative approach and whether they should be performed preferentially because of significant advantages.

Laparoscopy is possible in infants and children because of several technologic developments. As previously mentioned, the Hopkins rod lens telescopes have revolutionized pediatric endoscopy. These instruments range from 2 to 10 mm in diameter and are used most often in 0° or 30° lens configurations. We prefer to use 0° endoscopes because they cause less disorientation for the operating surgeon and are easiest for the novice to use. The 30° lenses are useful in specific instances, such as endoscopic suturing or when a structure must be assessed at an angle and placement of a second port is not desired. The right-angle or operating laparoscope is of little use for most of our laparoscopic procedures and if one is purchasing a new system, it is probably not worth the additional expense. The Hydrolaparoscope (Circon/ACMI, Stamford, CT), an instrument designed with a forward irrigation channel and a side (lens) irrigation channel, is useful in situations where there is purulent material or hemorrhage that may obscure the view. This instrument allows the surgeon to irrigate the end of the lens without having to remove the telescope from its port (Fig. 9-1). This convenient feature saves time on lengthy procedures.

Another essential is a lightweight video camera system. Discussion of the virtues of three-chip cameras and systems with the chip on the end of the endoscope is probably not as germane to laparoscopy in children as it is in adults. Because we tend to use the smaller endoscopes for many procedures on these small patients (but often use the larger endoscopes on older children), the lightest camera available that is adaptable to all sizes of

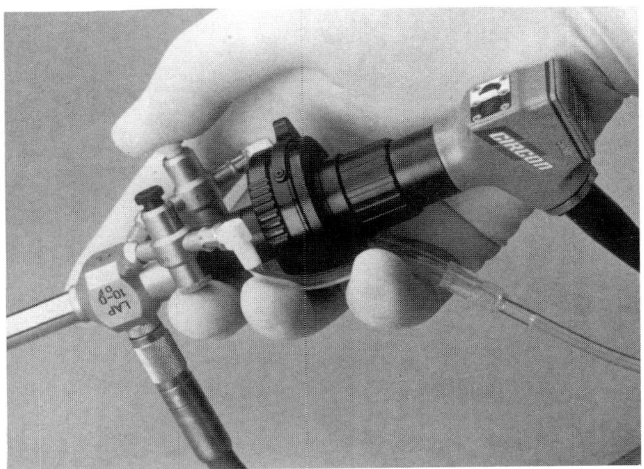

FIGURE 9-1. Hydrolaparoscope (Circon/ACMI, Stamford, CT).

endoscopes seems ideal. The weight becomes more of an issue when the smaller telescopes (2 to 5 mm) are used. Heavy cameras weight these telescopes down and tend to bend the shaft of the shorter 2-mm and 4-mm telescopes.

Another convenience, if one is concerned about image documentation, is a camera system with controls on the camera head. This convenient feature allows the camera operator to control the video printer or video recorder.

Laparoscopy in infants and children requires smaller port sets and more delicate instrumentation. The ideal trocar for the infant or small child is one that is about 2.5 cm in length and remains fixed in the peritoneal cavity until it is no longer required. There are several disposable devices that approach this configuration, being shorter than most adult cannulas and having an expandable flange that keeps them from slipping out of the abdomen after being inserted. The standard screw-type fixation devices tend to tear a child's skin, and they slip out easily because a child's abdominal wall is thin. Newer adhesive rings show some promise in holding the cannulas in place. Alternatively, one may use Steri-strips (3M, St. Paul, MN) to help secure the cannulas in place after insertion.

There has been an explosion in the development of instrumentation for endoscopic surgery. Most of the disposable devices are still too crude for use in small children. We prefer to use nondisposable instruments when delicate dissection is required, although we usually use a combination of the two types of instruments, depending on the procedure. Ideally, one should try to use as many 3- or 5-mm instruments as possible, avoiding the larger clamps and staplers except in those procedures in which they are essential. Most of the other instruments and accessories are the same as those used for adults.

Most laparoscopy in infants and children is performed under general anesthesia, with endotracheal intubation. Prophylactic antibiotics (preoperative) are recommended to prevent infections at the port sites.

All infants and children should have their stomach and bladder emptied just before beginning the procedure. The stomach can be emptied with a suction catheter and in most instances, the bladder can be emptied sufficiently by Credé's method.

The abdominal wall of the child is thin and elastic. This presents two problems. First, it is easy to introduce a needle or port into the subcutaneous space, thinking you are well into the peritoneal cavity; and second, it is easy to injure abdominal viscera during secondary port introduction. These problems, however, can be easily avoided.

A Veress needle can be used to establish a pneumoperitoneum in even the smallest infant. First, a stab wound is made in the skin of the inferior rim of the umbilicus, the length of which equals the diameter of the trocar to be introduced. The abdominal wall is then elevated by grasping it on either side of the umbilicus as the Veress needle is introduced. The Veress needle is introduced perpendicular to the long axis of the patient to avoid inserting the needle into the loose areolar subcutaneous tissue. The needle is best held by its shaft (like a dart) and the maneuver is a quick shallow thrust into the peritoneal cavity until the retractable blunt end of the needle is heard to "pop" free into the abdomen. When the insufflation tubing is connected, the flow of gas should be 0.5 L/minute or more; a lower rate of flow suggests that the needle is not in the proper location.

The total volume of gas introduced into the abdomen is variable. Because there is a significant variability in patient size, such rules are difficult to establish. It is preferable to set the pressure limits on pressure-regulated automatic insufflators. For infants, the pressure is set at 6 to 8 mmHg. For children, most procedures can be accomplished using pressures of 8 to 10 mmHg. Older children can better tolerate pressures of 10 to 12 mmHg.

After the abdomen is insufflated, the umbilical trocar is introduced. Ideally, a 5-mm trocar is used. Caution should be exercised when introducing the trocar. Despite abdominal insufflation, the abdominal wall is elevated as the trocar is introduced. A twisting motion on insertion permits better control. Downward force (with the shoulder rather than the hand) is applied. This technique lowers the probability of injury to adjacent viscera.

Insertion of secondary trocars can be more dangerous. One must always keep the tip in sight during the introduction while elevating the abdomen instead of relying on the insufflation to keep the abdominal wall away from the viscera.

Postoperatively, the port sites should be sutured in children. Because of the thinness of the abdominal wall,

TABLE 9-1
Laparoscopically Performed Procedures in Infants and Children

Appendectomy
Cholecystectomy
Trauma evaluation
Undescended testes
Varicocele
Small bowel obstruction
Abscess
Gallbladder shunts
Ventriculoperitoneal/Tenkoff catheters
Inguinal hernias
Pyloromyotomy
Nissen fundoplication
Tumor staging
Brachytherapy
Liver biopsy
Nephrectomy
Splenectomy
Bowel resection
Vagotomy
Pull-through for Hirschsprung's disease
Lymphadenectomy
Staging laparotomy
Vesicourethral reflux
Neonatal jaundice
Rectal prolapse
Acute pelvic inflammatory disease
Chronic pelvic pain correlation
Lysis of adhesions
Ovarian cyst
Adnexal torsion
Creation of neovagina

the likelihood of a hernia developing in a port site is present. We therefore close both the fascia and the skin with interrupted absorbable sutures. A Steri-strip or transparent occlusive dressing is also applied to each port site.

Patients who undergo operative procedures are placed on postoperative Reglan (A. H. Robins Co., Richmond, VA) to prevent nausea. In children older than 8 or 10 years of age, a patch of Transderm Scop (CIBA Pharmaceuticals, Edison, NJ) behind an ear is useful.

Children have fewer complaints of postoperative shoulder pain than do adults. (Some clinicians advocate leaving suction catheters in the peritoneal cavity for several hours to evacuate all the CO_2, as may be done after laparoscopy in adults.) Postoperative analgesic requirements vary and are best prescribed as necessary.

A wide variety of laparoscopic procedures can be accomplished in infants and children, as listed in Table 9-1.[6]

ACUTE PELVIC INFLAMMATORY DISEASE

Determining the incidence of acute pelvic inflammatory disease (PID) in adolescents is difficult. A 15-year-old girl who is sexually active has a 1 in 8 chance of acquiring acute PID (i.e., 10 times greater than for a woman 24 years of age).[7]

Fibrin trapping and sequestration of the bacterial inoculum by the omentum, intestinal distention, and tuboovarian complex localize the infection initially, with the subsequent result of abscess formation, making a laparoscopic approach effective. Fibrin deposits appear to be a barrier to in situ destruction by neutrophils, with resultant abscess formation.[8] Once an abscess is formed, it becomes difficult for antibiotics to adequately penetrate the abscess to correct the abnormality. By aggressively removing fibrin, exudate, and associated purulent material, the prognosis is improved. Henry-Suchet and coworkers evaluated 50 patients with tuboovarian abscess who were treated laparoscopically.[9] The efficacy of early aggressive laparoscopic management of acute PID was reemphasized (all received antibiotic therapy).

Copious amounts of irrigation fluid (ideally including Ringer's lactate solution) should be used to remove purulent material, fibrin, and exudate. Cultures should be obtained and appropriate antibiotic therapy administered. The patient is placed in a reverse Trendelenburg's position, with suctioning of the fluid in an effort to remove as much of the purulent material as possible.[10]

Intraovarian abscesses have been treated laparoscopically with aspiration and povidone-iodine lavage. Stubblefield reports a patient with prolonged morbidity in association with intraovarian abscess after acute PID, which was secondary to an intrauterine contraceptive device.[11] Laparoscopically guided needle aspiration of the abscess, with povidone-iodine lavage, proved effective in correcting the abscess process.[11] Fitz-Hugh-Curtis syndrome has been treated laparoscopically.[12]

Early aggressive operative laparoscopic intervention may well change the course of acute PID sequelae. Removal of fibrinous exudate and purulent material, complemented by appropriate antibiotic therapy, has proved to be effective with respect to less pelvic organ damage, infertility, and subsequent pelvic pain.

OVARIAN CYSTS

Imaging modalities enable an ovarian cyst to be diagnosed preoperatively. Abdominal pain in a child can be associated with an ovarian cyst. If necessary, large cysts can be decompressed laparoscopically with a needle. When malignancy is not suspected, such cysts can be excised completely or they can be fenestrated to avoid further problems. Oophorectomy is rarely indicated, except in cases of malignancy. When oophorectomy is required, it can be performed laparoscopically, in addition to omentectomy and other necessary procedures.

ADNEXAL TORSION

Increasing evidence attests to the role of detorsion from a laparoscopic approach. The surgeon should consider conservative "untwisting" with operative laparoscopy. Evaluation of the opposite adnexa is also recommended. An oophoropexy should be considered (especially if the adnexa is associated with a long mesosalpinx-mesovarium) in an effort to prevent subsequent torsion. Of interest, torsion is more frequent on the right side. There appears to be minimal evidence of thromboembolism associated with "untwisting" of the involved adnexa.

CHRONIC PELVIC PAIN

Frequently, pelvic pain assessment in the adolescent is clinically challenging and often poses a dilemma. Chronic pelvic pain (CPP) by definition requires 6 or more months of persistent lower abdominal pain. It is best subclassified as *primary,* in which there is no clear underlying etiology, or *secondary,* which is associated with an obvious cause.

Initially, a thorough history and physical examination is obtained. The former should include information regarding any gastrointestinal problems. When evaluating the genitourinary system, the physician should look for evidence of recurring cystitis or gynecologic disorders such as persistent vaginal discharge, which may lead to upper and lower reproductive tract infection. Dysmenorrhea should be inquired about. Pubertal milestones are also important, especially in an effort to determine any outflow-tract obstruction, which may be associated with hematocolpos, hematometra, hematosalpinx, and endometriosis—the latter a reflection of retrograde menstruation. Childhood diseases rarely cause pelvic pain. Entities such as mumps oophoritis, however, should be considered. A general physical examination is mandatory, complemented by a pelvic examination seeking evidence of a pelvic mass, tenderness, or uterine anomaly.

Laparoscopy is an integral part of the assessment of pelvic pain in the adolescent. In one series of 109 adolescent patients with CPP, endometriosis was noted to be present in 49 (45%); the youngest child was 10.8 years of age.[13] Findings include postoperative adhesions in 17 (16%) and congenital anomalies of the uterus in 10 (9%). Pelvic inflammatory disease and associated adnexal adhesions were identified in 9% and a chronic hemoperitoneum in 5%. Other sources of CPP are associated with functional ovarian cysts (5%); 10% were noted to have no pelvic abnormalities. The last category was miscellaneous for the remainder of the patients. Several studies have been published regarding the finding of endometriosis in the adolescent patient; these are addressed in Table 9-2. Endometriosis in association with an outflow-tract obstruction is correlated with 100% reversal of the endometriosis when an outflow tract is established.[14]

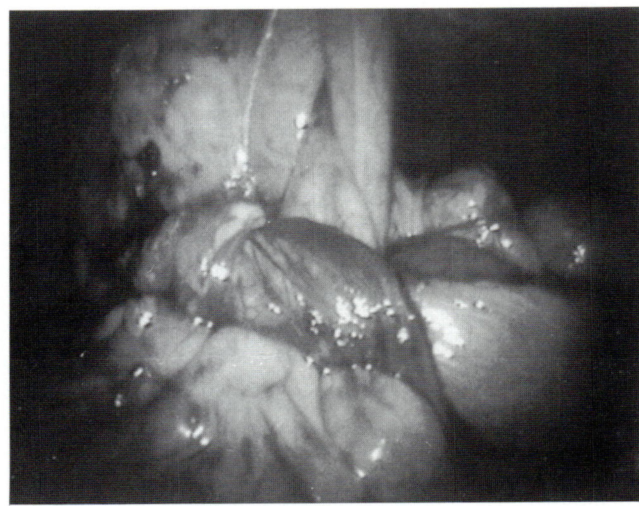

FIGURE 9-2. Adhesions causing a small bowel obstruction in a 2-year-old child. (Lobe TE: Evolving laparoscopic and thoracoscopic procedures in infants and children. Laparoscop Surg 1993;1:3)

LYSIS OF ADHESIONS

Pelvic or abdominal pain may be associated with complete intestinal obstruction, in which the abdomen is maximally distended; laparoscopy may be difficult or im-

TABLE 9-2
Laparoscopic Findings in Adolescents with Chronic Pelvic Pain

Study	No Visible Pathology No. (%)	Endometriosis No. (%)	Adhesions No. (%)	Chronic PID No. (%)	Ovarian Cyst(s) No. (%)	Pelvic Varicosities No. (%)	Myoma(s) No. (%)	Other No. (%)
Goldstein, et al[13] (n = 140)	19 (14)	66 (47)	18 (13)	10 (7)	5 (4)	0 (0)	0 (0)	22 (16)
Chatman & Ward (n = 44)	5 (12)	28 (65)	1 (2)	10 (23)	0 (0)	0 (0)	0 (0)	0 (0)
Vercellini, et al (n = 47)	19 (40)	18 (38)	2 (4)	1 (2)	1 (2)	0 (0)	0 (0)	6 (13)

PID, pelvic inflammatory disease.

possible. When the obstructed loops of bowel are partially decompressed, however, and it is possible to establish an adequate pneumoperitoneum, laparoscopy can be used to divide the adhesions that caused the obstruction (Fig. 9-2).

The open (or Hasson) technique to establish access to the peritoneal cavity is recommended.[15] After the initial inspection, it may be obvious where the source of obstruction is located. When this is not the case, one should insert one or two additional ports to "run the bowel." This maneuver facilitates evaluation and is best begun at either the ligament of Treitz or the ileocecal valve, whichever is easier to identify. Using two atraumatic graspers, the bowel is run until the point of obstruction is identified. When an adhesion has been located, it can be divided using electrosurgical techniques or it can be divided between clips or with a stapler. If a compromised loop of bowel is noted that requires resection, the surgeon can perform this laparoscopically.

MECKEL'S DIVERTICULUM

A Meckel's diverticulum can be managed laparoscopically. Generally, these patients fall into two categories: those who present with obstruction or inflammation and those who present with hemorrhage. Either group is usually diagnosed inadvertently at exploration. The diverticulum can be resected laparoscopically. Those who present with hemorrhage are usually diagnosed preoperatively by imaging studies that demonstrate either an acute hemorrhage or ectopic gastric mucosa.

When a Meckel's diverticulum is found, it can be resected in one of two ways. If it is broad-based and its aberrant gastric mucosa is in its tip—as opposed to its junction with the small bowel—it can be resected easily by transection across its base, using the linear stapler (Fig. 9-3). In these cases, it is imperative that the surgeon inspect the removed specimen to ensure that the offending aberrant tissue is removed in its entirety.

When the diverticulum is short and broad-based or aberrant tissue is suspected at its junction with the small bowel, a bowel resection is required. This is best accomplished by exteriorizing the diverticulum and performing the resection in a standard fashion or by laparoscopic techniques, using the linear stapler.

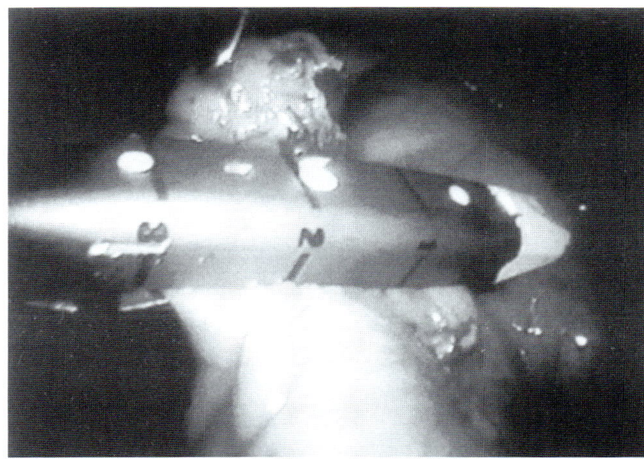

FIGURE 9-3. Resection of a Meckel's diverticulum, using an Endo-GIA stapler (U. S. Surgical Corporation, Norwalk, CT).

APPENDICITIS

As pediatric and general surgeons gain experience with laparoscopic techniques, it is apparent that one of its best applications is in the treatment of appendicitis.[16,17] Most of the arguments against approaching this disease laparoscopically are made by those unfamiliar with laparoscopic surgery.

There are two advantages to laparoscopic appendectomy: (1) a better cosmetic result, particularly in young girls, and (2) the early return to extracurricular activities after a brief recovery time (hours to days).

The complications of laparoscopic appendectomy include minor local wound infections that can be treated locally with antibiotics and an occasional intra-abdominal abscess, requiring drainage in association with a ruptured appendix.[18] After laparoscopic appendectomy for acute uncomplicated appendicitis, patients are discharged between 6 and 36 hours postoperatively and are allowed to return to unrestricted activity as soon as they are comfortable, usually within 72 hours. When dealing with a ruptured appendix requiring antibiotics, the advantages of laparoscopic appendectomy may not be as great. Some dispute this, however, and claim that the involved tissues are better inspected and the purulent material more easily and directly drained when using the laparoscopic approach. In the young adult who would like to "return to normal as soon as possible," the laparoscopic technique also offers the opportunity to treat the disease and allows return to a normal level of activity without restriction when antibiotic therapy is completed. In our opinion, this is the main advantage of laparoscopy in instances of ruptured appendicitis.

About 40% of our patients had a ruptured appendix at the time of laparoscopy. One suggested approach is to perform laparoscopy in patients who appear to have appendicitis that is uncomplicated by rupture or abscess formation.

There are several laparoscopic methodologies for performing an appendectomy. The procedure can be accomplished using a laser, surgical clips, linear stapling devices, endoscopic loops, or sutures, depending on the preference and expertise of the surgeon. The linear tissue stapler is our method of choice; however, because its use makes the procedure more expensive, some cen-

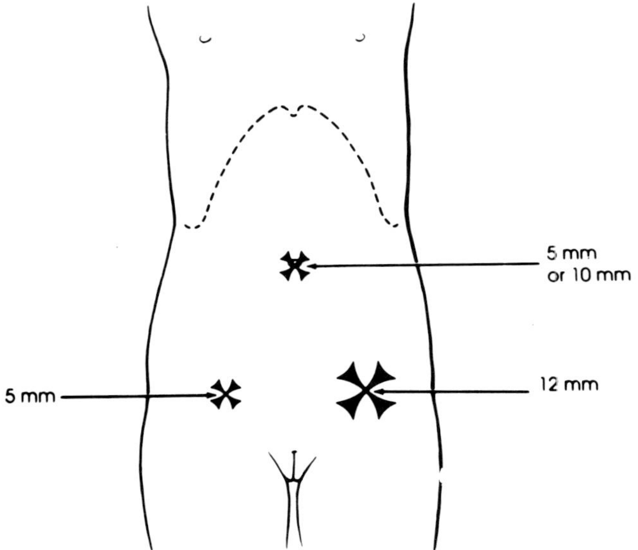

FIGURE 9-4. Trocar sites for pediatric laparoscopic appendectomy. (Lobe TE, Schropp KP, eds. Pediatric laparoscopy and thoracoscopy. Philadelphia: WB Saunders, 1993:117. With permission)

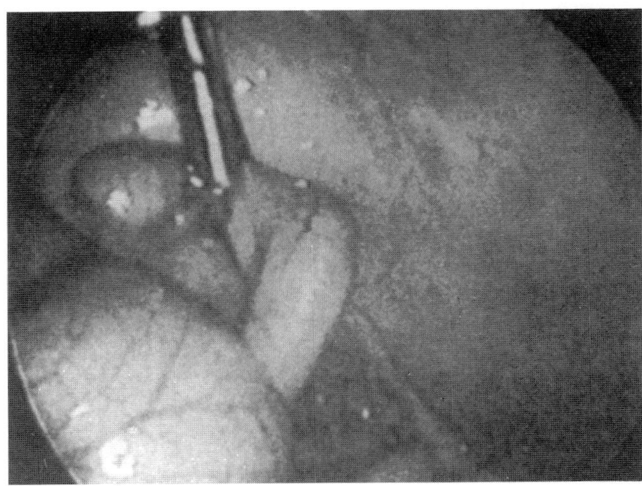

FIGURE 9-5. Appendix is held by endoscopic grasper.

ters are reverting to the use of clips (on the mesoappendix) and loops with pre-tied Roeder knots.

The initial approach to laparoscopic appendectomy requires placement of a nasogastric tube and a bladder catheter. The patient is placed supine in Trendelenburg's position for most of the procedure. Carbon dioxide pneumoperitoneum is established as described above and depending on the size of the patient, a 5- or 10-mm laparoscope is introduced through the umbilicus into the peritoneal cavity. We generally use a 5-mm laparoscope for patients younger than 10 to 12 years of age and find it acceptable to use a 10-mm laparoscope for older children.

On inspection of the peritoneal cavity, it is usually immediately obvious that there is some inflammation in the right lower quadrant. Occasionally, fluid is seen in the pelvis. We use two additional ports to complete the operation; their size and location depend on the technique. We prefer to place symmetric ports in the right and left lower quadrants below the "bikini line," lateral to the epigastric vessels on either side. One 5-mm port and one 12-mm port appear adequate (Fig. 9-4). To use an endoscopic GIA stapler, insert a 12-mm port in the left lower quadrant to ensure ample room for proper instrument placement and function. To mobilize the appendix, a 5-mm reducing cap must be used when 5-mm instruments are used with the larger port, so that the pneumoperitoneum is maintained.

One may begin with two tissue graspers, at least one of which has a ratcheted handle. With these graspers, the tissues are mobilized so that the tip of the appendix can be secured (in one of the graspers; Fig. 9-5). A closed grasper can serve as a blunt dissector in a manner similar to using a finger when doing an open procedure. This technique enables separation of inflammatory adhesions and fluid loculations to completely mobilize the appendix.

Occasionally, there are adhesions that need to be taken down sharply. Alternatively, Metzenbaum-style laparoscopic scissors can be used. Bipolar electrosurgery enables careful division of the adhesions while cauterizing blood vessels, thus minimizing bleeding. Once the appendix is mobilized and its junction with the base of the cecum is clearly identified, the mesoappendix and the appendix can be divided.

The stapler can be used to divide the mesoappendix and appendix individually. Use of vascular staples and replacement cartridges is feasible. The device is placed through a 12-mm left lower quadrant port and used to secure the mesoappendix and appendix down to the junction with the cecum. At the same time, one must be sure that the tip of the stapler is well identified and the line indicating the end of the cut is beyond the tissue (Fig. 9-6). If the mesoappendix and the appendix are divided in one application of the stapler and the tissues are too thick or inflamed, there may be a leak at the junction of the mesentery and the appendiceal stump when the two structures are not divided separately. The jaws of the stapler are then closed; the surgeon must check to be certain of its position and that there are no additional tissues or loops of bowel engaged in the device. Once the proper position is certain, the safety latch is released and the stapler fired.

With the appendix free, it can then be extracted through the left lower quadrant 12-mm port in such a manner that the inflamed or contaminated tissue never touches the port tract, thus avoiding possible infection. If the inflamed appendix is so thick that it cannot be removed through the port, a tissue sac or sterile condom-

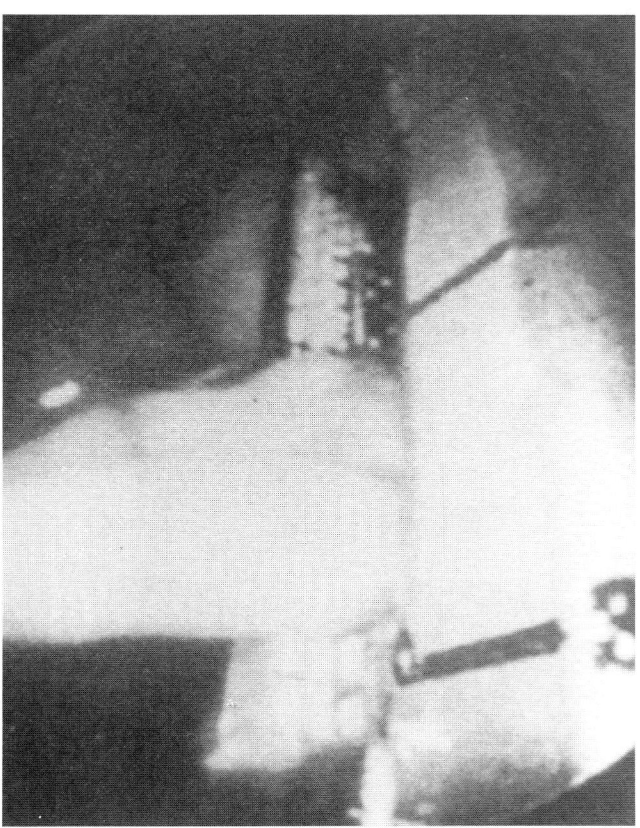

FIGURE 9-6. Laparoscopic view of Endo-GIA stapler applied to appendix, showing the "cut" mark beyond the tissues to be divided. (Lobe TE, Schropp KP, eds. Pediatric laparoscopy and thoracoscopy. Philadelphia: WB Saunders, 1993:118. With permission)

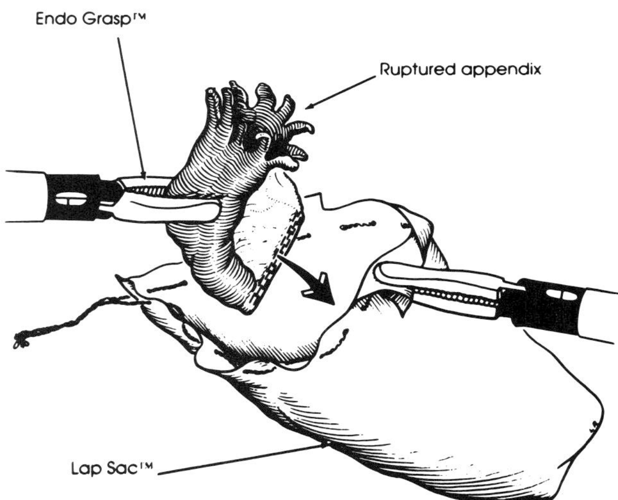

FIGURE 9-7. Extraction of the appendix, using a sac. (Lobe TE, Schropp KE, eds. Pediatric laparoscopy and thoracoscopy. Philadelphia: WB Saunders, 1993:118. With permission)

like sac can be inserted through the right lower quadrant port, the appendix placed within it, and the sac or condom withdrawn into the port to its point of resistance (Fig. 9-7). The port should be withdrawn completely, so that the neck of the sac or condom-like pouch is outside the abdominal wall. The sac or condom usually has enough lubrication from tissue fluids that it can easily slip out through the incision, thus minimizing contamination to the port tract. After the sac is removed, the left lower quadrant trocar and port are reinserted, and the surgical bed is inspected for hemostasis and irrigated as necessary.

If the surgeon feels uncomfortable leaving the appendiceal stump exposed, it can be inverted by placing a Z stitch or pursestring stitch, using standard laparoscopic suturing techniques.

With a ruptured or gangrenous appendix, the surgeon must take care to identify friable segments of the appendiceal wall, through which a fecalith may extrude. A fecalith lost in the peritoneal cavity may be a nidus for abscess formation, requiring subsequent intervention. In instances of a ruptured appendix in which an abscess is found, a Luken's trap is attached to the end of the suction device to obtain material for culture. At the end of the procedure, copious irrigation of the peritoneal cavity with normal saline and then antibiotic solution is recommended. In cases of intra-abdominal inflammation, such as appendicitis where frank pus is present and irrigation is used to help cleanse the peritoneal cavity, one should be aware of the dependent position of the diaphragm or pelvis, depending on the procedure. If one has a large quantity of irrigation fluid that is not adequately aspirated, there is a potential risk of loculation of the fluid and abscess formation. After laparoscopic appendectomy, when the appendix has ruptured and an abscess is drained and the abdomen irrigated, the patient is placed in a reverse Trendelenburg's position at the end of the procedure to allow the irrigation fluid to run into the pelvis, where it can be meticulously aspirated. Similarly, in cases of upper abdominal procedures wherein irrigation is used, the patient is placed in Trendelenburg's position at the end of the procedure and may even be rotated to the right or to the left in a semi-decubitus position, so that the fluid becomes dependent and can be completely aspirated.

The laparoscopic approach proves advantageous in cases of abdominal pain when the diagnosis is unclear. Ordinarily, an appendectomy is performed and one searches for other possible causes of the symptoms. It is often easier to explore the abdomen with the laparoscope than through the conventional right lower quadrant incision. In little girls, the ovaries and fallopian tubes can be atraumatically manipulated and inspected. The bowel can be inspected in its entirety, looking for a Meckel's diverticulum or other pathology, and the upper abdomen evaluated for cholecystitis or abscess formation.

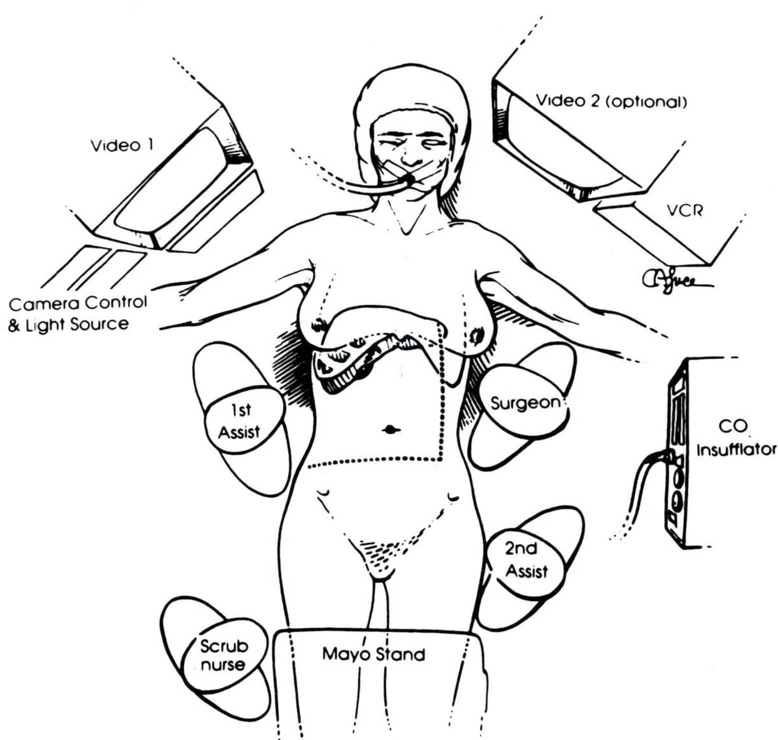

FIGURE 9-8. Operating room setup for laparoscopic cholecystectomy. (Schirmer BD, et al: Laparoscopic cholecystectomy: treatment of choice for symptomatic cholelithiasis. Ann Surg 1991;213: 665. With permission)

After the procedure has been completed, the ports are removed and the wounds closed. Patients whose appendix had ruptured remain on antibiotics and nasogastric suction, just as they would after open appendectomy. Patients with acute simple appendicitis are allowed regular diet and normal activity as tolerated and are discharged either on the day of surgery or as soon after as is feasible. Because there is no incision, patients may return to unrestricted activities immediately on discharge.

CHOLECYSTECTOMY

The results of laparoscopic cholecystectomy in children compares favorably with the procedure performed on adult patients.[19–23] The operating room setup is depicted in Figure 9-8.

The patient is prepared for a laparoscopic procedure and the pneumoperitoneum is created in the standard fashion. A four-port technique is preferred (Fig. 9-9). A 10-mm port is placed in the umbilicus for insertion of the laparoscope. Careful inspection of the liver and gallbladder allows optimal insertion of the three operating cannulas. Different functions are performed through each of the ports. The port in the mid-clavicular line (on the patient's right) is placed initially. A grasper is inserted through this port and the fundus of the gallbladder is grasped and displaced over the anterior edge of the liver. This exposes the triangle of Calot (Fig. 9-10). This port site may be altered, depending on the position of the gallbladder. It may be lower on the abdomen in the smaller child.

The second 5-mm cannula is placed in the anterior axillary position (on the patient's right). A grasper is positioned through this cannula and the gallbladder is grasped at the junction of the body and neck. When this instrument is directed in a caudal and lateral direction, it exposes the structures in the hepatocystic triangle (Fig. 9-11). As with the port in the mid-clavicular line, it may be necessary to adjust the position of this port for smaller patients. It is sometimes desirable to reverse the roles of the graspers in the anterior axillary and mid-clavicular ports when retracting the gallbladder. It is helpful to use ratcheted instruments to diminish the discomfort of the assistant.

The 10-mm port is placed in the subxiphoid position to the right of the falciform ligament in larger patients. The dissection and ligation of the cystic duct and artery are performed through this port and the gallbladder is removed through it. It is important that the instruments placed through this cannula intersect the cystic duct at a 60° or 90° angle. To obtain this angle, it may be necessary to place the port to the left of the falciform ligament in smaller patients. The dissector can be passed below the ligament or the falciform ligament can be divided. Adhesions to the gallbladder are dissected free. The cystic artery is then separated from the cystic duct. It is imperative that the surgeon clearly identifies the cystic artery, cystic duct, and right hepatic artery before any structure

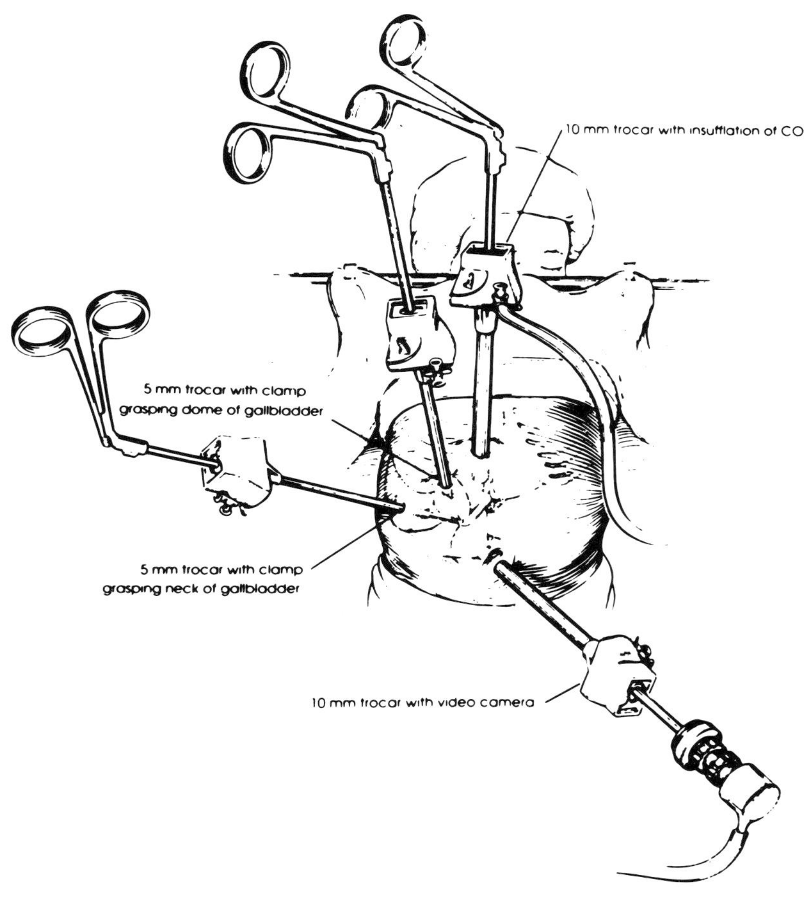

FIGURE 9-9. Port sites for laparoscopic cholecystectomy. (Davidoff AM, et al: The technique of laparoscopic cholecystectomy in children. Ann Surg 1992;215:186. With permission)

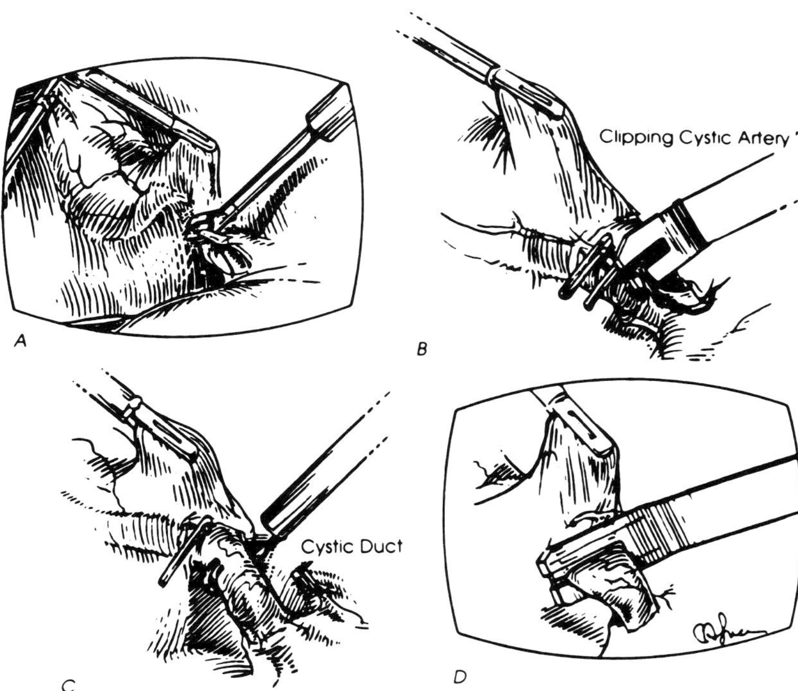

FIGURE 9-10. Exposure of the triangle of Calot. (Schirmer BD, et al: Laparoscopic cholecystectomy: treatment of choice for symptomatic cholelithiasis. Ann Surg 1991;213:665. With permission)

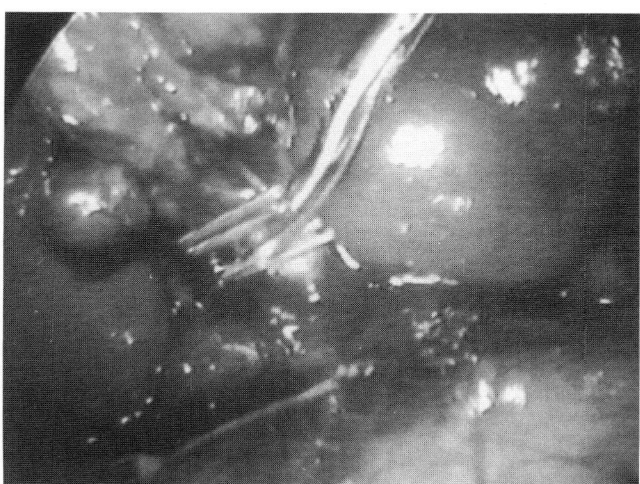

FIGURE 9-11. Exposure and division of the structures in the hepatocystic triangle. (Davidoff AM, et al: The technique of laparoscopic cholecystectomy in children. Ann Surg 1991; 215:186. With permission)

is divided. The cystic artery is ligated using four clips, then divided between the two sets of clips. The cystic duct is separated from the surrounding structures by blunt dissection. Two clips are then placed on the distal cystic duct in preparation for the cholangiogram.

Cholangiography may be performed by any one of several methods. Commercial catheters have been produced that can be passed through one of the ports but this results in a loss of exposure because one of the graspers must be removed. An 8- or 12-inch 16- to 18-gauge intravenous cannula (or the outer sheath of a Veress needle) can be placed directly through the abdominal wall, just below the edge of the liver between the anterior axillary and mid-clavicular ports. A cholangiogram catheter can be passed through this cannula. An incision is made in the exposed cystic duct and the catheter is advanced into its lumen. Clips are placed around the catheter to secure it in the duct. After the cholangiogram is obtained, the clips and catheter are removed. The clips are re-applied and the duct divided. Cannulation should be accomplished well away from the junctions of the common bile and cystic ducts.

After the cystic duct is ligated, the divided end is grasped and retracted toward the patient's right shoulder. The gallbladder is then dissected free from the liver, using a combination of laser or electrosurgery and blunt dissection. When dissection reaches the point at which only the peritoneum attaches the gallbladder to the liver, the ligated cystic artery and duct are carefully inspected and the gallbladder bed is examined for bleeding (Fig. 9-12). If this is not done before division of the peritoneal attachments, it is difficult to regain exposure of these areas. The intra-abdominal pressure should be lowered to less than 8 mmHg because venous bleeding may be tamponaded at higher pressures. The last of the peritoneal attachments are divided and the gallbladder is removed through the 10-mm subxiphoid cannula site. This is achieved by grasping the gallbladder at the cystic duct and pulling the gallbladder through the cannula. If this is not possible, the cannula is removed while maintaining the grasp on the cystic duct. The gallbladder can then be pulled through the fascial defect. If large stones are pres-

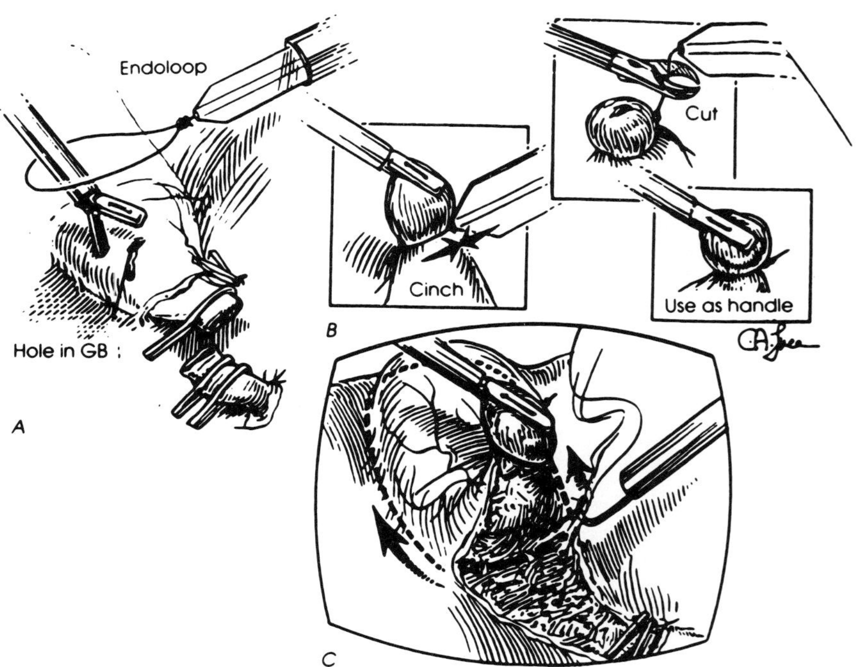

FIGURE 9-12. Examination of gallbladder bed for control of hemorrhage. (Schirmer BD, et al: Laparoscopic cholecystectomy: treatment of choice for symptomatic cholelithiasis. Ann Surg 1991; 213:665. With permission)

ent, the gallbladder may be opened and the stones crushed or removed with a large clamp, then removed.

UNDESCENDED TESTICLES

Laparoscopy for cryptorchid testes is rapidly becoming an accepted standard for this condition.[24–31] Patients with bilateral cryptorchidism or with a unilateral nonpalpable testis benefit from laparoscopy in several ways.

In unilateral disease, the differential diagnoses include undescended testis versus testicular atrophy. At laparoscopy, the surgeon can visualize the testicle in the inguinal canal or abdomen. In cases of testicular atrophy, the testicular vessels and vas deferens that end blindly just at the internal inguinal ring can be noted. This observation coupled with no palpable tissue in the inguinal canal or scrotum indicates that testicular atrophy has occurred. This is usually due to an intrauterine torsion. Laparotomy may not be required in this case. With bilateral disease, the surgeon can determine whether the testes are present and whether they lie in proximity to the inguinal canal or are in a high intra-abdominal location.

Carbon dioxide pneumoperitoneum is established, and a 5-mm umbilical cannula is placed for passage of the 4- or 5-mm laparoscope. In most cases, simple inspection of either or both internal inguinal rings provides the required information.

For the high intra-abdominal testis, one option is to perform a high ligation of the spermatic vessels and displace the testis downward to the internal inguinal ring, securing it with a clip or sutures for orchiopexy 6 weeks later. The patient is maintained in Trendelenburg's position and rotated, with the side opposite the cryptorchid testicle downward. The testicle and its pedicle can be identified. A small incision is made over the proximal spermatic vessels, just adequate to isolate them, and they are divided between surgical clips or suture-ligated, depending on the preference of the surgeon (Fig. 9-13). The peritoneum can then be sufficiently incised toward the pelvis to displace the testicle to the internal inguinal ring and secure it in position. This can either be accomplished by suture technique, or the gonad can be clipped or stapled in place (Fig. 9-14). Alternatively, a laser can be used to divide the testicular vessels without risking harm to adjacent structures.

After 6 weeks or more, sufficient vascular collateralization is likely to have occurred, so that an inguinal orchiopexy can be performed. Although it is too early to tell the long-term results of this technique, there is minimal disruption of the collateral vascular supply; therefore, this approach is appealing at this time. The available experimental data suggest that although the testis is viable after spermatic vessel ligation, its endocrine and reproductive capacity may be impaired. After simple in-

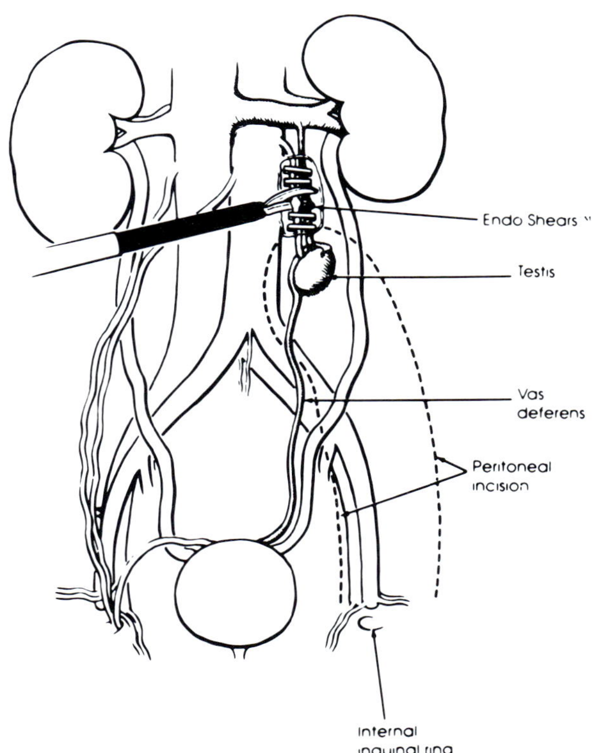

FIGURE 9-13. Endoscopic clip applied to testicular vessels below renal hilum. (Lobe TE, Schropp KP, eds. Pediatric laparoscopy and thoracoscopy. Philadelphia: WB Saunders, 1993: 137. With permission)

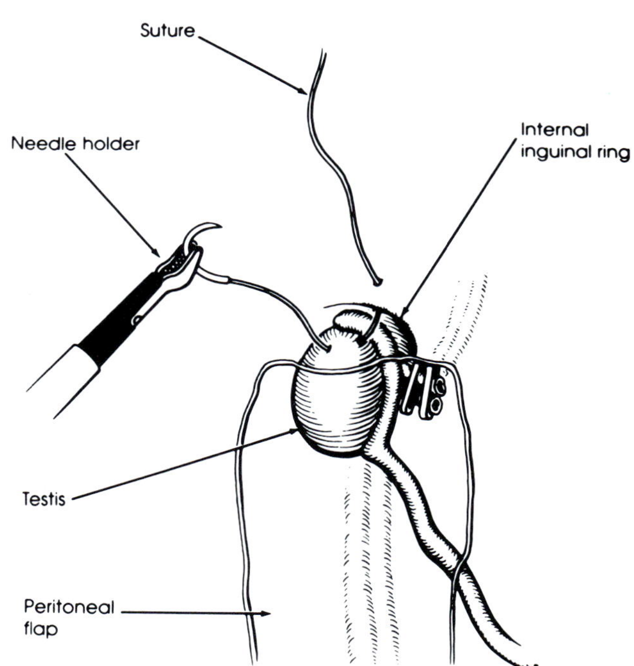

FIGURE 9-14. Gonad secured to internal inguinal ring. (Lobe TE, Schropp KP, eds. Pediatric laparoscopy and thoracoscopy. Philadelphia: WB Saunders, 1993:138. With permission)

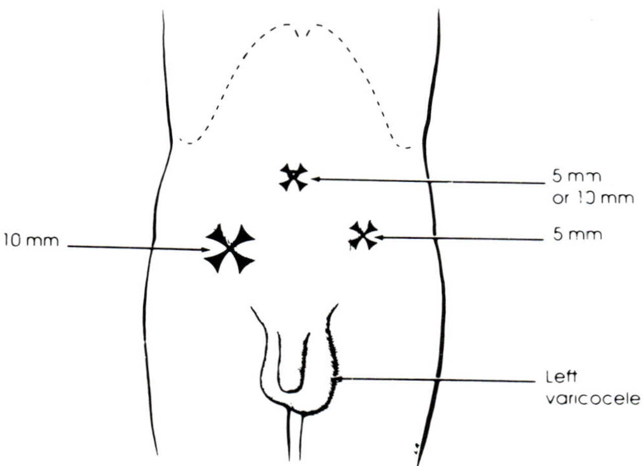

FIGURE 9-15. Port sites for left varicocele ligation. (Lobe TE, Schropp KP, eds. Pediatric laparoscopy and thoracoscopy. Philadelphia: WB Saunders, 1993:140. With permission)

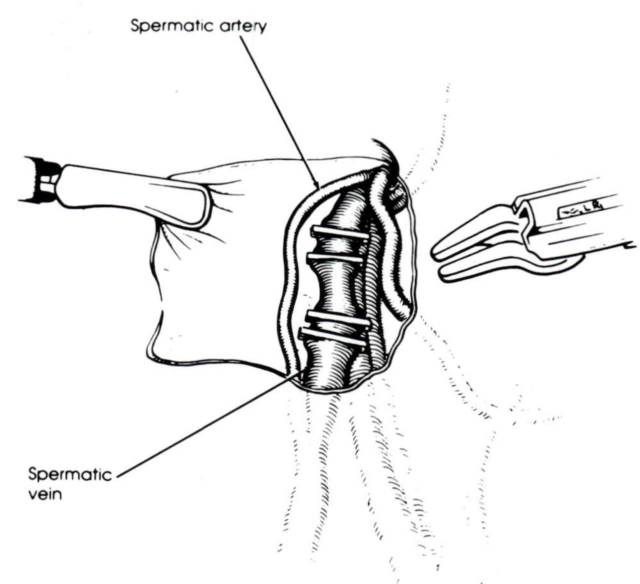

FIGURE 9-16. Clips on abnormal veins for varicocele ligation. (Lobe TE, Schropp KP, eds. Pediatric laparoscopy and thoracoscopy. Philadelphia: WB Saunders, 1993:140. With permission)

spection or relocation of the testis, the ports are removed and the wounds closed.

VARICOCELE

Pediatric surgeons often diagnose a varicocele in an older child or adolescent presenting with pain or concern over a bulging mass in the scrotum. The diagnosis is frequently obvious. Alternatives to management include operative ligation of the spermatic vein and the pampiniform plexus, venous immobilization using imaging techniques, and direct ligation through laparoscopy. Laparoscopic division of the veins is a simple procedure that can be performed as outpatient surgery, with minimal morbidity.[32] The technique is as follows. A CO_2 pneumoperitoneum is established, as outlined above. The patient is maintained in Trendelenburg's position, and the initial 5-mm port is placed through the umbilicus. Two additional ports are required: one 5-mm in the lower abdomen, in the quadrant on the side of the lesion, and the other either in the midline or in the opposite lower quadrant. This is usually a 10-mm port for passage of the clip applier (Fig. 9-15).

After establishing a pneumoperitoneum, the testicular vessels are identified as they enter the internal ring. The peritoneum over these vessels is gently incised and retracted, exposing the vas deferens and associated vessels. By using a fine-tipped dissector and positioning the end of the laparoscope close to the vessels, the artery and vein are dissected free from each other. Once the vein is identified and separated from the artery, it can be ligated with clips (Fig. 9-16) or sutured and then divided. Reperitonealization is not necessary. After making certain that there is no perioperative hemorrhage, the surgeon withdraws the cannulas and closes the abdominal incisions.

INGUINAL HERNIORRHAPHY

Many general surgeons believe that the laparoscopic repair of inguinal hernias in adults is an acceptable procedure. Although many of these procedures are being performed today, the technique has not withstood the test of time and may not be (as has been proposed) as durable as an open inguinal repair. The adult repair consists of incising the peritoneum anterior to the hernial defect; excising the sac; inserting a roll of polypropylene mesh into the inguinal defect; tacking a piece of polypropylene mesh over the defect, using a hernia stapler; and reperitonealizing the repair.

Routine laparoscopy usually proves useful in the management of inguinal hernias in children, to determine whether a hernia is present on the asymptomatic contralateral side.[33] A 3-mm port is inserted through an umbilical stab wound after insufflating the infant's abdomen to 8 to 10 mmHg with CO_2. A 2-mm 0° telescope (the same telescope used by pediatric surgeons for cystoscopy or bronchoscopy) can be used to inspect the lower abdomen (Fig. 9-17). Hernias are obvious when present. A patent processus vaginalis or the neck of a small hernia sac can also be identified when present (Fig. 9-18).

Inguinal hernias have been repaired laparoscopically, and this approach appears to be reasonable for

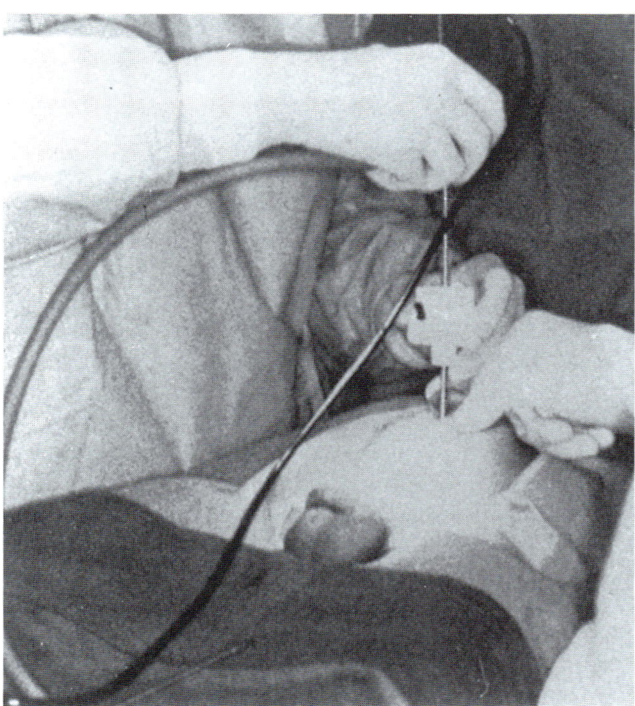

FIGURE 9-17. Two-millimeter 0° telescope, used for hernia exploration. (Lobe TE, Schropp KP, eds. Pediatric laparoscopy and thoracoscopy. Philadelphia: WB Saunders, 1993:157. With permission)

older children. Essentially the same principles are adhered to as for other repairs of indirect inguinal hernias in children, *viz* the hernia sac is divided and the neck of the sac obliterated.

Repair is carried out with the patient in Trendelenburg's position, and three ports are placed. An umbilical port is used for the laparoscope. Two other ports are inserted lateral to the rectus muscle, at or slightly above the level of the umbilicus—one on either side of the abdomen. The peritoneum is incised as in the adult repair. The hernia sac is then divided, taking care not to injure the cord structures, which are easily identified. The distal sac can either be removed or left in situ. The hernia defect is sutured closed, using interrupted nonabsorbable sutures. The peritoneum is then closed. Patients are discharged on the day of surgery and are instructed to return to unrestricted activities.

MESENTERIC CYSTS

Many mesenteric cysts can be diagnosed preoperatively with use of diagnostic imaging. When a cyst is identified and appears to be relatively free from other structures, it is amenable to laparoscopic intervention.

One begins with diagnostic laparoscopy through an umbilical cannula. If the cyst is large enough to obstruct the view and it is unlikely to be malignant, a needle is inserted through the abdominal wall directly into the cyst, allowing decompression. If the cyst is on a pedicle, it can usually be excised using laser or electrosurgical techniques, endoscopic sutures or loops, or mechanical devices such as clips or staplers.

Cysts buried in the mesentery or omentum can be dissected free and are similarly excised. Decompression of the cyst may help with its removal through the laparoscopic cannula. Rarely, a cyst can be so intimately involved with an adjacent loop of bowel that a bowel resection may be necessary to remove the cyst. This also can be accomplished laparoscopically, using the new linear staplers.

HEPATIC AND SPLENIC CYSTS

Occasionally, cystic lesions of the liver are observed, requiring intervention. As with other cystic lesions, they can either be excised or fenestrated, using the techniques already described. A laser can be used to unroof the cyst and then obliterate its lining. When infection is a consideration, cultures can be obtained by placing a drainage tube directly, using the laparoscope as a guide.

Although splenic cysts are uncommon, simple epidermoid cysts are ideal for laparoscopic correction. One such cyst in a teenage girl has been treated by the authors, using four ports to complete the procedure. A

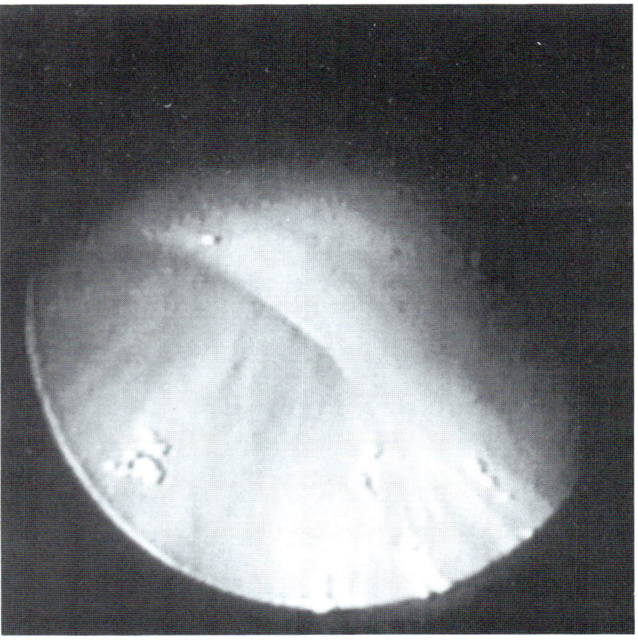

FIGURE 9-18. Patent processus vaginalis. (Lobe TE, Schropp KP, eds. Pediatric laparoscopy and thoracoscopy. Philadelphia: WB Saunders, 1993:158. With permission)

10-mm umbilical port was used to visualize the cyst. Two 5-mm ports were placed in the lower abdominal crease on either side of the rectus muscle to manipulate the tissues. To complete the procedure, an additional port was required. This was placed in the right mid-clavicular line, midway between the umbilicus and the costal margin.

Initially, the cyst was inspected. By all criteria, it appeared to be a simple cyst without evidence of infection. The Veress needle was placed through a separate stab wound immediately over the presenting portion of the cyst to puncture the wall and aspirate its contents. Serous fluid was removed, thus supporting the diagnosis of a simple cyst without infection. The cyst wall was then excised, using bipolar cautery to remove the lining at its junction with the spleen. The entire presenting wall of the cyst was removed. One segment of the posterior wall appeared to be thicker than the rest. This was transected using the Endo-GIA stapler. The lining of the cyst had many shallow trabeculations and appeared to overlie the splenic hilus. It was not thought worthwhile to attempt to strip the lining from the cyst for fear of inducing a hemorrhage that might necessitate a splenectomy.

NISSEN FUNDOPLICATION

The laparoscopic approach to Nissen fundoplication is not new. Dallemagne first performed a laparoscopic Nissen fundoplication at the Clinique Saint Joseph in Liege, Belgium, in January 1991.[34] Later that year, Geagea performed a similar procedure in Nova Scotia.[35]

Cuschieri and coworkers began performing laparoscopic antireflux surgery in 1989. They have described their results with this technique, used in eight elderly patients ranging in age from 60 to 79 years, with a mean follow-up of 11 months.[36]

Dallemagne has performed numerous procedures in patients ranging in age from 29 to 69.[34] His mean operative time is between 1.5 and 2 hours. Most patients resume a normal diet on the first postoperative day and are discharged on the second postoperative day. His results are similar to those achieved using laparotomy. Although some patients (adults) have early transient dysphagia, their postoperative course is described as benign and uneventful.

The indications for performing a laparoscopic antireflux procedure for gastroesophageal reflux in children are the same as those for the open approach. The theoretic advantages of the laparoscopic approach are related to the absence of an abdominal incision. In obese patients, a large incision is more likely to develop a wound complication, and it may impair postoperative pulmonary function. In the debilitated child, particularly those severely mentally handicapped or those who cannot follow instructions, the incision may impair pulmonary function and predispose the patient to atelectasis or pneumonia.

One accepted laparoscopic technique involves placing five ports in the abdomen: one for viewing with the telescope, one for retracting the liver, two for tissue manipulation, and one for suturing. The operation is identical to that performed by laparotomy: the liver is retracted away from the esophageal hiatus, the esophagus is mobilized, the diaphragmatic crura are approximated with sutures, the short gastric vessels are divided as necessary, a 360° fundoplication wrap is sutured into position, and a gastrostomy is placed as necessary.

The details of the procedure are as follows. Patients are best prepared for the operation by emptying the colon of gas and feces before the operation. Otherwise, the gas-distended colon is in the way, making the procedure difficult or impossible to perform. Under general endotracheal anesthesia, the bladder is catheterized or emptied using Credé's method and a nasogastric tube is passed. Some surgeons prefer to place the patient in the lithotomy position, so that the camera operator can stand between the patient's legs and be out of the way. This position is better suited to older or obese children or teenagers. Using sterile technique, a CO_2 pneumoperitoneum is established and maintained, and a 5- or 10-mm 0° laparoscope is placed in an umbilical port. A 5-mm port is placed below the right costal margin in the mid-clavicular line and another in the epigastrium. A 10-mm port is placed in the left mid-clavicular line below the costal margin, and a 5-mm port is located in the left anterior axillary line below the costal margin (Fig. 9-19). The liver is retracted by the epigastric port to expose the esophageal hiatus (Fig. 9-20). Although the port itself is sufficient to hold the liver out of the way in smaller patients, a retractor is necessary in larger patients. It may be easier in some patients to insert this retractor through the right lateral port, using the epigastric port for dissection and suturing. The short gastric vessels are divided between surgical clips as necessary (Fig. 9-21). Two medium length clips are applied to either side of the proposed line of division. The reticulating endoscopic dissector (U.S. Surgical Corporation, Norwalk, CT) is useful for isolating these vessels. The esophagus, with as large a bougie in place as it will accommodate, is mobilized and retracted using dissecting instruments passed through the right and left lateral ports. A short segment (about 6 inches) of umbilical tape is then passed behind the esophagus, as illustrated (Fig. 9-22). The exposed diaphragmatic crura are approximated to close the hiatus, using interrupted 2-0 silk sutures that have been lubricated with mineral oil. Extracorporeal knots are the easiest to tie under tension for a secure closure. Intracorporeal knot tying is an option if one is sufficiently skilled in this technique. The stomach is passed behind the esophagus from the patient's left to his right. With the stomach held in position, using an instrument passed

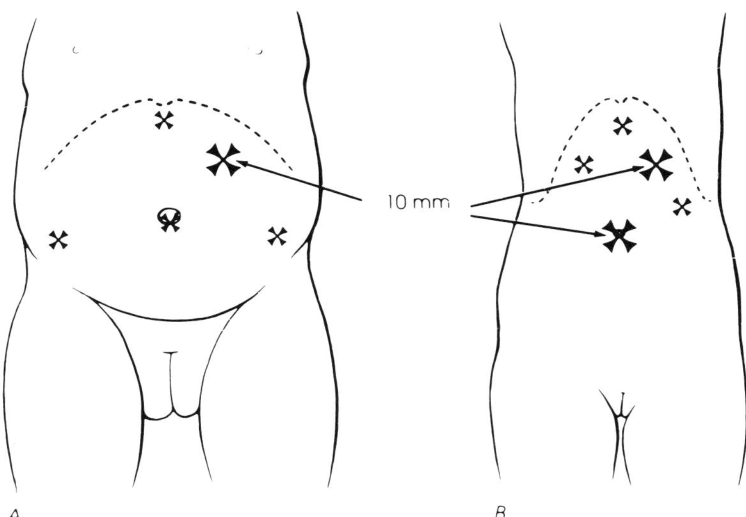

FIGURE 9-19. Port sites for Nissen fundoplication. (Lobe TE, Schropp KP, eds. Pediatric laparoscopy and thoracoscopy. Philadelphia: WB Saunders, 1993:169. With permission)

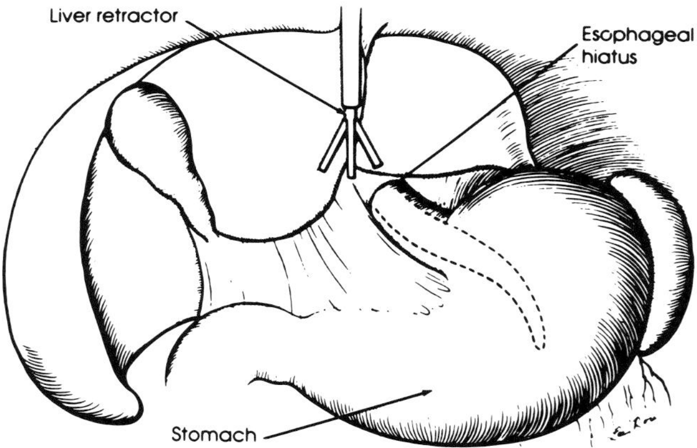

FIGURE 9-20. Exposure of esophageal hiatus for Nissen fundoplication. (Lobe TE, Schropp KP, Lunsford K: Laparoscopic Nissen fundoplication in childhood. J Pediatr Surg 1993;28:358. With permission)

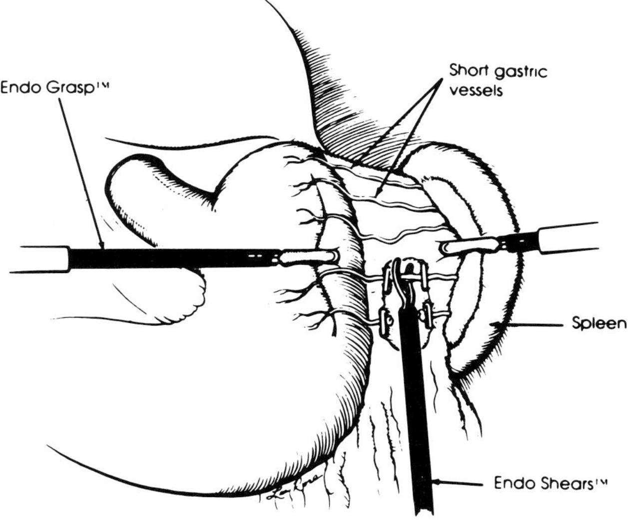

FIGURE 9-21. Division of short gastric vessels for Nissen fundoplication. (Lobe TE, Schropp KP, Lunsford K: Laparoscopic Nissen fundoplication in childhood. J Pediatr Surg 1993;28:358. With permission)

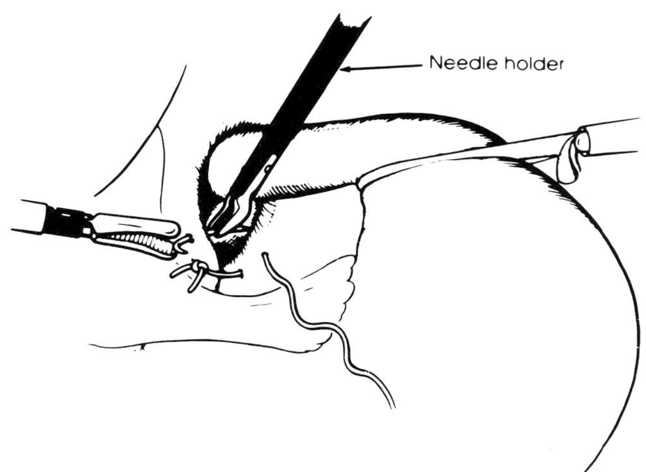

FIGURE 9-22. Umbilical tape around the esophagus, for control and mobilization of the esophagus for Nissen fundoplication to place sutures that close the hiatus. (Lobe TE, Schropp KP, Lunsford K: Laparoscopic Nissen fundoplication in childhood. J Pediatr Surg 1993;28:358. With permission)

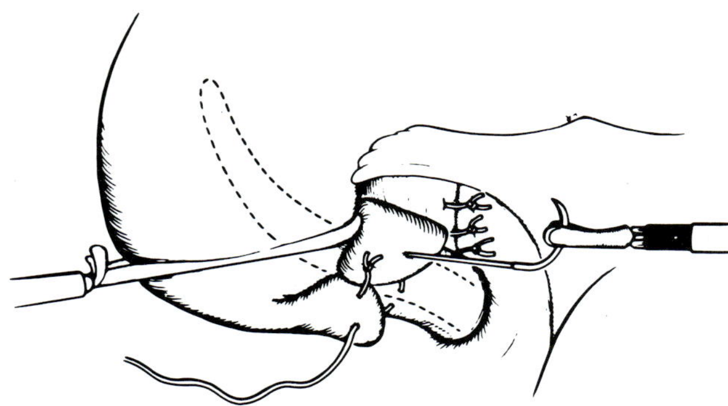

FIGURE 9-23. Sutures placed in stomach to secure 360° wrap. (Lobe TE, Schropp KP, Lunsford K: Laparoscopic Nissen fundoplication in childhood. J Pediatr Surg 1993;28:358. With permission)

from the right mid-clavicular line port, a back-handed suture is used to "snag" the stomach and complete the first (most distal) suture of the wrap. This maneuver saves having to put in another port. The 3- to 5-cm wrap is then secured in place, using interrupted 2-0 silk sutures, as for an open procedure (Fig. 9-23). The esophageal bougie and the port are then removed.

In a series of 12 laparoscopic Nissen fundoplications, the patients ranged in age from 3 months to 11 years of age and weighed from 2.5 to 53 kg. Two were female and ten were male. The first three procedures attempted were converted to open procedures because the proper instrumentation was not available (one case), a patient was discovered to have portal hypertension and the procedure was aborted (one case), and an opening was made in the posterior esophagus that was repaired using an open technique (one case). Since these initial three cases, none have required conversion to laparotomy.[37]

A gastrostomy was created for all but one patient. Initially, a percutaneous endoscopic technique was used while the stomach was observed through the laparoscope. The laparoscope is used to determine the optimal position for the gastrostomy, grasping the correct spot on the anterior gastric wall (Fig. 9-24) and externalizing the stomach through the subcostal mid-clavicular line trocar site. The gastrostomy tube is then sutured into place after the fundoplication is completed (Fig. 9-25). Because there is a lack of instruments small enough to use on infants weighing less than 3 kg, it is preferable to use the conventional approach for these patients.

Postoperatively, patients are fed liquids on the evening of their surgery and a full diet (by tube or by mouth) on postoperative day 1. Generally, they are discharged between 36 and 48 hours postoperatively, at which time they can return to unrestricted activities. Follow-up to 18 months showed the patients were all asymptomatic for gastroesophageal reflux and all of the fundoplications remained intact.

PYLORIC STENOSIS

Several pediatric surgeons around the world perform laparoscopic pylorotomy for idiopathic hypertrophic pyloric stenosis.[38] The technique is a relatively simple one. Umbilical access is achieved after CO_2 insufflation in the standard fashion. Another port is inserted laterally, to the left of the patient's midline. With the stomach decompressed, it is easy to identify the pyloric tumor. An elec-

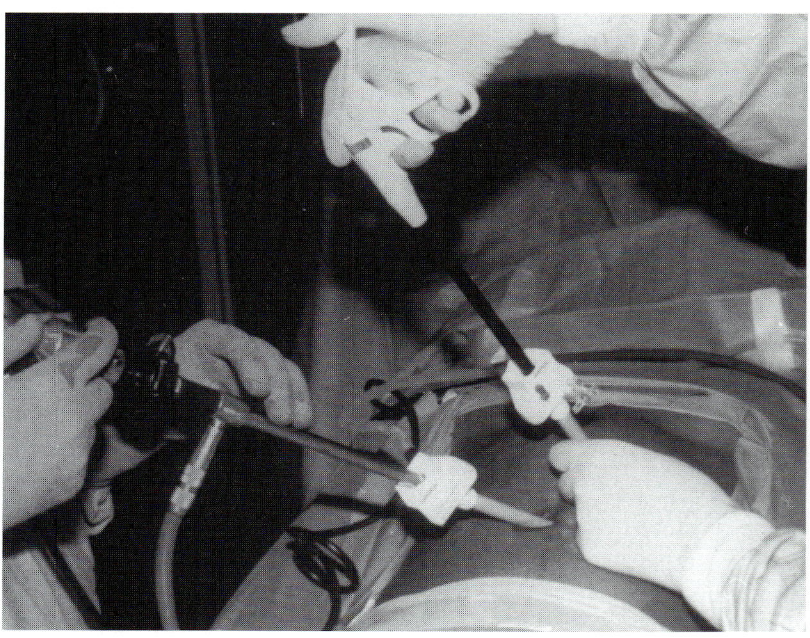

FIGURE 9-24. Identification of gastrostomy tube site, as viewed endoscopically.

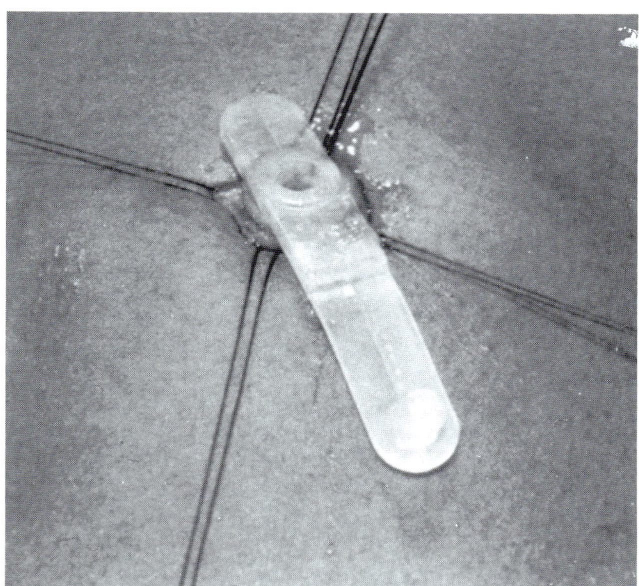

FIGURE 9-25. Gastrostomy tube being sutured in place after Nissen fundoplication.

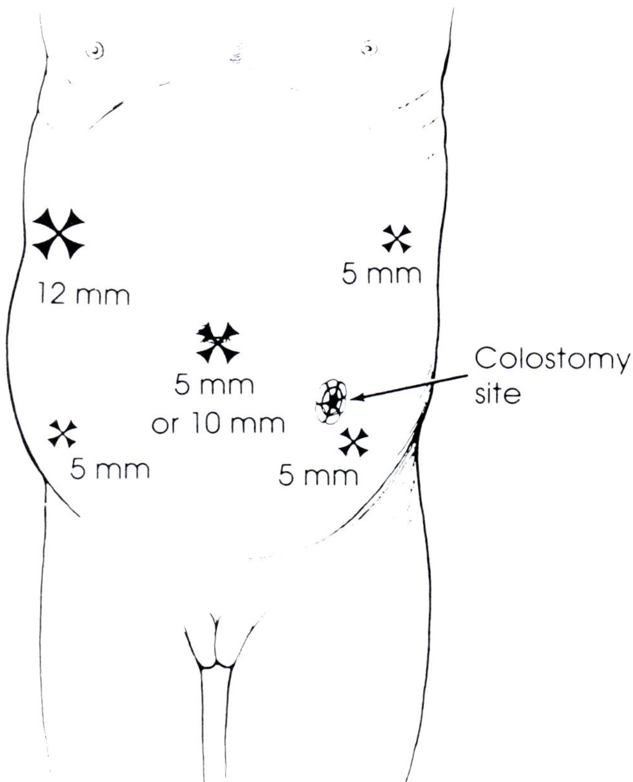

FIGURE 9-26. Cannula placement for a Duhamel pull-through. (Lobe TE, Schropp KP, eds. Pediatric laparoscopy and thoracoscopy. Philadelphia: WB Saunders, 1993:208. With permission)

trosurgical instrument for pylorotomy is used to incise the pyloric muscle down to the mucosa, along the length of the pylorus. Another instrument is then used to spread the muscle and separate its two halves. Surgeons adept at the technique can perform this procedure in 20 to 45 minutes. Overall, the surgeon appears to have relatively little control of the pylorus during the procedure. The high risk of perforation (nearly 10%) makes the procedure an investigative one.

PULL-THROUGH FOR HIRSCHSPRUNG'S DISEASE

A pull-through for Hirschsprung's disease can be safely performed laparoscopically. Although Swenson, Suave, and Duhamel procedures have all been reported, the Duhamel operation is preferred by the authors. The technique is as follows: patients are prepared for surgery, as for a standard Duhamel pull-through. In most instances, a leveling colostomy already exists. The stomach is emptied by nasogastric tube and a bladder catheter inserted. Because of the preexisting colostomy, the surgeon may prefer to use the open (Hasson) approach for placement of the initial port in the umbilicus. A CO_2 pneumoperitoneum is established and the laparoscope inserted through the umbilical cannula.

After the initial inspection with the patient in Trendelenburg's position, additional ports are inserted (Fig. 9-26). A 12-mm port is placed in the right side of the abdomen for application of a linear stapler. This stapler is used across the colostomy site, just at the level of the abdominal fascia, to take down the bowel from its attachment to the anterior abdominal wall. Two cannulas are then placed in the upper and lower quadrants of the patient's left side at the anterior axillary line lateral to the rectus muscle, and one additional cannula is placed on the right side. These can usually be 5-mm ports. Using the two left-sided cannulas, the bowel is elevated, exposing the mesentery. The peritoneum over the mesentery is incised and if necessary, the vessels are divided between the surgical clips. With the bowel intact, the colon is elevated and closed with an endoscopic stapler. An Endoscopic Kitner (OR Concepts, Inc., Roanoke, TX) is used to dissect distally and retrorectally to 1 cm from the mucocutaneous junction. The stapler is ideally suited to this task because its size approximates that of the proximal bowel to be pulled through. After the patient's bowel is prepped, the perineum is exposed on the surgical field, allowing access for anorectal dissection and anastomosis. Once the retrorectal dissection has been completed, the bowel can be transected, using one stapler at the peritoneal reflection and another proximal to the colostomy (Figs. 9-27 and 9-28).

Sutures are placed in the proximal staple line to pull the bowel through the retrorectal space. A transverse incision is made in the posterior rectum (1 cm proximal

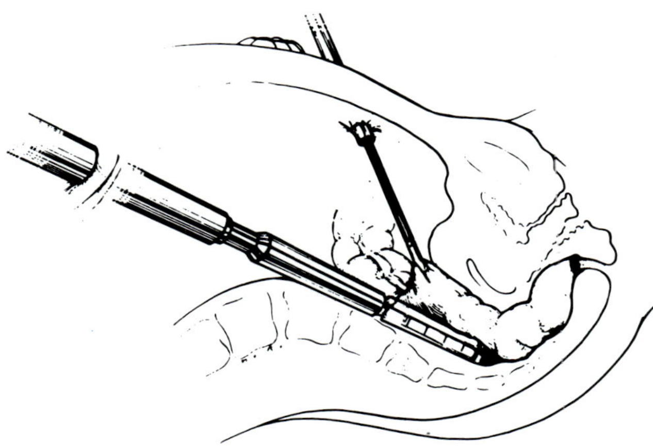

FIGURE 9-27. Retrorectal dissection for a Duhamel pull-through. (Lobe TE, Schropp KP, eds. Pediatric laparoscopy and thoracoscopy. Philadelphia: WB Saunders, 1993:209. With permission)

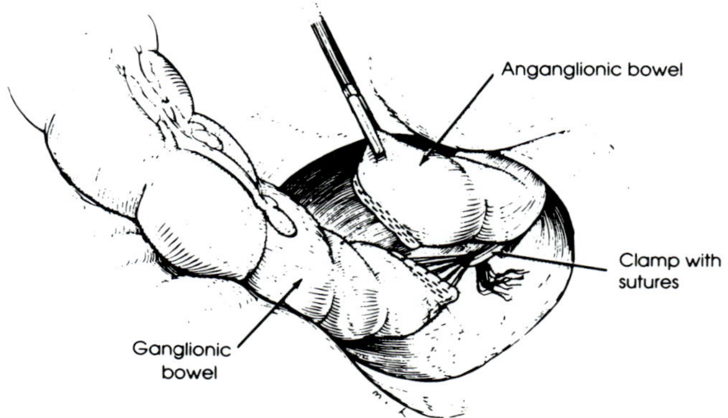

FIGURE 9-29. Pulled-through bowel in an endoscopic procedure. (Lobe TE, Schropp KP, eds. Pediatric laparoscopy and thoracoscopy. Philadelphia: WB Saunders, 1993:210. With permission)

to the mucocutaneous junction, as in a standard pull-through) and a curved clamp is inserted into the retrorectal space. The sutures are grasped and the bowel is pulled through (Fig. 9-29). A single layer of interrupted 4-0 absorbable sutures is used to complete the anastomosis in the standard fashion. The stapler is then inserted transrectally, its anterior limb in the anterior aganglionic pouch and its posterior limb in the posterior ganglionic bowel. The stapler is used to create the anastomosis between the two lumina (Fig. 9-30). Because the pneumoperitoneum has been lost, it is reestablished and additional staples can be applied with the Endo-GIA stapler

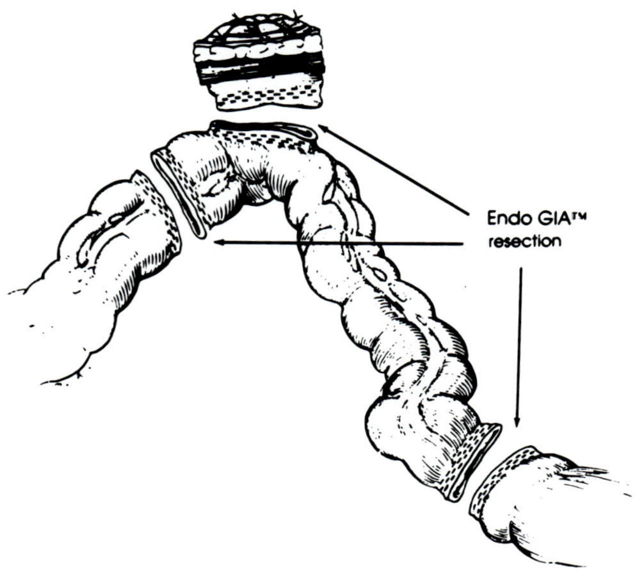

FIGURE 9-28. Endo-GIA transection of bowel for a laparoscopic Duhamel pull-through. (Lobe TE, Schropp KP, eds. Pediatric laparoscopy and thoracoscopy. Philadelphia: WB Saunders, 1993:209. With permission)

to ensure that the suture line is as close to the end of the anterior pouch as possible. Sutures can be placed to approximate the corners of the anterior pouch to the posterior intestine. If desired, a stapler can be used to create a single transverse suture line that includes the anterior wall of the anterior pouch and the anterior wall of the posterior pouch, thus eliminating any anterior spur that could accumulate stool (Fig. 9-31). The mesentery can be closed as desired, and all creases should be inspected for hemostasis.

The excised remnant of colon can be removed in one of two ways: it can either be brought out through the transrectal incision before the pull-through is accomplished or it can be removed at the end of the procedure at the time of excision of the residual colostomy.

At the end of the procedure, the colostomy (if present) is excised down to the fascia; the bowel segment removed through this fascial opening, if it has not already been removed; and the anterior abdominal wall closed in the standard fashion.

LYMPHADENECTOMY AND UROLOGIC PROCEDURES

Laparoscopic lymphadenectomy has been reported, especially in association with Hodgkin's disease and other entities, including neoplasms of the stomach, gallbladder, liver, and pancreas in addition to intestinal pathologic states requiring biopsy of lymph nodes or lymphadenectomy.[39] In addition, laparoscopic percutaneous transperitoneal lithotripsy on pelvic kidneys was reported in 1985.[39,40] A laparoscopic approach facilitated observation and displacement of loops of bowel during percutaneous access to the pelvic kidneys by retrograde nephrostomy. In a series of 16 patients aged 18 months to 38 years, nonpalpable testes were noted, six of which were bilateral cryptorchid patients, and 10 had a unilat-

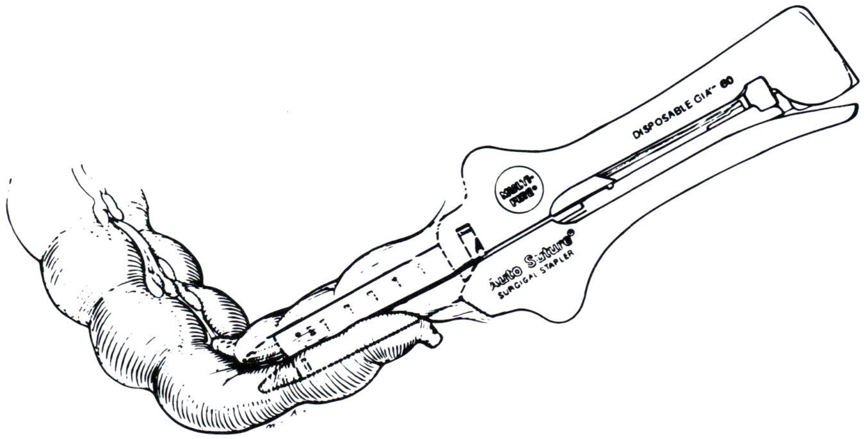

FIGURE 9-30. Endo-GIA application to complete rectal anastomosis for a laparoscopic Duhamel pull-through procedure. (Lobe TE, Schropp KP, eds. Pediatric laparoscopy and thoracoscopy. Philadelphia: WB Saunders, 1993:211. With permission)

eral nonpalpable gonad.[40] Furthermore, laparoscopic observation of the vas deferens and gonadal vessels in association with anorchia appears to be feasible in the pediatric and adolescent patient.

Laparoscopic ureterolysis has been reported in a 15-year-old female with a 2-month history of right flank pain.[41]

SPLENECTOMY

Another procedure that shows promise in the pediatric adolescent patient is laparoscopic splenectomy. Generally, these are performed on patients with hematologic disorders, the indications being determined by the primary disease. Patients are prepared as described for the fundoplication. They are vaccinated preoperatively with the appropriate polyvalent vaccines against pneumococcus and *Haemophilus influenzae*.

The procedure is as follows. A 5- or 10-mm laparoscope is placed through an umbilical port, its size depending on the size of the patient. A steep Trendelenburg's position is required. The patient is slightly rotated, with the left side elevated. Port placement is essentially a mirror image of that required for laparoscopic nephrectomy (Fig. 9-32). Two ports are placed: one 10-mm in the right mid-clavicular line in the upper abdomen and one 5-mm in the right mid-clavicular line, at or below the level of the umbilicus. The child is placed in a left lateral decubitus position, and two 5-mm cannulas are placed in the anterior axillary line, one just below the costal margin and one between the umbilicus and the iliac crest.

Initially, the greater curvature of the stomach is grasped gently with an atraumatic grasper or Babcock clamp, and the gastrosplenic ligament is retracted to expose the short gastric vessels. The vessels are then divided between surgical clips, with the clip applicator passed through the 10-mm mid-clavicular port (Fig. 9-33).

As the dissection progresses, it is helpful to rotate the patient to a more anterior position to allow the intes-

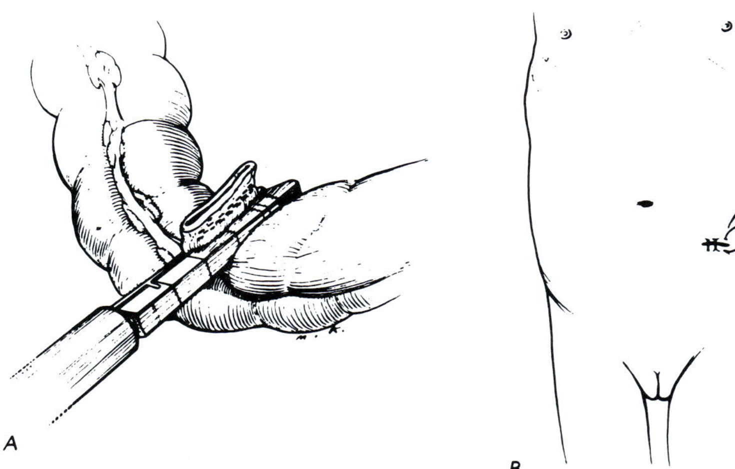

FIGURE 9-31. Endo-GIA stapler, used to eliminate the anterior spur for a Duhamel pull-through procedure. (Lobe TE, Schropp KP, eds. Pediatric laparoscopy and thoracoscopy. Philadelphia: WB Saunders, 1993:211. With permission)

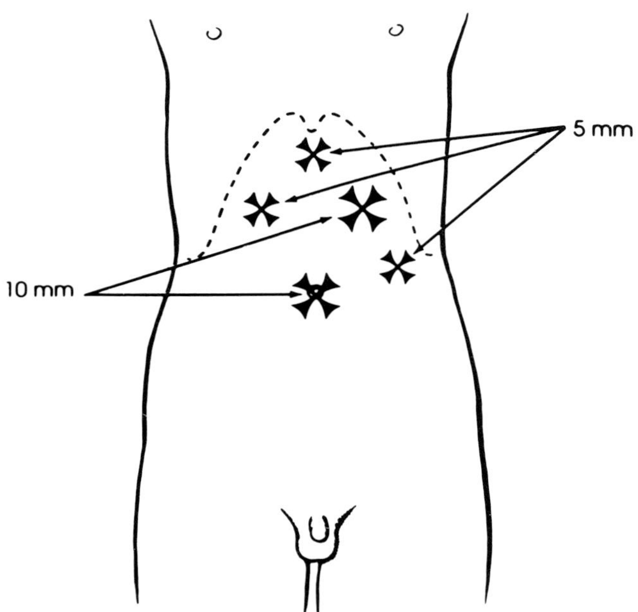

FIGURE 9-32. Port placement for laparoscopic splenectomy. (Lobe TE, Schropp KP, eds. Pediatric laparoscopy and thoracoscopy. Philadelphia: WB Saunders, 1993:191. With permission)

tines to fall out of the way. Using instruments passed through the lateral ports, the spleen is elevated and the splenic artery and vein at the hilum just beyond the tail of the pancreas is identified, using gentle dissection with a curved or right-angle dissector. The splenic hilum is then isolated and the vasculature controlled with a stapler, which is used to divide both vessels simultaneously (Fig. 9-34). This device provides excellent hemostasis and diminishes operative time significantly.

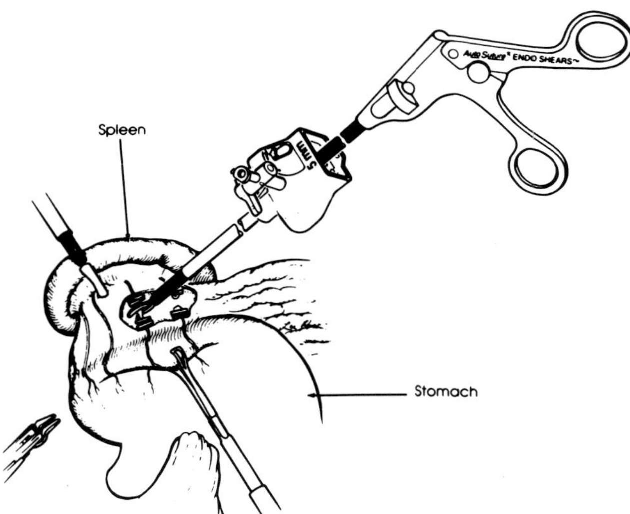

FIGURE 9-33. Division of short gastric vessels for laparoscopic splenectomy. (Lobe TE, Schropp KP, eds. Pediatric laparoscopy and thoracoscopy. Philadelphia: WB Saunders, 1993:191. With permission)

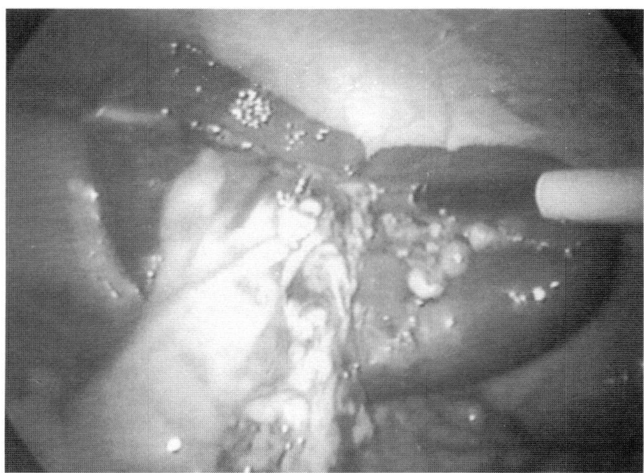

FIGURE 9-34. Exposure of the splenic hilum for a laparoscopic splenectomy.

After the major splenic vessels have been divided, there are often many ligamentous attachments that should be carefully divided using Metzenbaum-type endoscopic scissors. At this point, the spleen is completely mobilized and is free in the peritoneal cavity. A Lap Sac (Cook Urological, Spencer, IN) is then inserted through the 10-mm port. The sac is unfurled and the three tabs at the mouth of the sac are held open while the spleen is placed in it (Fig. 9-35). The neck of the sac is drawn up into a 10-mm cannula. When the entire neck is in the cannula, the sac should be withdrawn until the neck of the sac is exteriorized onto the anterior abdominal wall. The neck of the sac is opened and the tissue morcellator placed within the pouch. The organ can then be morcellated until it is sufficiently small, so that the entire pouch, with any residual tissue, can be withdrawn through the

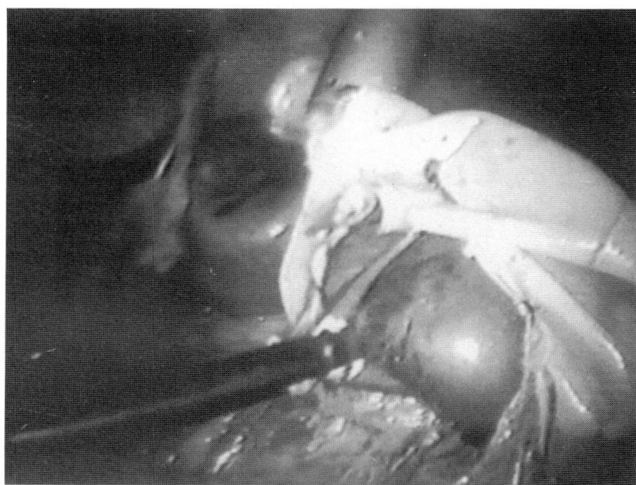

FIGURE 9-35. Placing the spleen in a Lap Sac (Cook Urological, Spencer, IN) for completion of laparoscopic splenectomy.

trocar site. The trocar and cannula are then reinserted and the pneumoperitoneum reestablished.

Depending on the indication for a splenectomy, a search should be made for an accessory spleen or spleens and these removed. Once it is established that there are no accessory spleens and that there is excellent hemostasis, the cannulas are removed and the incisions closed.

Thus far, 11 laparoscopic splenectomies have been performed by the authors on children age 18 months to 8 years. Four children had hereditary spherocytosis and three underwent a concomitant cholecystectomy. One child had sequestration crises from sickle cell disease. The other children had idiopathic thrombocytopenic purpura. All were offered clear liquids on the evening of surgery and returned to unrestricted activity by 48 hours postoperatively. There were no complications in the series.

NEPHRECTOMY

Nephrectomy for congenital abnormality or selected tumors can be performed laparoscopically. This technique appears to be most useful in the older child in whom a laparotomy would result in a longer and more morbid postoperative recovery. The technique requires a tissue morcellator to break the solid mass into sufficiently small pieces, so that it can be removed through a laparoscopic cannula.[42]

The procedure is initiated with the patient supine. Ports are inserted into (1) the umbilicus (for the laparoscope), (2) the mid-clavicular line on the side of the kidney to be removed, and (3) the anterior axillary line on the operative side. The patient is then placed in a lateral position. First, the colon is dissected to expose Gerota's fascia (Fig. 9-36). This fascia is then incised to

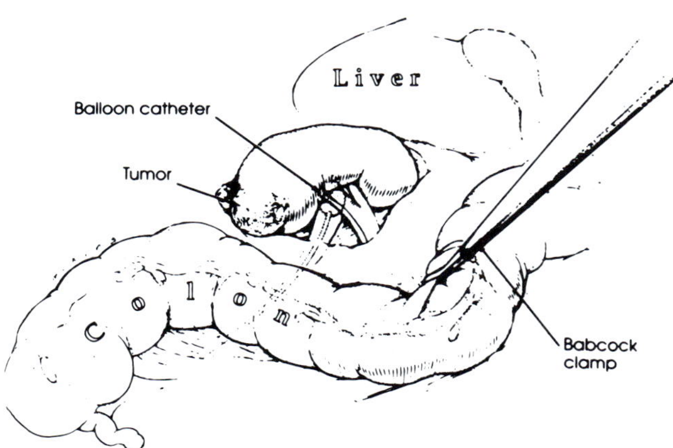

FIGURE 9-36. Mobilization of right colon to expose Gerota's fascia for a right nephrectomy. (Lobe TE, Schropp KP, eds. Pediatric laparoscopy and thoracoscopy. Philadelphia: WB Saunders, 1993:187. With permission)

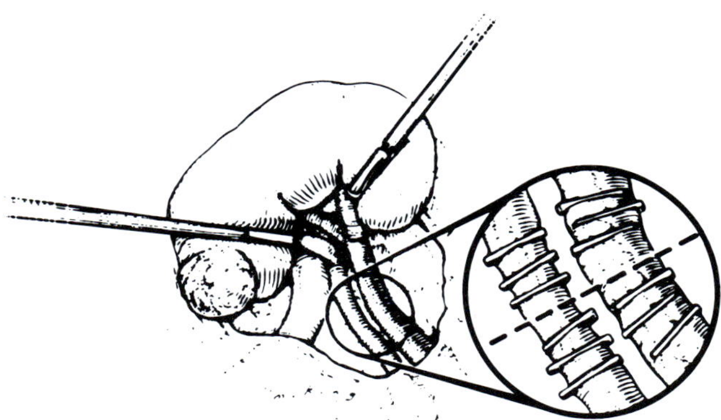

FIGURE 9-37. Kidney mobilized for a laparoscopic nephrectomy. (Lobe TE, Schropp KP, eds. Pediatric laparoscopy and thoracoscopy. Philadelphia: WB Saunders, 1993:187. With permission)

expose the kidney. Using the two most lateral ports, grasping instruments are used to elevate the kidney, so that the renal vessels can be dissected free and divided with either clips or a linear stapler. The ureter is then dissected as far distal as necessary and divided; the kidney is then freed from the renal fossa (Fig. 9-37).

The patient is then returned to a supine position. An endoscopic sac is inserted into the abdomen and opened. The kidney is placed into the sac, the neck of which is withdrawn from the abdomen through a 10- or 12-mm trocar site. The tissue morcellator is then inserted into the sac and the tissue extracted. After careful inspection of the abdomen for hemostasis, all instruments are removed. Patients can usually be returned to full diet and unrestricted activity within 48 hours.

SUMMARY

The surgeon must be cognizant of the extensive applications of laparoscopic surgery in the pediatric or adolescent patient. The ability to provide surgical care in association with either outpatient or short-stay surgery appears to be cost-effective and is appropriate state-of-the-art medical care. As the array of surgical instruments continues to evolve, new and innovative laparoscopic procedures will continue to become increasingly available for the pediatric patient.

References

1. Semm K: Verres Weitere Entwicklungen in der gynakologischen Laparoskopie, Pelviskopie, Wysteroskopie, Fetoskopie. Baltimore-Munich: Urban and Schwarzenburg, 1978.
2. Semm K: History. In: Operative gynecologic endoscopy. Sanfilippo JS, Levine RL, eds. New York: Springer-Verlag, 1989:1.
3. Gans SL, Berci G: Advances in endoscopy of infants and children. J Pediatr Surg 1971;6:199.

4. Gans SL, Berci G: Peritoneoscopy in infants and children. J Pediatr Surg 1973;8:399.
5. Gans SL: A new look at pediatric endoscopy. Postgrad Med J 1977;62:91.
6. Lobe TE: The applications of laparoscopy and lasers in pediatric surgery. Surg Annu 1993;25(Pt 1):175.
7. Westrom L: Incidence, prevalence and trends of acute pelvic inflammatory disease and its consequences in industrialized countries. Am J Obstet Gynecol 1980;138:880.
8. Reich H: Endoscopic management of tuboovarian abscess and pelvic inflammatory disease. In: Operative gynecologic endoscopy. Sanfilippo JS, Levine RL, eds. New York: Springer-Verlag, 1989:107.
9. Henry-Suchet J, Soler A, Loffredo V: Laparoscopic treatment of tuboovarian abscesses. J Reprod Med 1984;29:579.
10. Jacobson L, Westrom L: Objectivized diagnosis of acute pelvic inflammatory disease. Am J Obstet Gynecol 1969; 105:1088.
11. Stubblefield PG: Intraovarian abscess treated with laparoscopic aspiration and povidone-iodine lavage. A case report. J Reprod Med 1991;36(5):407.
12. Owens S, Yeko TR, Bloy R, Maroulis GB: Laparoscopic treatment of painful perihepatic adhesions in Fitz-Hugh-Curtis syndrome. Obstet Gynecol 1991;78(3 Pt 2):542.
13. Goldstein D, DeCholnoky C, Emans SJ: Adolescent endometriosis. J Adolesc Health Care 1980;1:37.
14. Sanfilippo J, Wakim NG, Schikler K, Yussman MA: Endometriosis in association with a uterine anomaly. Am J Obstet Gynecol 1986;154:39.
15. Hasson M: Open laparoscopy in operative gynecologic endoscopy. Sanfilippo J, Levine R, eds. In: Operative gynecologic endoscopy. New York: Springer-Verlag 1989:57.
16. Gotz F, Pier A, Bacher C: [Laparoscopic appendectomy. Indications, technique and results in 653 patients.] Chirurg 1991;62:253.
17. Ure BM, Spangenberger W, Hebebrand D, Eypasch EP, Troidl H: Laparoscopic surgery in children and adolescents with suspected appendicitis: results of medical technology assessment. Eur J Pediatr Surg 1992;2:336.
18. Gilchrist BF, Lobe TE, Schropp KP, et al: Is there a role for laparoscopic appendectomy in pediatric surgery? J Pediatr Surg 1992;27:209.
19. Moir CR, Donohue JH, van Heerden JA: Laparoscopic cholecystectomy in children: initial experience and recommendations. J Pediatr Surg 1992;27:1066.
20. Ware RE, Kinney TR, Casey JR, Pappas TN, Meyers WC: Laparoscopic cholecystectomy in young patients with sickle hemoglobinopathies. J Pediatr 1992;120:58.
21. Davidoff AM, Branum GD, Murray EA, et al: The technique of laparoscopic cholecystectomy in children. Ann Surg 1992;215:186.
22. Holcomb GW III, Olsen DO, Sharp KW: Laparoscopic cholecystectomy in the pediatric patient. J Pediatr Surg 1991; 26:1186.
23. Newman KD, Marmon LM, Attorri R, Evans S: Laparoscopic cholecystectomy in pediatric patients. J Pediatr Surg 1991; 26:1184.
24. Diamond DA, Caldamone AA: The value of laparoscopy for 106 impalpable testes relative to clinical presentation. J Urol 1992;148(2 Pt 2):632.
25. Plotzker ED, Rushton HG, Belman AB, Skoog SJ: Laparoscopy for nonpalpable testes in childhood: is inguinal exploration also necessary when vas and vessels exit the inguinal ring? J Urol 1992;148(2 Pt 2):635.
26. Heiss KF, Shandling B: Laparoscopy for the impalpable testes: experience with 53 testes. J Pediatr Surg 1992; 27:175.
27. Waldschmidt J, Schier F: Surgical correction of abdominal testes after Fowler-Stephens using the neodymium: YAG laser for preliminary vessel dissection. Eur J Pediatr Surg 1991;1:54.
28. Doig CM: Use of laparoscopy in children with impalpable testes. Int J Androl 1989;12:420.
29. Bloom DA, Ayers JW, McGuire EJ: The role of laparoscopy in management of nonpalpable testes. J Urol (Paris) 1988; 94:465.
30. Garibyan H: Use of laparoscopy for the localization of impalpable testes. Neth J Surg 1987;39:68.
31. Castilho LN, Ferreira U: Laparoscopy in adults and children with nonpalpable testes. Andrologia 1987;19:539.
32. Peters CA: Laparoscopy in pediatric urology. Urology 1993;41(1 Suppl):33.
33. Lobe TE, Schropp KP: Inguinal hernias in pediatrics: initial experience with laparoscopic inguinal exploration of the asymptomatic contralateral side. J Laparoendosc Surg 1992;2:135.
34. Dallemagne B, Weerts JM, Jehaes C, Markiewicz S, Lombard R: Laparoscopic Nissen fundoplication: preliminary report. Surg Laparosc Endosc 1991;1:138.
35. Geagea T: Laparoscopic Nissen's fundoplication: preliminary report on ten cases. Surg Endosc 1991;5:170.
36. Cuschieri A, Shimi S, Nathanson LK: Laparoscopic reduction, crural repair, and fundoplication of large hiatal hernia. Am J Surg 1992;163:425.
37. Lobe TE, Schropp KP, Lunsford K: Laparoscopic Nissen fundoplication in childhood. J Pediatr Surg 1993;28:358.
38. Alain JL, Grousseau D, Terrier G: Extramucosal pylorotomy by laparoscopy. J Pediatr Surg 1991;26:1191.
39. Das S, Amar AD: The impact of laparoscopy on modern urologic practice. Urol Clin North Am 1988;15(3):537.
40. Eshghi AM, Roth JS, Smith AD: Percutaneous transperitoneal approach to a pelvic kidney for endourological removal of staghorn calculus. J Urol 1985;134:525.
41. Kavoussi LR, Clayman RV, Brunt LM, Soper NJ: Laparoscopic ureterolysis. J Urol 1992;147(2):426.
42. Clayman RV, Kavoussi LR, McDougall EM, et al: Laparoscopic nephrectomy: a review of 16 cases. Surg Laparosc Endosc 1992;2:29.

Chapter 10

Laparoscopic Surgery: An Atlas for General Surgeons, edited by Gary C. Vitale, Joseph S. Sanfilippo, and Jacques Perissat. J. B. Lippincott Company, Philadelphia, © 1995.

Operative Laparoscopy During Pregnancy

Marcello Pietrantoni
Joseph S. Sanfilippo

Evaluation of abdominal pain in the pregnant patient is frequently a challenge for the general surgeon and the obstetrician-gynecologist. Common nonobstetric problems usually involve acute appendicitis or acute cholecystitis. Nonetheless, concerns of a more obstetric and gynecologic nature may include torsion of an adnexa, adnexal mass (i.e., teratoma, luteoma, endometrioma), or rupture of a hemorrhagic corpus luteum cyst. Cognizance of the pertinent changes and alteration of anatomic landmarks and related physiology that is affiliated with these clinical problems is paramount during pregnancy.

Laparoscopy, as both a diagnostic and therapeutic modality, has a prominent place in gynecologic practice. A similar role for this technique is evolving in general surgery. Laparoscopic cholecystectomy and appendectomy are included in the "minimally invasive" surgical category.[1] This surgical approach has several potential advantages over the conventional and traditional laparotomy. Total operative time is significantly less and postoperative convalescence is undoubtedly shorter.[2] De novo adhesion formation is less likely, and shorter hospital stays may translate into substantial economic advantages.[3,4,5]

MATERNAL–FETAL CONSIDERATIONS

Pregnant women are vulnerable to all the potential surgical maladies, as are their counterparts who are not pregnant. Major medical complications are observed in about 15% to 20% of pregnancies but surgical problems are relatively uncommon (1% to 2%).[6] Medical and surgical evaluations call for prompt diagnosis and appropriate operative intervention.

Paramount is a thorough history and physical examination of the pregnant patient when she presents with what appears to be a nonobstetric surgical problem.[7] Particular attention should be focused on the maternal history, emphasizing any medical complications (e.g., cardiac disease, diabetes mellitus, chronic hypertension, Rh status, asthma, sickle cell disease, prior pelvic inflammatory disease, chronic pelvic pain, and anomalies, especially if the fetus is aneuploid). If there is vaginal bleeding, identification of placental location (central previa) is significant. Abruptio placentae, chorioamnionitis, pyelonephritis, preeclampsia, ectopic pregnancy, and rarely, an abdominal pregnancy (10.9 per 100,000 live births) are also of significance because they often are associated with abdominal pain.[8]

Secondly, one must obtain pertinent laboratory analyses (Table 10-1). Although uncommon, patients have been known to present with obstipation or with pseudocyesis or cancer of the ovary or uterus. If one is considering an operative procedure, accurate assessment by ultrasound for fetal viability and anomalies is compulsory (comprehensive ultrasound). Anatomic alterations caused by encroachment of the gravid uterus up to the mid- and upper abdominal quadrants must be noted.

Contraindications for pursuing a laparoscopic approach in the removal of either the appendix or gallbladder are being evaluated. Advanced disease, abdominal sepsis, ileus, bleeding disorders, and late second- or third-trimester pregnancies are considered to be contraindications to endoscopic surgery.

The gestational age at which the uterus would limit laparoscopic access to the abdominal cavity is of concern and is still debated among researchers. There are many advantages to the closed laparoscopic technique: (1) the patient's postoperative course is shortened with minimal

TABLE 10-1
Hematologic Alterations in Pregnancy

Laboratory tests	*Normal Values* Nonpregnant	*Normal Values* Pregnant
Total protein (g/dL)	6.5–8.6	6.8
Serum albumin (g/dL)	3.5–5.0	2.5–4.5
Blood urea nitrogen (mg/dL)	10–25	5–15
Glucose (mg/dL)	70–110	65–100
Serum calcium (mEq/L)	4.6–5.5	4.2–5.2
Serum phosphate (mg/dL)	2.5–4.8	2.3–4.6
Alkaline phosphatase (IU/L)	35–48	35–150
Cholesterol (mg/dL)	120–290	177–345
Triglycerides (mg/dL)	33–166	130–400
Hemoglobin (g/dL)	12	>11
Hematocrit (%)	36	33
Platelets (Plt/L)	$140–440 \times 10^9$	Unchanged
Fibrinogen (mg/dL)	150–300	250–600
Serum creatinine (mg/dL)	0.6	0.8

use of analgesia, (2) there is a reduced risk of atelectasis from postoperative hypoventilation respiratory problems, and (3) there is less decrease in fetal activity. Patients are able to eat a regular diet on the day of surgery and are usually discharged within 24 hours. Earlier ambulation afforded by the laparoscopic method decreases the risk of thromboembolic disease, to which pregnant patients are predisposed because of the increase in coagulation factors.[9]

The surgeon should evaluate the pregnant woman literally as two patients. Fundamental operative maternal–fetal considerations regarding surgical and anesthetic risks are related to those of the altered maternal anatomy and physiology:

- Circulatory system
  45% increase in plasma volume
  33% increase in erythrocytes
  10% to 20% increase in cardiac volume
  30% increase in resting stroke volume and cardiac output
  15% to 20% increase in heart rate

- Respiratory system
  Increased tidal volume
  Increased minute ventilatory volume
  Increased minute oxygen uptake
  Decreased functional residual volume (Table 10-2)[10–13]

The gastrointestinal system must be considered, with the most important concerns being delayed gastric emptying, decreased esophageal tone, and incompetence of the esophageal–gastric sphincter.[14]

One must also consider fetal viability. If the fetus is greater or equal to 24 weeks, but less than 34 weeks gestation with preterm contractions, corticosteroid (betamethazone 12 mg intramuscularly every 12 hours for 4 doses), and thyroid releasing hormones (TRH; 400 μg intramuscularly every 12 hours for 4 doses) should be given for fetal lung maturation. The initial maternal perioperative assessment is recommended (documenting vital signs, consideration for placement of an intravenous line, transcutaneous oximeter, complete blood count, type and screen, and crossmatch if blood transfusion is a distinct probability). Serum electrolytes, liver enzymes, electrocardiogram, urinalysis and culture, clotting profiles, and autologous blood donation may be considered, depending on the circumstances.[15]

Perioperative prophylactic broad-spectrum antibiotics should be administered to those patients at risk for infection (e.g., those with diabetes mellitus, heart disease).[16] Although rare, rheumatic heart disease remains the most common cause of "heart disease" throughout the world. Those patients with heart disease should receive ampicillin (2 g intravenously) plus gentamicin (1.5 mg/kg intravenously), 30 to 60 minutes before surgery, with the dose repeated twice thereafter at 8-hour intervals. Prophylactic low-dose heparin (8000 U subcutane-

TABLE 10-2
Criteria to Evaluate Ventilatory Status

	Normal Values	*Abnormal Values*
PULMONARY		
Respiratory rate	16	>35
Vital capacity (mL/kg)	3310	<15
Maximum inspiratory force (cm H_2O)	97	<25–35
OXYGENATION		
PaO_2, room air (torr)	76–100	<65
Alveolar–arterial O_2 diff – 100% O_2 (torr)	30–70	>350
$PaCO_2$ (torr)	30	>50

ously) for the morbidly obese patient should be considered. Full heparinization is required for patients with prior documented pulmonary embolism or thrombophlebitis.[17] Serial determination of the activated partial thromboplastin time is used to guide the heparin dose. In addition, a Kleihauer-Bethke test is recommended, even in cases with minor trauma, to evaluate any maternal–fetal bleeding.[18] It is important that 300 μg of Rh immune globulin be administered after any invasive procedures, such as abdominal surgery either by laparoscopy or laparotomy, in the unsensitized Rh-negative mother. The volume required to produce sensitization is generally considered to be large; however, as little as 0.1 mL of Rh-positive erythrocytes appears to be sufficient to result in sensitization of an Rh-negative individual.[19]

The optimal time for elective nonobstetric surgery is during the early second trimester because there is a higher incidence of spontaneous abortion during the first trimester and pre-term labor in the mid- to late second and third trimesters. Tocolysis should be a consideration for either elective or emergency surgery at 24 or more weeks' gestation. Fetal heart-rate monitoring can provide objective data, not only preoperatively but intra- and postoperatively. The fetal heart-rate monitoring enables the surgical team to detect onset of premature labor or fetal distress. In addition, pregnant women in a supine position may have compression of the inferior vena cava and aorta; this affects the venous circulation by diversion of the venous blood, resulting in a decreased amount of regional anesthetic required. It may also cause hypotension and fetal distress. These patients should be placed in the left lateral decubitus position, with their right hip elevated.

The surgical principles that apply to laparotomy also apply to operative laparoscopy despite their technical differences. A few of the technical limitations of laparoscopy include loss of depth perception, inability to directly palpate tissue, limitation of the number of instruments that can be used simultaneously, restriction of the angles available to approach the surgical field, and the increased distance from the surgical field to the surgeon's hands, which intensifies motion, making fine movements more laborious.

Obstetric Anesthesia

Anesthetic complications have the potential to result in significant maternal morbidity and mortality (Table 10-3).[19a] The mortality rate due to anesthetic complications is about 0.6 per 100,000 live births. General anesthesia is the preferred method for most obstetric surgical emergencies. A concern over the use of general anesthesia is its potential to induce fetal–neonatal depression (incidence, 3%), in addition to spontaneous abortion in the first trimester.[20] General anesthesia involves a rapid-sequence induction (sodium pentothal or Propofol-Diprivan; Stuart Pharmaceuticals), followed by nitrous oxide. When general anesthesia is indicated, agents that produce maternal tachycardia must be avoided, particularly in patients with cardiac disease. Halothane, enflurane, and isoflurane are used to supplement nitrous oxide during maintenance of general anesthesia. Nitrous oxide crosses the blood–placenta barrier; however, it does not accumulate in fetal tissues, as do other anesthetics. Halothane is less commonly used because it is associated with an increased incidence of hepatitis and cardiac arrhythmias, secondary to the release of catecholamines.[21] Enflurane and isoflurane are contraindicated in those patients having or suspected of having impaired renal function.

TABLE 10-3
Maternal Mortality and Morbidity From Anesthetic Complications

Anesthetic Complications	*Deaths per 100,000 Live Births*
Failed endotracheal intubation	4.3
Aspiration	2.1
Sepsis	1.1
Hemorrhage	4.7
Cardiac arrest or cerebral anoxia	1.6

Several concerns related to anesthesia must be addressed when treating the pregnant patient (Table 10-4). The respiratory center of the fetus is highly vulnerable to sedative and anesthetic medications. They rapidly traverse the placenta and may result in respiratory depression in the newborn infant. Naloxone hydrochloride (Narcan) is a narcotic antagonist capable of reversing respiratory depression. It is administered subcutaneously, intravenously, or intramuscularly to the full-term neonate at a dose of 10 μg/kg.

Difficulty with tracheal intubation appears to be the most frequent contributing factor to anesthetic-related maternal deaths.[22] Carbon dioxide is the gas most often selected to establish a pneumoperitoneum. Studies on the possible effects of excessive exposure are few. Fetal cardiac defects have been noted when pregnant rats were exposed to a concentration as low as 3%, and dental maldevelopment when levels as high as 30% were administered.[23,24] Vertebral defects in the offspring of rabbits exposed to 8% carbon dioxide for a few days have also been reported.[25] Carbon dioxide rapidly forms carbonic acid on the parietal peritoneum, which results in considerable maternal pain. Using nitrous oxide for peritoneal insufflation causes less irritation of the diaphragm. Nitrous oxide, when administered over a long period (1 to 2 days) at 50% concentration, has been associated with increased spontaneous abortions, skeletal deformities, and babies who are small for gestational age.[26]

A major fatality that may follow general anesthesia is pulmonary aspiration of gastric contents. Administering

TABLE 10-4
Identifying Anesthetic Risks in Pregnant Surgical Patients

Systems

GASTROINTESTINAL

- Gastric contents left longer in stomach
- Contents pushed upward
- Prolonged gastric emptying time
- Increased risk for aspiration and regurgitation
- Antacids preoperatively—elevate pH of gastric juices (pH>2.5); less risk with intubation
  - Intra-abdominal pressure

CARDIOVASCULAR

- Inferior vena cava (IVC) and aortic compression
  - Complete IVC obstruction occurs in 90% of women at term when in the supine position
- ECG changes from heart displacement and upward compression
  - Premature ventricular contractions
  - Sinus tachycardia
  - Paroxysmal supraventricular tachycardia—increased
- Decreased peripheral vascular resistance
- Increased cardiac output and vasodilatation
- Blood loss of 30%–35% has a significant adverse effect on fetus
- Blood volume expanders (e.g., Ringer's lactate) recommended

RESPIRATORY

- Breathing—diaphragmatic, not costal
- Oxygen consumption increases
- Relaxing cricopharyngeal sphincter
- Hyperventilation—compensation
- Swelling—nasopharynx; intubation difficult
- Tidal volume increased by 40%
- Respiratory rate increases by 15%
- Alveolar ventilation increases by 70%

Common Anesthetics

INHALATION AGENTS

- Nitrous oxide
  - Crosses blood–placenta barrier
  - Significant accumulation in fetus
  - Increased incidence of spontaneous abortions
  - Skeletal deformities
  - Smaller offspring
- Halothane
  - Congenital deformities in operating-room personnel
- Enflurane
  - Teratogenesis
  - Increased heart rate
  - Hypotension
  - Decreased seizure threshold
  - Arrhythmias
- Isoflurane
  - Teratogenicity unknown

INTRAVENOUS AGENTS

- Diazepam
  - Cleft palate
- Thiopental sodium
  - No associated congenital anomalies

MUSCLE RELAXANTS

- Succinylcholine
  - Non-depolarizing muscle relaxant
    - No adverse effect on fetus
    - Prolonged duration of action; decrease in serum cholinesterase during pregnancy

LOCAL/REGIONAL ANESTHESIA

- Bupivacaine (Marcaine) 0.75%–cardiac arrhythmias after rapid IV injection
- Lidocaine
  - Accidental intravascular injection: adverse effects on fetal central nervous system and myocardium
  - Greatest risk with surgery: first trimester

antacids shortly before induction of anesthesia has dramatically decreased mortality, more so than any other practice.[27] The use of nonparticulate antacids like 30 mL of 0.3 mol/L sodium citrate with citric acid (Bicitra) is suggested to neutralize the acidity (pH of 1.0) of the gastric contents. Gibbs and Banner report that Bicitra neutralizes about 70 mL of gastric acid in nearly 90% of women undergoing cesarean section when prescribed 45 minutes preoperatively.[28] It is documented that maternal deaths comprise 5% of all anesthetic-related problems. Magnesium hydrochloride is also effective in neutralizing gastric juice but it has a short duration and because of the particulate matter, it has been shown to cause pneumonitis. Cimetidine is often given but it requires a 60-minute interval to decrease gastric acidity when parenterally administered.

Preoperative airway assessment with use of a modified Mallampati test is recommended to evaluate the oropharyngeal structures, which are visible on maximal mouth opening.[29] Visualization of the airway is also more difficult during pregnancy. Engorgement of the mucosal surface due to increased capillary blood flow may cause edema of the pharynx and larynx. Other potential risk factors associated with difficult intubation include obesity; short neck; missing, protruding or single maxillary incisors; receding mandible; facial edema; and swollen tongue.

Thus, in summary, (1) the patient should be given antacids as prophylaxis against aspiration; (2) a rapid sequence induction of anesthesia should be performed; (3) a tenuous airway should be secured, with the patient awake and breathing spontaneously; (4) anesthesia should include monitoring of pulse oximetry and end-tidal CO_2 to confirm proper placement of endotracheal tubes and adequacy of ventilation (Table 10-5).

During surgery, it is an imperative fundamental ob-

TABLE 10-5
Central Hemodynamic Parameters in Nonpregnant and Pregnant Women

	Nonpregnant	*Pregnant*
Central venous pressure (mmHg)	1–10	1–10
Pulmonary artery pressure (mmHg)	9–16	9–16
Pulmonary capillary wedge pressure (mmHg)	3–10	3–10
Pulmonary vascular resistance (dyne × sec × cm^{-5})	20–120	78
Systemic vascular resistance (dyne × sec × cm^{-5})	770–1500	1210
Cardiac output (L/min)	4–7	6.2

jective that provisions be made for adequate oxygenation to meet the needs of maternal and fetal tissues because failure to do so may result in substantial cell injury or cellular death. Oxygen demand and consumption are the same as in the healthy nonpregnant individual. In the critically ill patient, however, oxygen transport may be impaired by three processes: impairment of hemoglobin concentration (anemic hypoxia), decreased hemoglobin oxygen saturation (hypoxic hypoxia), and reduced cardiac output (stagnant hypoxia).[30] Demand for oxygen is minimized by eliminating factors that increase the metabolic work of the cell (e.g., fever, pain, labored breathing, malnutrition, and infection). These adverse effects, although rarely serious, provide a good argument for the preferential administration of a regional anesthetic (e.g., epidural or spinal) when surgery is indicated in the early to middle second trimester. Ideally, the patient's stomach should be emptied before any emergency procedure is undertaken. With extensive intra-abdominal surgery, a nasogastric tube should not be removed postoperatively until there is evidence of normal bowel function. An indwelling urinary catheter is also recommended because it provides useful information regarding vascular perfusion and blood volume. Hypotension (systolic blood pressure less than 100 mmHg) has been reported to occur, with an incidence ranging from 8% to 13% after regional anesthesia.[31]

Postoperative Management

Continuous electronic fetal heart-rate monitoring is advocated postoperatively. This may be accomplished by monitoring for suspected pre-term labor through the use of the external tocodynamometer and cervical examinations. Many different protocols for tocolysis exist but a common principle of initial management is ensuring adequate maternal hydration. Attempts to arrest premature labor may be accomplished with either intravenous magnesium sulfate (6 g load and more than 2 g/hour for maintenance) or indomethacin (loading dose of 50 to 100 mg rectal suppository and 25 mg orally for maintenance every 6 hours for 48 hours), provided the fetus is fewer than 32 weeks' gestation with normal amniotic fluid volume. If indomethacin is used for longer than 48 hours, Doppler-flow ultrasound studies of the ductus arteriosus are suggested.[32] Long-term use of β-mimetics such as terbutaline (Brethine, Geigy Pharmaceuticals) or ritodrine hydrochloride (Yutopar, Astra Pharmaceuticals) are not recommended because of their significant metabolic and cardiovascular side effects (i.e., hyperglycemia, hypokalemia, fetal–maternal tachycardia, chest pain, pulmonary edema, shortness of breath, cardiac dysrhythmia, and electrocardiogram "ischemic" changes [ST-wave inversions]). Short-term use of β-mimetics such as terbutaline in doses of 0.25 mg every 20 minutes for not more than three doses may be prescribed. β-Sympathomimetic agents should not be used when there is active infection, multiple gestation, or hydramnios because of the increased risk of pulmonary edema. Analgesic relief for minor discomfort can be controlled with acetaminophen.

For pain that cannot be controlled by minor pain relievers, acetaminophen plus codeine or plain codeine should also be considered. Acetaminophen is a category B drug, which means there is no evidence of any adverse fetal risks from animal studies but no controlled studies in pregnant women are available.[33] Long-term use of nonsteroidal anti-inflammatory agents is not recommended during pregnancy; however, short-term use is a relative contraindication. Narcotics offer excellent relief for severe pain but are known to cause neonatal depression if administered within 1 to 2 hours before delivery.

ACUTE APPENDICITIS

With an incidence of one in 2000 pregnancies, acute appendicitis is the most common surgical condition during pregnancy. There is equal distribution, with respect to incidence in each of the three trimesters and in the puerperium.[34,35] Frequently the diagnosis is delayed, with obvious adverse sequelae. Perhaps this is due partly to the confusing picture of nausea, vomiting, and abdominal discomfort also observed with the pregnancy per se, complemented by a normal physiologic leukocytosis (about 10,000 to 12,000/mL). A high index of suspicion for appendicitis is preeminent in making the diagnosis. It is important that the surgeon be aware of the constant change in location of the appendix during the progres-

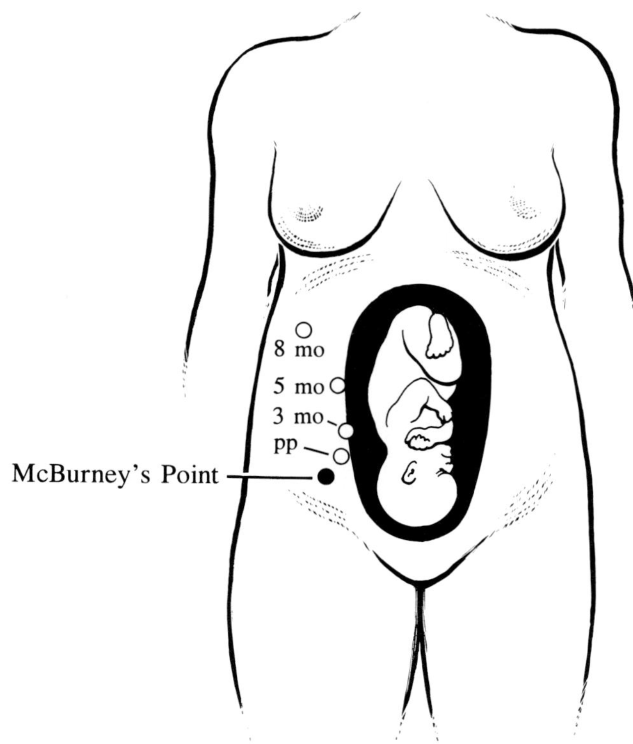

FIGURE 10-1. Migration of the appendix during pregnancy at various gestational ages. PP, postpartum.

sive enlargement of the uterus during gestation (Fig. 10-1). Differential diagnoses include round ligament pain (spasm), adnexal torsion, and other gastrointestinal and genitourinary abnormalities (e.g., pyelonephritis). Dysuria occurs in up to 25% of pregnant women who have appendicitis in the third trimester.[36]

Diagnosis

The initial visceral pain is typically gradual in onset, with an associated colicky pattern (due to smooth muscle contractions), which may reflect obstruction (fecalith or calculus). Classically, the pain is often referred to the epigastrium or periumbilical area and is often dull and diffuse in nature. During pregnancy, the enlarged uterus causes displacement of the appendix. The upward displacement of the appendix by the uterus is also accompanied by a rift of the inflamed appendix from the abdominal wall. Such displacement tends to minimize the signs of peritoneal irritation. Fewer than half of pregnant patients have peritoneal signs.

With respect to specifics for each trimester, during the first trimester the pain is primarily (65% to 90% of the time) in the area of McBurney's point and 30% of the time in the pelvic area.[37,38] During the second trimester, the pain is associated with the lateral upward displacement of the appendix; frequently, the point of maximal tenderness is above the iliac crest (75%). During the third trimester, pain and tenderness may be localized to the right costal margin (37%). This occurs during pregnancy because of the progressive increase in size of the gravid uterus, which displaces the base of the appendix. Anorexia, accompanied by nausea and vomiting, often precedes onset of pain by several hours; however, up to 75% of patients present with this symptom.[39]

Independent of the trimester, right lateral rectal tenderness is commonly noted; about 50% of patients have abdominal muscle spasm or guarding.[40] The uterus, because of its size and encroachment on the appendix, often intensifies pain during the physical examination process. The pain is localized primarily to the area around the appendix (see Fig. 10-1). It becomes paramount that pain associated with uterine origin be differentiated from that of appendicitis. Uterine pain can frequently be alleviated by placing the patient in the left lateral (decubitus) position and providing adequate fluid hydration. Both Alder's sign (fixed tenderness) and Bryan's sign (tenderness in the right lateral position) may be used to differentiate uterine pain origin from that of appendicitis.[41] Temperature elevation (low-grade, less than 100.5°F) may also be associated with acute appendicitis. The latter sign usually implies an intact vermiform appendix. Sterile pyuria or hematuria may occur when the inflamed appendix lies in the vicinity of the ureter.

Management

If the appendix ruptures, peritonitis often ensues and the uterus attempts to wall off the abscess; assertive, proper drainage minimizes any maternal–fetal complications. In many cases, premature labor results, again underscoring the importance of early and appropriate diagnosis. Fetal morbidity and mortality significantly increase after appendiceal perforation.[42] The diagnostic error in pregnant women is about 25% to 40%.[43] The mortality rate associated with nonperforated appendicitis in the general population is 0.1%.[44] In comparison, mortality in the first trimester is about 0.9% and may approach 7.3% for women in the third trimester.[39,45] Appendiceal perforation occurs with an incidence of up to 41% in pregnant women, in contrast to an incidence of 10% to 15% in the general population.[36,43] Therefore, early "aggressive" use of laparoscopy repeatedly has proved to be helpful in management of suspected appendicitis in the pregnant patient.

A series of 150 patients undergoing laparoscopic appendectomy was reported by Schreiber.[46] This series included six pregnant patients in all stages of gestation. The overall complication rate for the 150 patients was 0.75% and there were no complications among the pregnant patients, thus attesting to the efficacy of a laparoscopic approach to acute appendicitis.

CHOLECYSTITIS

The incidence of acute cholecystitis during pregnancy is 1 to 6 per 10,000; that is, it is more common in pregnancy, due partly to the marked alteration in gallbladder physiology during this period.[47] The saturation of cholesterol in bile increases while the circulating bile salt pool is decreased, resulting in production of more lithogenic bile. Acute cholecystitis is one of the most common nonobstetric causes of an acute abdomen in pregnancy, second only to appendicitis. There appears to be an association with advanced maternal age, obesity, diet, diabetes mellitus, ethnicity, familial hyperlipoproteinemia, hypertriglyceridemia (type IV), increased gravidity, rapid weight loss during the puerperium, and a history of previous episodes of cholecystitis.[47] Preexisting gallstones are not often a cause of cholecystitis in pregnancy, partly because the ability of the gallbladder to contract is inhibited by the increased circulating levels of progesterone. This hormone produces smooth muscle relaxation, which causes decreased gallbladder contractility and emptying, complicated by bile duct hypotonia. Progesterone also inhibits the gallbladder's contractile response to cholecystokinin.

It is estimated that up to 15% of the population of the United States have gallstones (20 million); however, because about 50% of gallstones are asymptomatic, the actual prevalence is difficult to estimate.[47] Only 1% to 4% per year of previously asymptomatic patients with stones develop symptoms or a complication of gallstone disease. In the second and third trimesters, fasting and residual volumes are twice as great as in the nonpregnant state, and the rate and percentage of bile expelled after stimulation diminish. Gallbladder emptying is significantly slowed in the second and third trimesters.[48] There is evidence that biliary cholesterol saturation is increased and that the proportion of chenodeoxycholic acid is decreased. Thus, there is a predisposition to gallstone formation, which is often symptomatic. Cholecystectomy is performed in 3 to 8 per 10,000 pregnant women, the cause of more nonobstetric surgery in pregnancy than any other procedure except appendectomy. Gallstones are the most common and most costly digestive system disease, with an annual estimated overall cost of more than $5 billion.[49]

Diagnosis

The obstetrician and general surgeon should be well acquainted in the various modes of clinical presentation of gallbladder disease among pregnant patients. Many times, acute cholecystitis–cholelithiasis presents initially with biliary colic (misnamed *colic*), manifest by nausea and associated vomiting and lasting up to 3 to 4 hours. Pain persists if the common bile duct is obstructed by a stone, and there is often radiation to the subscapular area, right flank, or shoulder. Right subcostal tenderness associated with temperature elevation and increasing leukocytosis is characteristic. Ultrasonography appears to be efficacious (90% of cases) in diagnosing the presence of stones (they are echodense) or dilation of the common bile duct. Murphy's sign is often positive; however, a positive Murphy's sign (severe pain under the right costal margin, elicited with deep inspiration) and a palpable gallbladder occur in only 5% of pregnancies.[49,50] Oral cholecystogram and intravenous cholangiography are contraindicated in pregnancy. Technetium 99m–iminodiacetic acid scan of the gallbladder has been used in pregnancy, with minimal risk of radiation exposure.[51]

Management

Conservative treatment is less effective in the puerperium, when acute cholecystitis has been reported to be more frequent and severe. Therapeutic measures that are not recommended in pregnancy are endoscopic papillotomy with stone extraction, intrabiliary solvent infusion systems, and medical dissolution with chenodeoxycholic acid or ursodiol or methyl terbutyl ether or monoctanoin.[52]

As with acute appendicitis, there is a higher incidence of premature labor with fetal loss after the operative procedure.[53] Ideally, first-trimester patients are treated conservatively until the second trimester, at which time a cholecystectomy is electively performed. Laparoscopic cholecystectomy in patients in the first trimester of pregnancy is controversial because of the unknown effects of carbon dioxide pneumoperitoneum on the developing fetus.[54] Carbon dioxide may cause hypercarbia and acidosis. During the second trimester, patients are best treated surgically as soon as the pancreatitis subsides; ideally, third-trimester patients are managed medically until the puerperium, when definitive surgery is performed because of the risk of damage to the uterine musculature during the procedure. Any patient who does not improve with medical management should undergo surgical intervention, regardless of gestational age of the fetus. There is a 0.05% mortality in low-risk individuals.[52] The efficacy of cholecystectomy during pregnancy without fetal loss has been established, partly because of advances with respect to early diagnosis and anesthesia management, along with the use of tocolytic agents.[55]

Laparoscopic cholecystectomy is a relatively new operation. It was first performed in France in 1987 and in the United States in 1988.[52] About 80% of all cholecystectomies are performed using this innovative procedure. Most patients with symptomatic cholelithiasis are candidates for laparoscopic cholecystectomy if they are able to tolerate general anesthesia and have no serious cardiopulmonary disease. As a rule, indications for laparoscopic cholecystectomy are similar to those for open cholecystectomy.

TABLE 10-6
Cholecystectomy During Pregnancy

Study	Design	Patients	Comments
Schreiber[46]	Laparoscopic appendectomy; six pregnant at various stages	6	Complication rate 0.75%, none of which occurred in the pregnant population
McKellar, et al[55]	Evaluated high incidence of fetal loss during first trimester and premature labor in third trimester in association with cholecystectomy	22	Elective abortion not recommended, even when intraoperative cholangiogram was obtained; tocolytic agents most efficacious
Weber, et al[56]	First reported laparoscopic cholecystectomy during pregnancy	1	
van Beek, et al[57]	Gallstone disease evaluated in women <30 years of age; correlation between age, pregnancy, obesity, and oral contraceptive use (retrospective study)	885	All underwent cholecystectomy; relative risk 1.6 for pregnancy-related gallstone disease requiring cholecystectomy
Bloch and Kelly[58]	Acute pancreatitis during pregnancy or postpartum	21	Acute pancreatitis associated with pregnancy; "gallstone pancreatitis"
Baillie et al[59]	Extrahepatic biliary obstruction by gallstones	5	Four had acute cholangitis, one had gallstones, pancreatitis; treatment: endoscopic sphincterotomy
Basso et al[62]	Prospective antenatal study of oral contraceptives	512	Early gestation, age at menarche had no significant effect; higher incidence of cholelithiasis in older women and patients with dysmenorrhea; positive trend of cholelithiasis in patients with history of symptomatic gallstones

In a series of 22 patients, the incidence of biliary stone disease during pregnancy was 0.05%.[55] Nine required cholecystectomy during pregnancy, with no specific preponderance of surgical intervention during any one trimester. Common bile duct exploration was required in three of the nine patients. In addition, three others had intraoperative cholangiography. Delay of appropriate surgical intervention does not appear to be warranted.

Weber and coworkers reported the first laparoscopic cholecystectomy during pregnancy.[56] The recovery time was significantly shortened, compared with a laparotomy. Little is published regarding gallstone management in the postpartum period.[57] Bloch and Kelly, however, report a 22-year study in which acute pancreatitis developed in 21 women during pregnancy, 10 cases of which occurred fewer than 6 weeks after delivery.[58] Gallstones were the cause of the pancreatitis in each patient. The recommended surgical treatment included cholecystectomy and exploration of the common bile duct without operative cholangiography (Table 10-6).

Sphincterotomy

It is estimated that up to 15% of patients undergoing cholecystectomy have common duct stones. These stones are a major source of morbidity; therefore, their detection and removal before a planned laparoscopic cholecystectomy is mandatory—especially if there is evidence of jaundice, recent pancreatitis, or a dilated common duct.

The procedure of endoscopic sphincterotomy is reported by Baillie and coworkers.[59] In this study, extrahepatic biliary obstruction occurred in association with gallstones during pregnancy. Five patients (four with acute cholangitis and one with gallstone pancreatitis) were treated by endoscopic sphincterotomy. Of interest, all patients proceeded to deliver at term. The efficacy of endoscopic retrograde cholangiopancreatography and sphincterotomy must be considered. The success rate of endoscopic common duct stone extraction approaches 90% to 95% in expert hands.

SUMMARY

The literature pertaining to the ever-expanding indications for operative laparoscopy consists predominantly of descriptive studies. Few randomized controlled trials have been performed. In 1988, the American Association of Gynecologic Laparoscopists reported a serious complication rate of 15 per 1000 procedures and mortality of 5 per 100,000.[61] Therefore, the general surgeon must recognize the limitations of his or her capabilities. Experience is increasing with the laparoscopic approach for the pregnant patient who requires surgical intervention for acute appendicitis or cholecystectomy. This technique avoids increased morbidity, prolonged hospital stay, and the recovery complications associated with the more traditional approach (celiotomy). Additionally, there is no consensus as to the gestational age at which the uterus would limit laparoscopic access to the abdominal cavity. If the laparoscopic procedure is traditional (closed laparoscope), 18 to 20 weeks' gestational age would be the upper limits for performing this technique, although laparoscopic appendectomy has been reported to be successful as late as 25 weeks' gestation.[46] The uterine fundus in relation to the umbilicus must be assessed because as gestational age advances, the risk is greater for injury. Careful consideration of an "open laparoscopic technique" is appropriate to minimize trauma to the internal viscera. This technique is especially useful and appropriate when adhesions are suspected, which increase the probability of visceral injury.

Acknowledgment

We would like to acknowledge the technical assistance of Ms. Sandra G. Nevitt.

References

1. Wolfe BM, Gardiner B, Frey CF: Laparoscopic cholecystectomy: a remarkable development. Editorial. JAMA 1991; 265:1573.

2. Azziz R, Steinkampf MP, Murphy A: Postoperative recuperation: relation to the extent of endoscopic surgery. Fertil Steril 1989;51:1061.

3. Lundorff P, Hahlin M, Kallfelt B, Thorburn J, Lindblom B: Adhesion formation after laparoscopic surgery in tubal pregnancy: a randomized trial versus laparotomy. Fertil Steril 1991;55:911.

4. Levine RL: Economic impact of pelviscopic surgery. J Reprod Med 1985;30:655.

5. Chung RS, Broughan TA: The phenomenal growth of laparoscopic cholecystectomy: a review. Cleve Clin J Med 1992;59:186.

6. Barron WM: The pregnant surgical patient: medical evaluation and management. Ann Intern Med 1984;101:683.

7. Hampton JR, Harrison MJG, Mitchell JRA, et al: Relative contributions of history-taking, physical examination, and laboratory investigation to diagnosis and management of medical outpatients. Br Med J 1975;2:486.

8. Atrash HK, Friede A, Hogue CJ: Abdominal pregnancy in the United States: frequency and maternal mortality. Obstet Gynecol 1987;69:333.

9. Talbert LM, Langdell RD: Normal values of certain factors in the blood clotting mechanism in pregnancy. Am J Obstet Gynecol 1964;90:44.

10. Ueland K: Maternal cardiovascular dynamics. VII. Intrapartum blood volume changes. Am J Obstet Gynecol 1976; 126:671.

11. Schrier RW, Dur JA: Pregnancy: an overfill or underfill state. Am J Kidney Dis 1987;9:284.

12. Clark SL, Cotton DB, Lee W, et al: Central hemodynamic assessment of normal term pregnancy. Am J Obstet Gynecol 1989;161:1439.

13. Gilroy RJ, Mangura BT, Lavietes MH: Rib cage and abdominal volume displacements during breathing in pregnancy. Am Rev Respir Dis 1988;137:668.

14. O'Sullivan GM, Sutton AJ, Thompson SA, Carrie LE, Bullingham RE: Noninvasive measurement of gastric emptying in obstetric patients. Anesth Analg 1987;66:505.

15. Andres RL, Piacquadio KM, Resnik R: A reappraisal of the need for autologous blood donation in the obstetric patient. Am J Obstet Gynecol 1990;163:1551.

16. Hemsell D: Prophylactic antibiotics in gynecologic and obstetric surgery. Rev Infect Dis 1991;(Suppl 10):S821.

17. Hyers TM, Hull RD, Weg JG: Antithrombotic therapy for venous thromboembolic disease. Chest 1986;89 (2 Suppl):26s.

18. Virgilio LA, Simon NV: Measurement of fetal cells in the maternal circulation. Obstet Gynecol 1977;50:364.

19. Bowman JM: Hemolytic disease (erythroblastosis fetalis) maternal blood group immunization. In: Creasy RK, Resnik R, eds. Maternal-fetal medicine: principle and practice. 3rd ed. Philadelphia: WB Saunders, 1993:711.

19a. Sachs PB, Oriol NE, Ostheimer GW, et al: Anesthetic-related maternal mortality, 1954 to 1985. J Clin Anesth 1989;1:333.

20. Knill-Jones RP, Newman BJ, Spence AA: Anaesthetic practice and pregnancy. Lancet 1975;2:807.

21. Farrell G, Prendergast D, Murray M: Halothane hepatitis. Detection of a constitutional susceptibility factor. N Engl J Med 1985;313:1310.

22. Rocke DA, Murray WB, Rout CC, Gouws E: Relative risk analysis of factors associated with difficult intubation in obstetric anesthesia. Anesthesiology 1992;77(1):67.

23. Haring OM: Cardiac malformations in rats induced by exposure of the mother to carbon dioxide during pregnancy. Circ Res 1960;8:1218.

24. King CTG, Wilk A, McClure FJ: Carbon dioxide-induced acidosis in pregnant rats and caries susceptibility of their progeny. Proc Soc Exp Biol Med 1962;11:486.

25. Shepard TH: Catalog of teratogenic agents. Baltimore: Johns Hopkins University Press, 1986:262.

26. Pedersen H, Finster M: Anesthetic risk in the pregnant surgical patient. Anesthesiology 1979;51(5):439.

27. Roberts RB, Shirley MA: The obstetrician's role in reducing the risk of aspiration pneumonitis. With particular reference to the use of oral antacids. Am J Obstet Gynecol 1976;124:611.

28. Gibbs CP, Banner TC: Effectiveness of Bicitra as a preoperative antacid. Anesthesiology 1984;61:97.

29. Mallampati SR: Clinical sign to predict difficult tracheal intubation (hypothesis). Can Anaesth Soc J 1983;30:316.

30. Barcroft J: Anoxaemia. Lancet 1920;2:485.

31. Jouppila R, Jouppila P, Karinen JM, Hollmen A: Segmental epidural analgesia in labour: related to the progress of labour, fetal malposition and instrumental delivery. Acta Obstet Gynecol Scand 1979;58:135.

32. Moise KJ Jr: Effect of advancing gestational age on the frequency of fetal ductal constriction in association with maternal indomethacin use. Am J Obstet Gynecol 1993; 168:1350.

33. Briggs GG, Freeman KR, Yaffe SJ, eds: Drugs in pregnancy and lactation. A reference guide to fetal and neonatal risk. 3rd ed. Baltimore: Williams & Wilkins, 1990:2/a.

34. Brant HA: Acute appendicitis in pregnancy. Obstet Gynecol 1967;29:130.

35. Black WP: Acute appendicitis in pregnancy. Br Med J 1960; 5190:1938.

36. Masters K, Levine BA, Gaskill HV, Sirinek KR: Diagnosing appendicitis during pregnancy. Am J Surg 1984;148:768.

37. Sarason EL, Bauman S: Acute appendicitis in pregnancy: difficulties in diagnosis. Obstet Gynecol 1963;22:382.

38. Baer JL, Reis RA, Arens RA: Appendicitis in pregnancy with changes in position and axis of the normal appendix in pregnancy. JAMA 1932;98:1359.

39. Cunningham FG, McCubbin JH: Appendicitis complicating pregnancy. Obstet Gynecol 1975;45:415.

40. Hibbard LT: Cesarean section and other surgical procedures. In: Gabbe SG, Niebyl JR, Simpson JL, eds. Obstetrics. Normal and problem pregnancies. New York: Churchill Livingstone, 1986.

41. Alders N: Sign for differentiating uterine from extrauterine complications of pregnancy and puerperium. Br Med J 1951;2:1194.

42. Spitzer M, Kaiser IH: Perforative appendicitis in the third trimester of pregnancy. NY State J Med 1984;84:132.

43. Weingold AB: Appendicitis in pregnancy. Clin Obstet Gynecol 1983;26:801.

44. Schwartz SI: Appendix. In: Schwartz SI, Shires GT, Spencer FC, eds. Principles of surgery. New York: Blakiston, 1989.

45. Babler EA: Perforative appendicitis complicating pregnancy: with report of a successful case. JAMA 1908;51:1310.

46. Schreiber JH: Laparoscopic appendectomy in pregnancy. Surg Endosc 1990;4:100.

47. Simon JA: Biliary tract disease and related surgical disorders during pregnancy. Clin Obstet Gynecol l983;26:810.

48. Braverman DZ, Johnson ML, Kern F Jr: Effects of pregnancy and contraceptive steroids on gall bladder function. N Engl J Med 1980;302:362.

49. Hill LM, Johnson CE, Lee RA: Cholecystectomy in pregnancy. Obstet Gynecol l975;46:291.

50. O'Neill JP: Surgical conditions complicating pregnancy. I. Acute appendicitis—real and simulated. Aust NZ J Obstet Gynaecol 1969;9:94.

51. Marcus CS, Mason GR, Kuperus JW, Mena I: Pulmonary imaging in pregnancy. Maternal risk and fetal dosimetry. Clin Nucl Med 1985;10(1):1.

52. Gallstones and laparoscopic cholecystectomy. NIH consensus development panel on gallstones and laparoscopic cholecystectomy, NIH Consensus Conference, Bethesda MD. JAMA 1993;269:1018.

53. Greene J, Rogers A, Rubin L: Fetal loss after cholecystectomy during pregnancy. Can Med Assoc J 1963;88:576.

54. Ostman PL, Pantle-Fisher FH, Faure EA, Glosten B: Circulatory collapse during laparoscopy. J Clin Anesth 1990;2(2):129.

55. McKellar DP, Anderson CT, Boynton CJ, Peoples JB: Cholecystectomy during pregnancy without fetal loss. Surg Gynecol Obstet 1992;174(6):465.

56. Weber AM, Bloom GP, Allan TR, Curry SL: Laparoscopic cholecystectomy during pregnancy. Obstet Gynecol 1991;78(5 Pt 2):958.

57. van Beek EJ, Farmer KC, Millar DM, Brummelkamp WH: Gallstone disease in women younger than 30 years. Neth J Surg 1991;43(3):60.

58. Bloch P, Kelly TR: Management of gallstone pancreatitis during pregnancy and the postpartum period. Surg Gynecol Obstet 1989;168(5):426.

59. Baillie J, Cairns SR, Putman WS, Cotton PB: Endoscopic management of choledocholithiasis during pregnancy. Surg Obstet Gynecol 1990;171(1):1.

60. Classen M, Hagenmuller F, Knyrim K, Frimberger E: Giant bile duct stones—non-surgical treatment. Endoscopy 1988;20:21.

61. Peterson HB, Hulka JF, Phillips JM: American Association of Gynecologic Laparoscopists' 1988 membership survey on operative laparoscopy. J Reprod Med 1990;35:587.

62. Basso L, McCollum PT, Darling MR, Tocchi A, Tanner WA: A study of cholelithiasis during pregnancy and its relationship with menarche, breast feeding, dysmenorrhea, oral contraception and a maternal history of cholelithiasis. Surg Obstet Gynecol 1992;175(1):41.

Chapter 11

Laparoscopic Surgery: An Atlas for General Surgeons, edited by Gary C. Vitale, Joseph S. Sanfilippo, and Jacques Perissat. J. B. Lippincott Company, Philadelphia, © 1995.

Laparoscopy for Non-Gynecologic Abdominal Emergencies

Denis Collet
Pierre J. Testas
Jean Christophe De Watteville

Laparoscopy is rapidly becoming an integral part of the evaluation and treatment process of acute abdominal disorders. As with open surgery, a laparoscopic procedure performed for diagnostic reasons can be converted easily to a definitive procedure for some abdominal emergencies. One must realize, however, that the surgical team assembled for an emergency procedure is frequently not one that usually works together. Under these circumstances, it may be difficult to perform effectively the most ordinary procedures. Because laparoscopic treatment of emergencies can be technically difficult, extensive experience in routine laparoscopic surgery is necessary before undertaking emergency laparoscopic surgery. This chapter does not discuss acute complications of biliary stones, which is described in a number of chapters.

BASIC PRINCIPLES

Instrumentation

In addition to the basic operative laparoscopy equipment, we recommend that the following be present as well:

- 10-mm aspirator—for those cases requiring a complete peritoneal lavage
- 10-mm digestive clamps with nontraumatic jaws—useful to grasp and maneuver the inflamed or distended bowel, reducing the risk of injury
- 10-mm nontraumatic liver retractor—for elevating the liver or retracting the bowel; the tip of the retractor can be covered with a Penrose drain to prevent additional visceral injury
- 10-mm needle holder
- Several liters of warm physiologic saline or Ringer's lactate solution
- Instruments for open surgery

Patient Positioning

The surgeon should face both the operating field and the television (TV) monitor. If the operating field is in the upper quadrant or quadrants of the abdomen, we recommend that the patient be placed in pelvic exenteration stirrups, with the surgeon standing between the patient's legs. The TV monitor should be behind either the patient's right or left shoulder. If the operating field is situated in the right lower quadrant, the surgeon must stand on the patient's left side, with the TV monitor on the right, and vice versa if it is in the left lower quadrant. Whatever the position, the patient must be properly secured to the table to allow maximal table rotation intraoperatively (for collecting abdominal fluids or exposing the operating field).

A Foley catheter should be placed in the bladder because it is impossible to know preoperatively where the trocars will be inserted. Finally, the patient's position must be such that should a rapid switch to an open procedure become necessary, it can be done easily.

Creation of a Pneumoperitoneum

Because the bowel is frequently distended, due to either ileus or an obstruction, insertion of the Veress needle must be done carefully. Locating the digestive gases on the preoperative roentgenograph can help the surgeon determine the proper site for needle insertion. One should be aware that the left hypochondrium is frequently a suitable area. All the standard safety measures must be taken before insufflation: the tip of the needle must be moved gently, to be certain that it is in a free space; gentle suction must not draw either blood or digestive contents; and the saline in a syringe connected to the needle must flow spontaneously into the abdominal cavity. After creating an adequate pneumoperitoneum, the first trocar is placed where there is likely to be free space on the abdomen wall. Afterward, the other trocars are placed under direct vision with the laparoscope in place.

The open laparoscopic technique may be useful, especially in a patient with prior laparotomy. A mini-incision is performed in a free area of the abdomen wall. All the layers of the abdominal wall must be opened under direct vision, including the peritoneum. A free space can then be found in the abdomen and checked with a finger or a Kelly forceps. A 10-mm Hasson-type cannula is then placed and connected to the insufflator. The peritoneum and fascia are closed around the cannula, using a pursestring suture.

Exploration of the Abdominal Cavity

One of the major advantages of laparoscopy over laparotomy is the ability to perform a more complete exploration of the abdomen: the entire peritoneal cavity can be carefully examined through a 10-mm incision. In these emergency cases due to bowel distention and inflammation, injuries usually consist of entering with the tip of the trocar the bowel lumen or causing bleeding of the mesentery. Thus, it is important to be gentle, to progress slowly, to separate the viscera with irrigation solution rather than by pulling or dissection, and to rotate the table to gain access to specific areas. Injuries often have minimal consequences if diagnosed immediately. The operation can always be converted to an open procedure or the injured viscera can be exteriorized through a small laparotomy incision and repaired externally.

At the end of the exploration, the surgeon should be able to answer three questions:

1. What is the primary pathology?
2. Do complications exist?
3. Can the treatment be performed safely through the laparoscope?

If there is even a little doubt, the procedure must be converted to an open procedure without any hesitation.

Insertion of one or two additional 5-mm trocars is necessary. Most often, the first trocar is inserted directly in the suprapubic area, facilitating inspection of the pelvic organs. The second trocar is inserted either in the left or right lower quadrant (most often in the right), facilitating inspection of the peritoneal cavity above and below the transverse colon. Each trocar is inserted under direct visualization to avoid vascular or visceral injury. At the beginning of the inspection of the peritoneal cavity, one should determine the presence or absence of peritoneal fluid. If present, all of it should be aspirated for cytologic examination. The patient should then be placed in Trendelenburg's position, to visualize the pelvic organs. After the sigmoid colon and the small bowel are displaced, they are carefully inspected for inflammatory or pelvic adhesions, ovarian cysts, and other visceral or peritoneal disorders.

One should next evaluate the cecum, including the appendix. The entire small bowel is inspected, viewing first the ileum and then the jejunum. An atraumatic forceps is used to gently grasp the small bowel near the mesenteric side. Occasionally, such as when there is bowel distention, this maneuver may be difficult. In this instance, the patient should be placed in reverse Trendelenburg's position. During this inspection, adhesions between the omentum and the small bowel and on the abdominal wall are identified. They can usually be incised after bipolar coagulation if that is deemed necessary.

The patient should be tilted to the right side for inspection of the sigmoid colon and the left colon. During the next step, one should inspect the area above the transverse colon with a blunt probe, facilitating examination of the liver, spleen, subdiaphragmatic peritoneum, gallbladder, duodenum, and hiatal area. For this inspection, it is recommended that a 10-mm trocar be inserted 2 or 3 cm above the umbilicus. The posterior wall of the stomach and the anterior segment of the pancreas are systematically inspected. Incision of the gastrocolic omentum may be necessary inferior to the greater curvature of the stomach for insertion of the laparoscope in the lesser sac.

DIAGNOSTIC EMERGENCY LAPAROSCOPY

Right Iliac Pain

Right lower quadrant abdominal pain is the most frequent indication for laparoscopy to confirm the diagnosis of acute appendicitis. After a careful inspection of the peritoneal cavity and especially of the pelvic organs in female patients, the surgeon should inspect the cecal area to visualize the appendix. The appendix appears 2 or 3 cm below the cecum and should be visualized from the cecum to its distal segment. If the appendix is in a retrocecal position, the cecum is elevated with atraumatic forceps, peritoneal attachments are lysed, and the laparoscope is passed behind the right colon to visualize and release the appendix. Only when the appendix is visualized entirely can one determine whether acute appendicitis is present.

If the appendix appears to be normal, one may conclude that acute appendicitis is not present and other pathology should be sought (eg, mesenteric adenitis or Meckel's diverticulum). If after careful inspection of the peritoneal cavity one cannot determine an etiology for the abdominal pain and there is still a question of whether the appendix is normal, it is recommended that an appendectomy be performed. In our experience, this approach reduces the incidence of unnecessary appendectomy by nearly a third.

Peritonitis

Laparoscopy enables one to diagnose acute peritonitis and frequently allows the surgeon to initiate appropriate surgical treatment. Perhaps the most important diagnosis that can be made laparoscopically is that of a perforated peptic ulcer. Laparoscopy can reveal a defect in the anterior wall of the duodenum, often close to the gallbladder. Sometimes after division of the gastrocolic omentum, a perforated ulcer on the posterior wall of the stomach can be identified.

Laparoscopy facilitates identification of ischemic bowel perforation injury with pelvic inflammatory disease. When peritonitis is associated with appendicitis, the laparoscopist is able to identify a purulent-appearing appendix, with or without perforation.

Bowel Obstruction

When bowel obstruction is suspected, the laparoscopic approach enables the surgeon to identify adhesions. Often, they are difficult to identify, especially when they are near the posterior peritoneum and "bound down." It is recommended that two additional 5-mm trocars be inserted to displace the small bowel, which may be obscuring the obstructing point. If the lesions cannot be identified, laparotomy must be performed. Laparoscopy also enables the surgeon to identify bowel neoplasm or inflammatory bowel stenosis, which may necessitate bowel resection. In some cases, laparoscopy may reveal specific pathology, which may be approached using a small incision in the abdominal wall directed laparoscopically, with exteriorization of the involved bowel. The pathology can then be identified and often treated by segmented bowel resection.

Abdominal Trauma

Laparoscopic inspection of the abdominal cavity in trauma allows precise diagnosis and avoidance of unnecessary laparotomies but is not a substitute for peritoneal lavage and computed tomography scanning. If a hemoperitoneum is suspected, laparoscopy can clearly reveal lacerations on the anterior surface or dome of the liver. If present, a subcapsular hematoma can also be easily identified. Laparoscopy is useful diagnostically near a penetrating injury of the parietal peritoneum, and injury to the adjacent abdominal organs can usually be either excluded or confirmed. If the peritoneum is breached, the entire bowel and mesentery must be inspected to identify bleeding, serosal injury, or signs of bowel perforation. Prospective randomized trials are necessary to determine the use of laparoscopy for evaluation of penetrating trauma.

Splenic injuries may not be a good indication for a laparoscopic approach. Further experience is necessary but massive bleeding and clotting obscure anatomy and may delay control of bleeding, compared with an open approach.

LAPAROSCOPIC TREATMENT OF PERFORATED ULCER

A perforated ulcer is usually best approached with the patient placed in the supine position, with legs apart. The operator stands between the legs, allowing equal access to instruments placed through all ports. The pneumoperitoneum created by the perforated ulcer facilitates the insertion of the Veress needle and the trocars. Normally, four trocars are necessary:

- 10-mm in the umbilicus, for the laparoscope
- 10-mm in the right hypochondrium, for the liver retractor
- 10-mm in the left hypochondrium, for the aspirator, grasper, and needle holder
- 10-mm in either the right hypochondrium or the right flank, for forceps, scissors, and grasper (Fig. 11-1)

A trocar placed suprapubically may be useful to clear any accumulated fluid in the pouch of Douglas and the pelvis. In most patients, these areas cannot be reached from the upper part of the abdomen with standard instruments.

The first step is exploration of the peritoneal cavity. Usually, the perforation is situated on the anterior aspect of the duodenal bulb. Frequently, the edge of the liver adheres to the duodenum and the omentum is thickened, making the perforation difficult to identify. It is important to progress slowly from the stomach to the duodenum, dividing the adhesions with hydrostatic pressure to avoid injury to the liver (Fig. 11-2). Frank bleeding or even a constant oozing of blood may make the operation difficult, if not impossible. Once the perforation has been identified, it is essential to identify its posi-

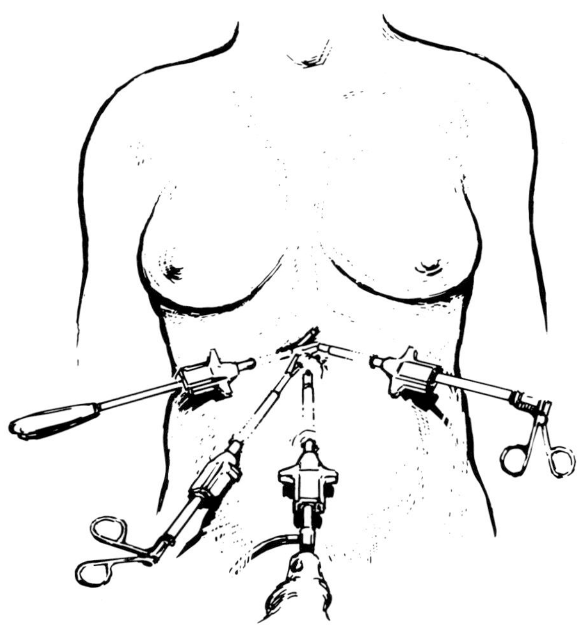

FIGURE 11-1. Port placement for perforated ulcer.

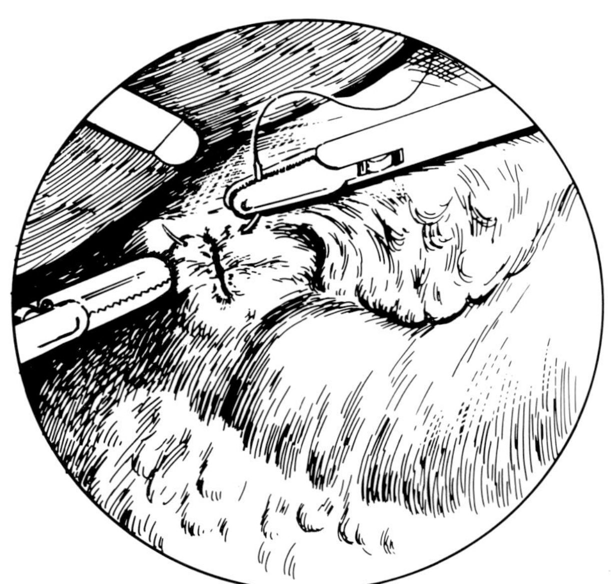

FIGURE 11-3. Suture closure of perforated ulcer.

tion relative to the pylorus. If the stomach is perforated, the possibility of malignancy must be considered. This finding should lead to either a large biopsy of the perforated area or preferably to a laparotomy for consideration of partial gastrectomy.

One has several options for treating the lesion:

1. It may be closed with separate stitches (Fig. 11-3). This is the simplest method but technically one of the most difficult because it requires technical expertise in laparoscopic suturing, maintaining tension. Furthermore, the edematous duodenum is fragile and tends to tear.
2. The perforation can be plugged with omentum that is coated with fibrin sealant (Fig. 11-4). Although this is an easy solution, some technical points must not be underestimated. The omentum is sometimes so thick that it does not remain (spontaneously) over

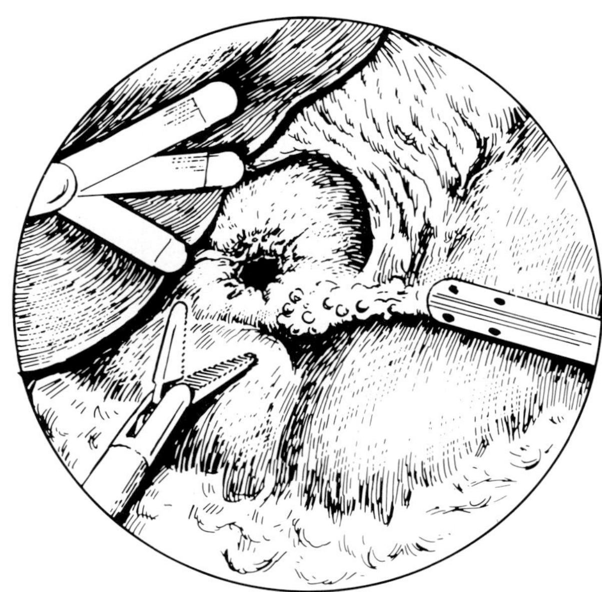

FIGURE 11-2. Perforated ulcer. Dissection and irrigation of perforation site.

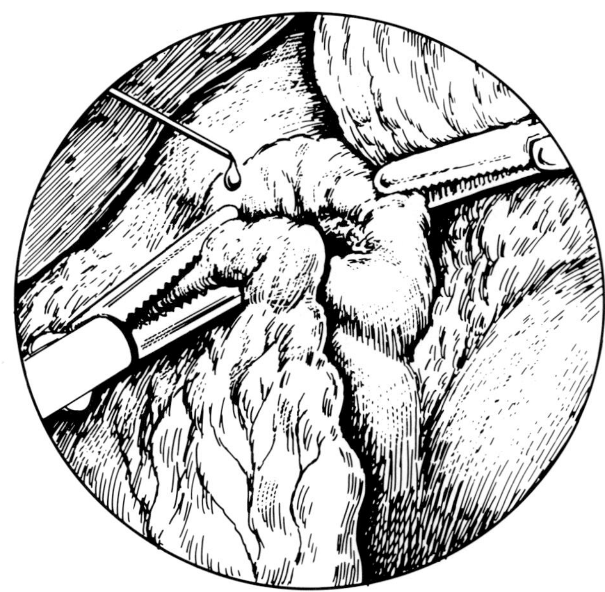

FIGURE 11-4. Omental patch of large ulcer, with application of fibrin glue.

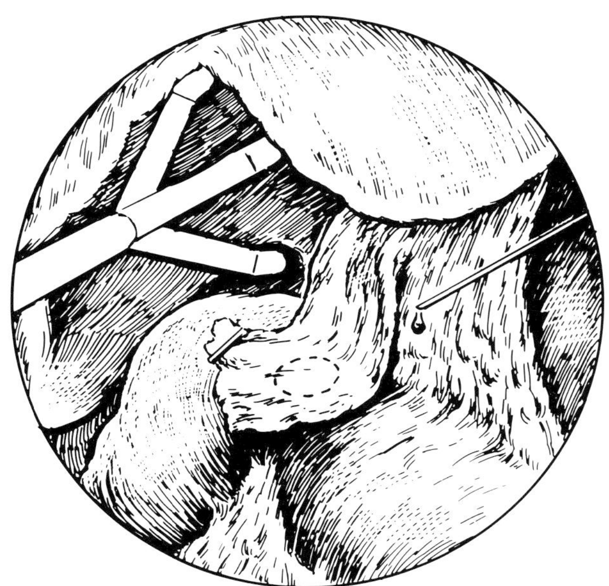

FIGURE 11-5. Repair of perforated ulcer using ligamentum teres.

the perforation. The inflamed tissue constantly releases serous fluid, which makes the sealant inefficient. If the greater omentum is not available, one can use the round ligament after dividing it near its umbilical attachment (Fig. 11-5). Another solution consists of pulling the omentum into the lumen of the duodenum with a flexible endoscope, introduced perorally intraoperatively. A biopsy forceps or a Dormia basket is then passed into the operating channel from the duodenum through the perforation, permitting one to grasp and pull the omentum into the duodenum (Fig. 11-6). It is then fixed with sutures, fibrin sealant, or both, laparoscopically (Fig. 11-7). This technique has some advantages. It is possible to evaluate both the duodenum and the stomach during the operation to assess whether the repair is of good quality. Success of the repair can be checked by the bubble test at the end of the operation by gently inflating the duodenum after filling the abdomen with normal saline. It requires another endoscopic technique, however, and a surgeon skilled in flexible endoscopy.

3. If the omentum is firmly adherent to the perforation and seals the hole, it may not be worth freeing these involved adhesions. The operation consists exclusively of a complete lavage of the abdominal cavity, with drainage of the subhepatic space.

After closing the ulcer, the final step is an extensive peritoneal lavage. The entire cavity must be inspected and cleared, including the subdiaphragmatic spaces, subhepatic space, gutters, and the pouch of Douglas (Fig. 11-8). The false membranes must be gently pulled away as much as possible. It may take a significant amount of time and may require 10 to 15 L of warm normal saline. It is absolutely essential to have the abdominal cavity as clean as possible on completion of the operation. A closed suction drain may optionally be left adjacent to the perforation.

Postoperatively, the nasogastric tube must be con-

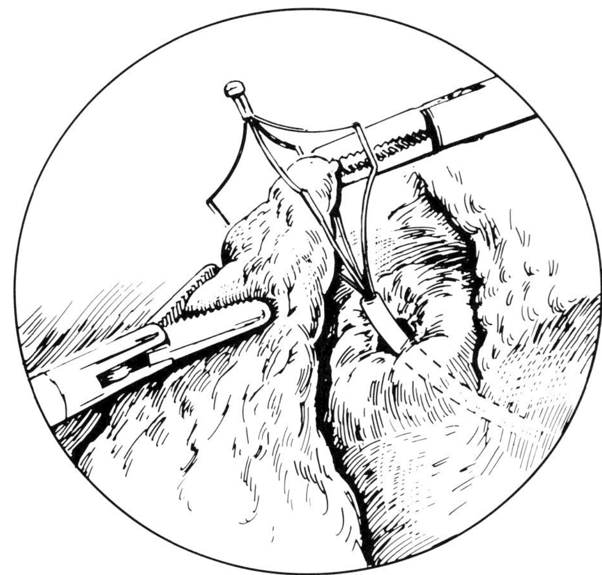

FIGURE 11-6. Use of basket placed endoscopically through perforation to assist in pulling the omentum into the stomach.

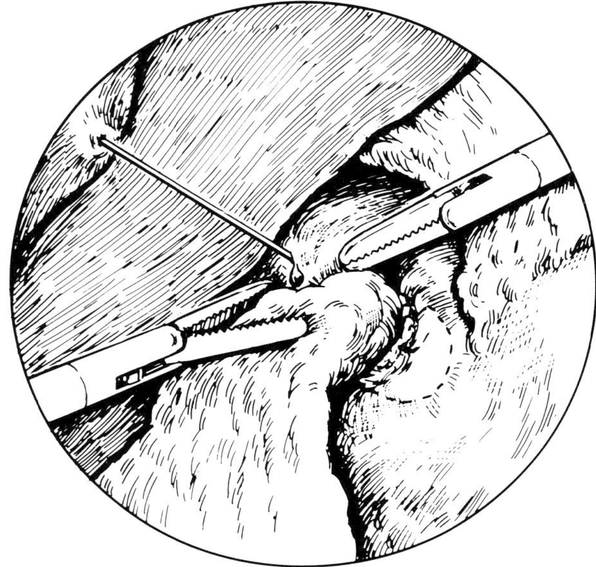

FIGURE 11-7. Fibrin glue is placed on omentum stuffed into ulcer.

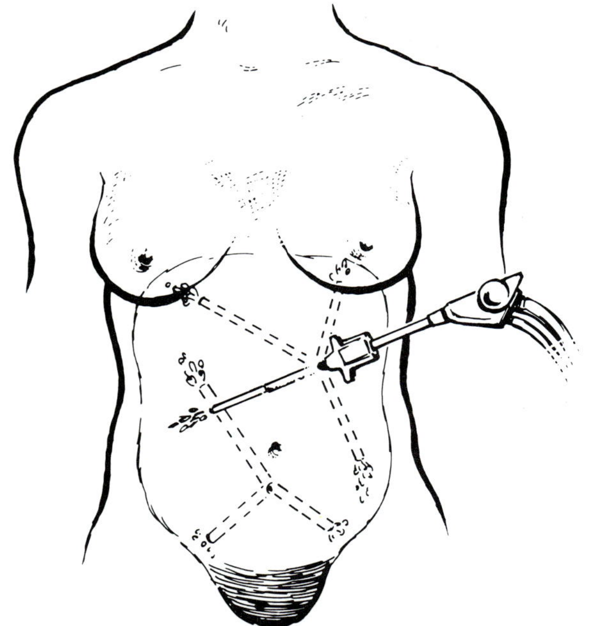

FIGURE 11-8. Technique of extensive irrigation for perforated views.

nected to suction until a Gastrografin upper gastrointestinal series is performed on the sixth postoperative day. If there is no leakage, the nasogastric tube can be removed. The suction drain can be removed 1 or 2 days later, if used. Oral feeding can be resumed gradually.

If a vagotomy is necessary, one has several options. A truncal vagotomy can be performed. The risk of spasm of the pylorus, however, necessitates either a pyloroplasty or a balloon dilation of the pylorus, performed endoscopically.

It is theoretically possible to do either a highly selective vagotomy or a posterior truncal vagotomy with an anterior seromyotomy. These procedures require extensive experience in laparoscopic surgery. Additionally, dissecting the vagus nerve in the hiatal orifice in such septic conditions makes risk of contamination of the mediastinum a concern. If vagotomy is thought to be necessary, it can be delayed for several weeks. It can be performed either laparoscopically or, preferably, thoracoscopically.

LAPAROSCOPIC TREATMENT OF SMALL BOWEL OBSTRUCTION

This type of obstruction usually occurs in patients who have abdominal adhesions from a prior laparotomy. Any scar can provide such a complication, regardless of when the operation was performed. For these patients, there are two main points to consider relative to laparoscopy.

First, one must not wait for extensive dilation of the bowel before deciding to operate. Extensive dilation of the bowel makes it impossible or dangerous to introduce the trocars and the instruments.

Second, the insertion of the Veress needle and the first trocar can be hazardous. One must avoid the area of scarring and any dilated bowel. This means that the laparoscope should be inserted into nontraditional locations. The technique of open laparoscopy is particularly advantageous here.

If a prior midline incision has been made, which is the most common situation, we recommend placing the laparoscope laterally, in either the right or the left flank, and inserting the instruments on the same side, above and below the first port. If the scar is in the right lower quadrant (previous appendectomy), the laparoscope is inserted in the umbilicus; one trocar is inserted below the xiphoid and another suprapubically. Usually, these ports are sufficient, but in any given case, one or two additional ports may be necessary to adequately expose the adhesions and the bowel (Fig. 11-9).

Actually, there are no absolute rules for the position of the ports but they must be placed in such a manner that the surgeon faces the adhesions. In this position, the surgeon can divide the adhesions from above to below (or vice versa), using both hands while the laparoscope is held by the first assistant. Bipolar electrocautery is recommended because it minimizes the risk of thermal injury to the bowel. The adhesions must be divided as far as possible from the bowel wall. Once the deep aspect of the scar is exposed, the causal agent of the obstruction must be found. With this in mind, all of the bowel must

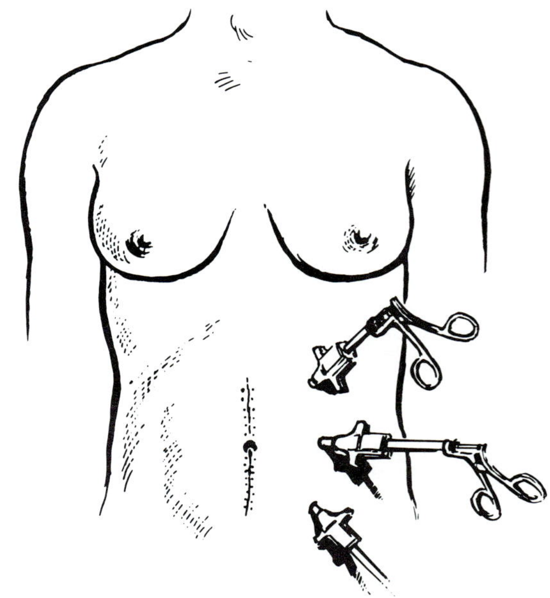

FIGURE 11-9. Port placement for small bowel obstruction.

be carefully inspected. Often, one finds a single strangulating adhesion at the junction of the dilated and collapsed bowel. We recommend clipping or ligating the adhesion before dividing it (Fig. 11-10). Control of bleeding later, if necessary, is difficult to accomplish once the edges of the cut adhesions retract among the dilated intestinal loops. The entire bowel must be carefully inspected.

One has several options if an injury to the bowel occurs during the dissection. The injured loop may be pulled out of the cavity through a small incision in the abdominal wall, using the laparoscope to aid in selecting the best location for the lesion. The injured loop may be sutured laparoscopically or one can convert to an open operation (Figs. 11-11 and 11-12). The choice depends on the surgeon's experience in laparoscopic surgery and the severity of the adhesions. At the end of the procedure, the cavity must be washed with warm normal saline.

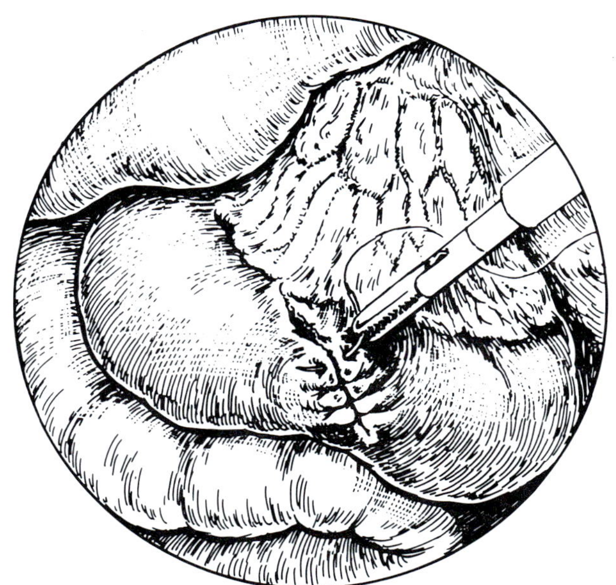

FIGURE 11-11. Laparoscopic repair of small bowel injury.

COLONIC EMERGENCIES

In patients with colonic obstruction, laparoscopy can be performed to establish the diagnosis. A colostomy can be created if a future multistage surgical intervention is planned.

A perforated diverticulum can be treated by a proximal colostomy, associated with drainage of the left lower quadrant and the pouch of Douglas. Laparoscopic access permits one to completely clear the abdominal cavity and to mobilize a proximal colonic segment to the abdominal wall, without having the problem of a proximal laparotomy wound. Because this procedure is not definitive and leaves the infected colon behind, it must be performed only in very ill patients who would otherwise not tolerate an emergency colectomy.

Laparoscopic colectomy in an emergency setting with acute inflammation is technically difficult, requiring a great amount of experience in laparoscopic surgery. A Hartmann's procedure, using an auto-stapler for closure

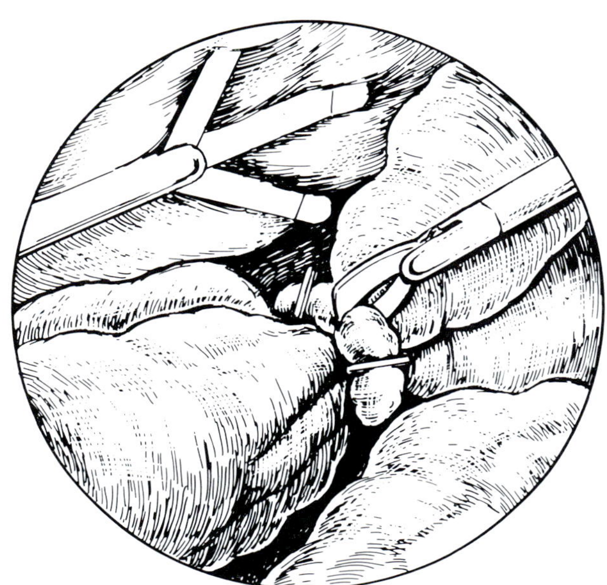

FIGURE 11-10. Lysis of adhesive bank, causing small bowel obstruction.

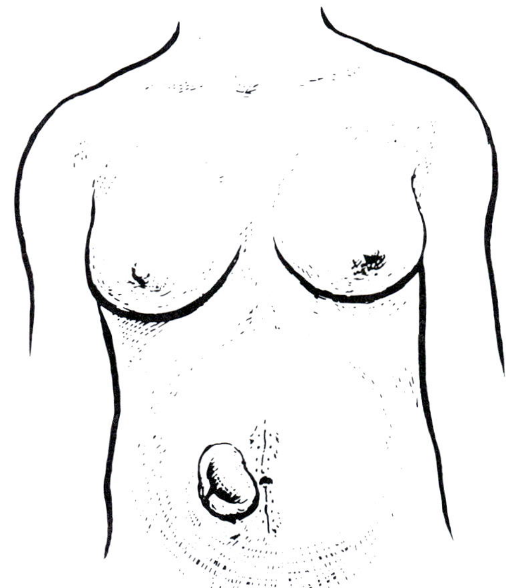

FIGURE 11-12. Exterior repair of small bowel injury.

of the rectal stump, may be used. Ultimately, the advantages of laparoscopic access over laparotomy must be demonstrated in these situations because prolonged operative time with an aseptic abdomen may be detrimental. Suture or staple closure of a colonic perforation occurring during a colonoscopy with a prepped colon is an excellent application of laparoscopic technique.

OTHER EMERGENCIES

In acute pancreatitis, an exploratory operation of the abdominal cavity can be performed initially to confirm the diagnosis and to establish the proper staging. Moreover, a cholecystectomy and cholangiogram, or in selected cases a cholecystostomy, may be performed laparoscopically. A jejunostomy for internal feed or peripancreatic drains for peritoneal lavage can be placed laparoscopically.

Laparoscopy may be used in cases of suspected small bowel ischemia (for both initial resection and for a second look) to check the viability of the remaining bowel and the anastomosis. If the first operation is performed as an open procedure, the second can be performed laparoscopically. At the end of the open operation, a 10-mm trocar is left in place, its distal extremity inserted under the peritoneum. For the second look, one must only withdraw the cannula 2 or 3 mm until the abdominal tip is free in the peritoneal cavity. The insufflator may then be hooked up to the cannula and the laparoscope inserted. Should further exploration be necessary, the tip of the cannula is reinserted (at the same site) and left in place. If further exploration is not warranted, the cannula is removed and the fascia closed.

Suggested Readings

Bruhat MA, Dubois F: La chirurgie abdomino-pelvienne par coelioscopie. Rapport présenté au 94ème Congrès Français de Chirugie. Paris: Springer-Verlag 1992.

Berci G, Sackier JM, Paz-Partlow M: Emergency laparoscopy. Am J Surg 1991;161:332.

Mouret P, François Y, Vignal J, Barth X, Lombard-Platet R: Laparoscopic treatment of perforated peptic ulcer. Br J Surg 1990;77:1006.

De Watteville JC, Testas P: La coelioscopie dans les urgences digestives. In: Testas P, Delaitre B, eds. Chirurgie digestive par voie coelioscopique. Paris: Maloine 1991;170.

Wood D, Berci G, Morgenstern L, Paz-Partlow M: Mini-laparoscopy in blunt abdominal trauma. Surg Endosc 1988; 2:184.

Laparoscopic Surgery: An Atlas for General Surgeons, edited by Gary C. Vitale, Joseph S. Sanfilippo, and Jacques Perissat. J. B. Lippincott Company, Philadelphia, © 1995.

Chapter 12

Complications of Advanced Laparoscopic Surgery

Harry Reich

Most of the data on complications from advanced laparoscopic procedures are garnered from questionnaires or case reports. Usually, the response rate to questionnaires is low. Many of the institutions or individuals who do not respond choose not to participate because of a higher than normal incidence of injuries. In addition, many of the injuries that are reported are attributed to the inexperience of the surgeon.

Theoretically, the incidence of injuries should be the same at laparoscopy or laparotomy. At laparotomy, however, most surgeons are able to repair any injury immediately; injuries repaired at laparotomy are rarely reported. Surgeons often need to perfect their laparoscopic suturing techniques. When this is achieved, injuries to bowel and most other organs can be repaired endoscopically. Most surgeons cannot suture well laparoscopically, necessitating a conversion to laparotomy for repair of injury to visceral organs. Extensive adhesions must be properly assessed and the presence of bowel carefully detected (Figs. 12-1 and 12-2).

HERNIA

The incidence of incisional hernias of the anterior abdominal wall after operative laparoscopy is greatly increased if 10-mm or larger trocars are placed at extraumbilical sites. These sites should be closed with sutures. If the incision is lateral to the rectus muscle, the deep fascia is located, elevated with skin hooks, and suture-repaired. If the incision is through the rectus muscle, the peritoneal defect is closed with a laparoscopically placed suture.[1]

INFECTION

Infection is exceedingly rare after laparoscopic surgery. There is a theoretic risk that bacterial infection can be disseminated throughout the peritoneal cavity by extensive use of aquadissection. Bacteria grow poorly in Ringer's lactate solution, however.[2] Infections of an umbilical incision are usually prevented by burying the knot of the suture below the deep fascia. Infection is detected by pain, swelling, and erythema of the overlying skin. Treatment consists of warm compresses, drainage, and appropriate antibiotic coverage. Infection rarely occurs in 5-mm trocar sites, especially after closure without suture. In more than 2000 procedures, this author has experienced only one rectus muscle infection that required drainage.

DISSEMINATION OF CANCER

A theoretic risk also exists for dissemination of cancer cells when a cyst is aspirated. In our experience, there has been no recurrence with early ovarian serous cystadenocarcinoma (two cases) or endometrial adenocarcinoma (four cases) treated laparoscopically. Hysterectomy performed 1 month after a laparoscopic myomectomy resulted in a diagnosis of sarcoma, which was negative for residual disease. When a suspicious lesion is excised, consideration should be given to leaving 1 L of sterile water in the peritoneal cavity at the close of the procedure to lyse free cells. Because this usually results in a marked increase in urinary output, the patient should be carefully observed postoperatively for urinary retention.

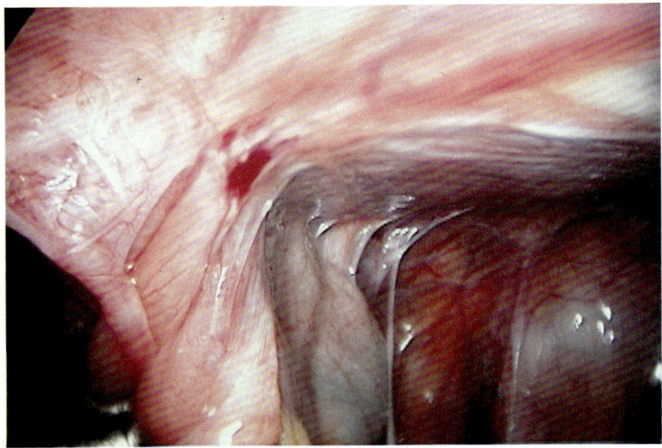

FIGURE 12-1. Extensive anterior abdominal wall small bowel adhesions.

Cutaneous seeding of carcinoma of the gallbladder has been reported after laparoscopic cholecystectomy.[3] Thus, cysts or organs with or without possible malignant excrescences should not be pulled through tight incisions. The LapSac (Cook Ob/Gyn, Spencer, IN) is ideal in this instance; cysts should be placed in it before their aspiration and later removal.

FLUID OVERLOAD

Fluid overload is possible when using large amounts of irrigation solution (e.g., Ringer's lactate or normal saline) during a lengthy procedure. Most long laparoscopic surgical procedures are performed on relatively healthy patients. The fluid, in physiologic balance with body fluids, is absorbed through the peritoneal surfaces during and after the laparoscopic procedure and is mainly excreted through the kidneys. Loosely approximating umbilical and second-puncture incisions provide an easy exit for excess fluids (i.e., when the patient's intra-abdominal pressure rises, leakage from umbilical and lower quadrant incisions is common and usually ceases within 12 hours). Pulmonary edema is a possibility; it occurred in four of this author's last 1000 cases. Treatment is with furosemide (Lasix) and supplemental oxygen. Oxygen saturation is monitored with a pulse oximeter. For most long laparoscopic procedures, lactated Ringer's solution should be infused at 4 to 5 mL/kg/hour, which in a 70-kg woman results in 280 to 350 mL of fluid per hour.

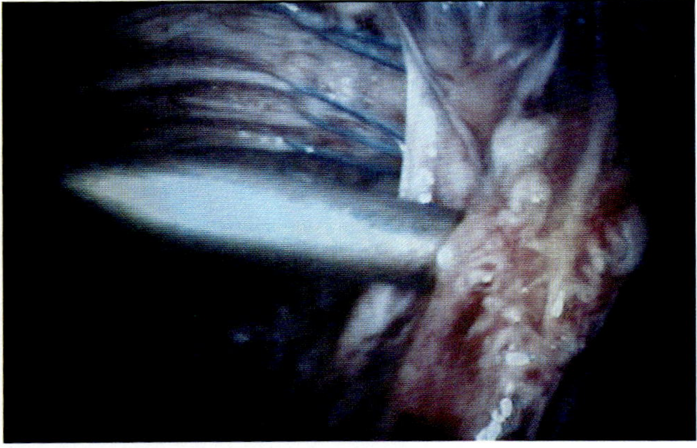

FIGURE 12-2. Manipulation around adhesions reveals small bowel to be stuck to Marlex mesh and Prolene sutures. Patient had over 10 laparotomies and repair of a large incisional hernia.

SUBCUTANEOUS AND SUBFASCIAL EMPHYSEMA AND EDEMA

Other complications relate to distribution of fluid in tissues and potential spaces outside the peritoneal cavity. (Accumulation of fluid in tissue is edema; accumulation of gas in tissue is emphysema.) Areas commonly affected are the subcutaneous and subfascial spaces. Often, both subcutaneous emphysema and edema exist concurrently, with edema more prominent in the dependent areas.

Instrument manipulation often loosens the parietal peritoneum surrounding the point of entrance into the peritoneal cavity. Carbon dioxide (CO_2) then infiltrates the loose areolar tissue of the body, and crepitant areas can sometimes be palpated in the shoulder and fascial regions. This swelling subsides within a few hours after the end of the procedure. Subfascial edema of the labia can often be expressed through the lower quadrant incisions by putting pressure on the labia. Similar pressure on the anterior abdominal wall pushes CO_2 out through the umbilical incision during or after the procedure.

When the vulva is affected by this fluid–gas mixture, marked vulvar swelling can occur, and an indwelling Foley catheter may be necessary. The amount of facial edema, including periorbital and scleral edema, is proportional to the length of the procedure and the degree of the Trendelenburg's position that the patient was in. It rapidly resolves within 2 to 4 hours postoperatively (i.e., usually by the time of discharge). In rare cases, pleural effusion may be present. This should be ruled out with an upright abdominal radiograph when persistent upper abdominal "gas pain" is present.

VESSEL AND VISCUS INJURY

Veress needle and trocar-induced vascular or viscus injury can result in life-threatening complications in advanced laparoscopic surgical procedures. A fourth of the respondents to a survey of board-certified Canadian gynecologists had each induced at least one sharp trocar or needle injury; half of the injuries required laparotomy for correction.[4] Inadvertent traumatic perforation to the bowel or large vessels during initial trocar placement is a known risk of laparoscopy, which often is beyond the control of the surgeon. These injuries, although rare, cannot be prevented all the time because trocar insertion is a blind procedure that involves a forceful thrust with a sharp instrument. An open laparoscopic approach may not reduce the risk of bowel trauma if the small bowel is stretched and fused to the anterior abdominal wall beneath the entry site. Shielded disposable trocars produce the same type of injury as their reusable counterparts; they are not safer.

Vessel Injury

Injury to a large vessel (e.g. aorta or iliac) usually signifies the need for an immediate laparotomy. Fatalities have been reported, however, due to slow bleeding into the retroperitoneal space that went unnoticed by the surgeon at the time of laparoscopy.[5] Increased intra-abdominal pressure (10 to 15 mmHg, secondary to insufflation of CO_2); decreased venous pressure (from the use of Trendelenburg's position); and retroperitoneal hematoma formation may temporarily tamponade a large vessel injury. As soon as the pressure gradients return to normal, bleeding may start, which may eventually lead to hypovolemic shock.

To detect this deadly complication, it is essential to examine the course of the large vessels at the start and on completion of the endoscopic procedure. When an injury has occurred, it is usually possible to detect a defect in the peritoneum overlying the site of a retroperitoneal entry. The operator can differentiate between a Veress-needle (small, round) or trocar (triangular) injury. If one is absolutely certain that the wound was made by the Veress needle, consideration may be given to not intervening immediately but to observing the patient instead.

Should a hematoma be present, its overlying peritoneum can be opened, using laparoscopic scissors or CO_2 laser. The hematoma is evacuated by alternating suction and irrigation (aquadissection) in the retroperitoneal space. Blood in areolar or adipose tissue is desiccated. Laparotomy should be performed if there is any evidence of an expanding hematoma or persistent bleeding. Ideally, at laparotomy a vascular surgeon does the exploration. The aorta and common iliac vessels should be isolated with vascular tourniquets before exploration of the area of the suspected laceration.

EPIGASTRIC VESSELS

Injury to the deep epigastric vessels can be avoided by observing them directly with the laparoscope because one can usually see the venae comitantes adjacent to the obliterated umbilical ligaments of the anterior abdominal wall. The deep epigastric artery has two branches that emanate from the external iliac artery near its transition into the femoral artery and lie in the medial peritoneal fold of the internal inguinal ring. The round ligament curls around these vessels on entrance into the inguinal canal. Superficial epigastric vessels are identified by transillumination. Both direct observation and transillumination should be performed in every case. Because the deep epigastric vessels lie beneath the lateral margin of the rectus muscle, lateral insertion also avoids muscle bleeding.

Should bleeding ensue from a second puncture site, rotating the second puncture sleeve through 360° often results in vessel tamponade. Thereafter, pressure on this site for 5 to 10 minutes may control the bleeding. During this time, intraperitoneal manipulation can be performed through another port. If this procedure does not control the bleeding, long Kleppinger bipolar forceps inserted through the operating channel of an operating laparoscope are used to desiccate the vessels above the parietal peritoneum cephalad and caudad to the trocar (Fig. 12-3). If a subfascial hematoma is present at the end of the procedure, the peritoneum at one side of the hematoma, usually in the flank, is opened and the hematoma evacuated by alternating irrigation with suction until clear effluent is obtained.

Although bipolar desiccation is almost always satisfactory, other methods are available. Tamponade of the vessel at the site of injury can be obtained by inserting a Foley catheter through the second port, removing the cannula after inflating the Foley catheter, and bringing the distended Foley balloon into pressurized contact with the laceration. The balloon is held in this position by putting traction on the Foley catheter and placing a hemostat on it at its exit site from the abdominal cavity.

Suture occlusion of the vessels may be considered. A Keith straight needle can be inserted into the peritoneal cavity on one side of the vessel and out the opposite side to perform ligation. Large curved needles can be used full thickness through the abdominal wall under laparoscopic observation.

OVARIAN OR UTERINE VESSELS

Bipolar desiccation can control bleeding from ovarian or uterine vessels. Collateral circulation to the pelvic organs ensures that ischemic changes do not occur.

Viscus Complications

Gastrointestinal injuries can occur during any laparoscopic procedure but especially laparoscopic adhesiolysis. The surgeon should be familiar with early detection and management of these injuries. In many cases, lapa-

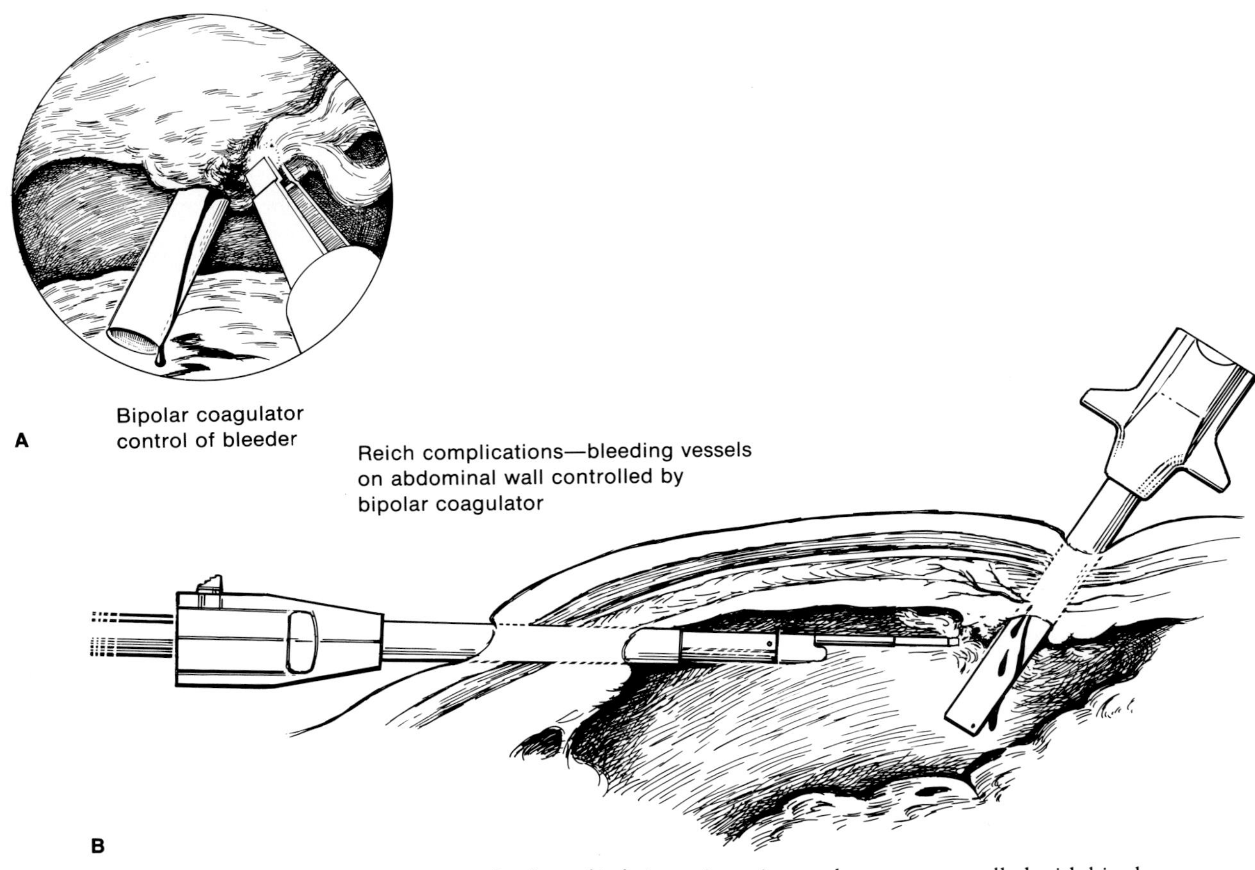

FIGURE 12-3. (**A**) Laparoscopic view of inferior epigastric vessel trauma controlled with bipolar coagulation. (**B**) Overall view (sagittal) of coagulation of deep epigastric vessels using bipolar forceps through the operating channel of an operative laparoscope.

rotomy is not required. Laparoscopic repair of small and large bowel injuries is reported.[6,7]

STOMACH

Routine use of an orogastric tube is recommended to reduce the possibility of a trocar injury to the stomach and to increase operating space by limiting gaseous distention of the stomach and small bowel. Should such an injury occur, however, a laparoscopic view of the inside of the stomach is evident. Treatment consists of a laparoscopically placed pursestring or figure-eight suture in the seromuscular layer surrounding the defect and nasogastric tube drainage for 2 days.

BOWEL

Trocar Insertion Injury. Perforation of the intestine may occur either at the time of Veress needle or umbilical trocar insertion or later on. Injury by Veress needle probably occurs more often than is diagnosed. These injuries often go unnoticed when intestinal loops adhere to the anterior abdominal wall and can seal off the perforation promptly. Insufflation of an intestinal loop occurred eight times in 500 procedures in one reported series.[8,9] The emanation of foul-smelling gas through the pneumoperitoneum needle is a helpful diagnostic sign; expectant management without laparotomy is recommended.

Injury during insertion of the first trocar (usually umbilical) may represent a diagnostic challenge, and recognition of this complication at the time of laparoscopy is crucial. When a segment of bowel (usually the transverse colon) adheres to the abdominal wall, the trocar can pierce the entire lumen of the bowel (Figs. 12-4 and 12-5). The bowel remains fixed around the sleeve of the trocar during the entire procedure, so the accident may not be noticed unless the operator carefully examines the entire abdominal cavity. Again, recognition of the complication at the time of laparoscopy is most important. If perforation of the transverse colon is suspected, the trocar sleeve and the laparoscope inside it are retracted slowly. If pierced, the bowel lumen comes into view during this maneuver. The recommended treatment is laparotomy for suture repair of the perforation or resection of the bowel segment. If an experienced laparoscopic surgeon is available, laparoscopic suture or a laparoscopic stapler can be used to close the defect. If the

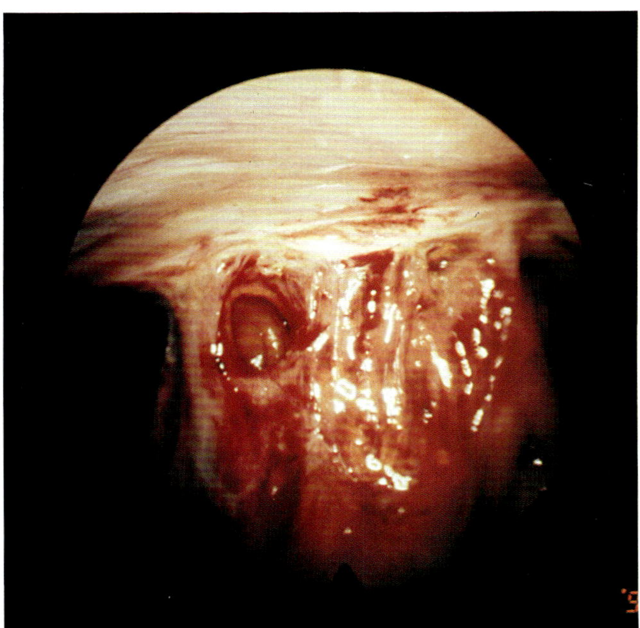

FIGURE 12-4. Small bowel enterotomy that occurred while using the laser to divide the adhesions.

perforation has occurred in a bowel segment other than the transverse colon, it may be beneficial to leave the trocar in situ until the affected segment is identified and clamped. Colostomy is rarely indicated.

When there are extensive small bowel adhesions, a small bowel perforation that occurs may not be recognized until later in the procedure, when omental and small bowel adhesions are freed from the anterior abdominal wall. If these adhesions are not freed, a perforation may not be recognized. Thus, when finding extensive adhesions surrounding the umbilical puncture, the surgeon should consider finding another higher primary puncture site that provides a panoramic view of the entire peritoneal cavity (e.g., the left costal margin in the mid-clavicular line). The adhesions can then be freed down to and just beneath the umbilicus, clearing the umbilical portal for further work. If CO_2 insufflation is not obtainable through the umbilicus, Veress needle puncture in the left ninth intercostal space, anterior axillary line, is recommended.[7]

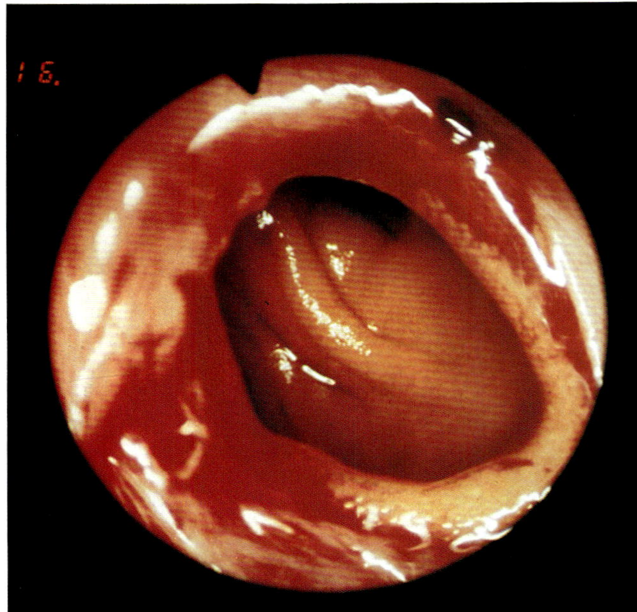

FIGURE 12-5. Close-up of Figure 12-4.

A "safety" shield component of some disposable trocars may become momentarily stuck at the level of the fascia. Its release can result in a direct violent force that may cause a crush injury to retroperitoneal vessels or the intestines located between the applied force and the lumbosacral spine. Mutilation of the mesentery and large gaping bowel rents may also occur.

A small bowel perforation is repaired transversely, using 3-0 Vicryl, silk, or polydioxanone (PDS) and a taper SH needle (Figs. 12-6 through 12-9). The repair is made transversely, using interrupted sutures that are tied either externally or with intracorporeal instruments. Sterile milk is instilled into the bowel lumen before the closing of the last suture to detect any leakage from the laceration or occult perforations near the small bowel mesentery (Fig. 12-10).

Bowel resection and primary enteroenterostomy is indicated if (1) the length of an enterorrhaphy exceeds half the bowel diameter, (2) there are multiple injuries in proximity, or (3) a segment of bowel is devascularized. The choice of single layer, double layer, or stapled method of repair is best determined by the surgeon. Peritoneal drainage after small bowel injury is not indicated.

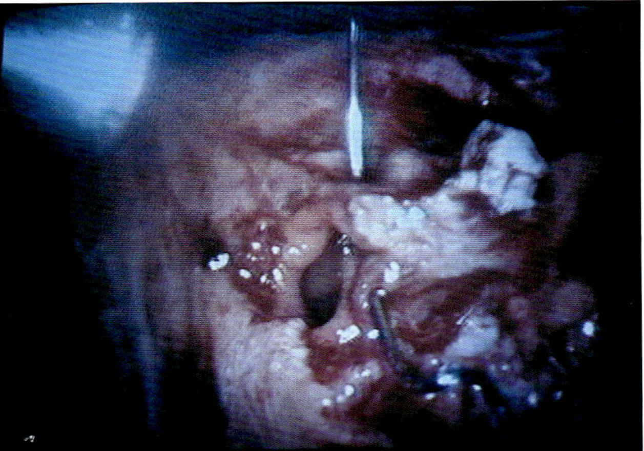

FIGURE 12-6. 3-0 Vicryl on a taper needle is used to repair defect. Three interrupted sutures are required. The first suture is placed.

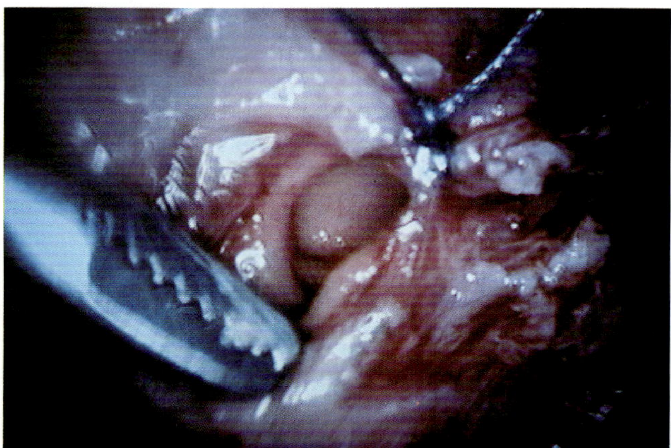

FIGURE 12-7. The first suture is tied.

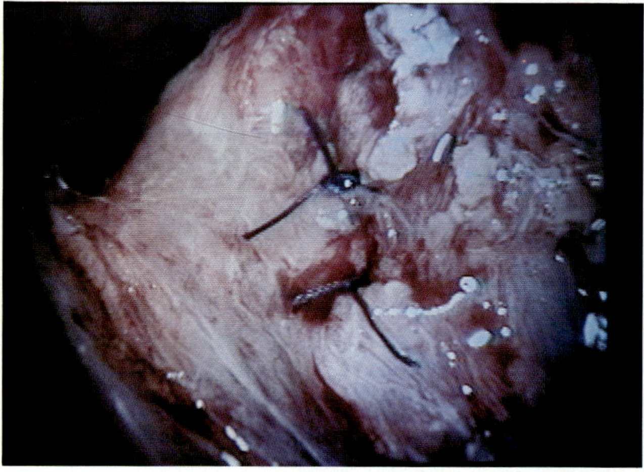

FIGURE 12-9. The first two sutures are tied. Before inserting the last one, the small bowel is filled with sterile milk to detect any leak after closure.

Antibiotics are routinely administered as the surgical repair begins and postoperatively for three doses when intestinal injury has occurred. In most cases, nasogastric decompression is avoided after laparoscopic repair.

Non-Trocar Injury. Small bowel perforation during surgery for pain from adhesions that resulted from multiple previous surgeries is common, occurring in more than 25% of these procedures (author's unpublished observation). Despite the application of traction and countertraction to each adhesion, as these adhesions are carefully cut, it is inevitable that a few bowel punctures are made. Repair is simple, as just described; a nasogastric tube is rarely indicated. Superficial thermal injuries to the bowel can be treated prophylactically by placing a laparoscopic pursestring suture beyond the thermally affected tissue.

Large bowel injury during surgery occurs most often at the level of the rectosigmoid or in the deep cul-de-sac. Detection and careful inspection of the injury are critically important. Superficial lesions can be managed by careful postoperative observation. Defects involving the full thickness of the wall require surgical repair by an experienced surgeon, either laparoscopically or by laparotomy. Resection with or without colostomy is rarely indicated.

In the bowel-prepped patient, injury to the anterior rectum can usually be repaired laparoscopically. Full-thickness penetration of the wall of the rectum may occur during excision of rectal endometriosis nodules. After excision of the nodule and identification of the rent in the rectum wall, a single- or double-layered repair is

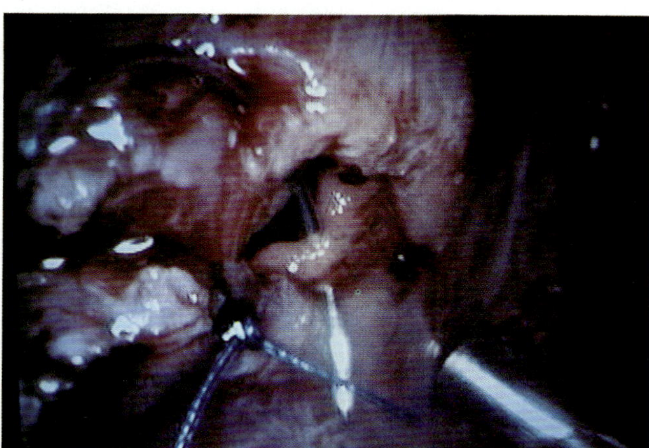

FIGURE 12-8. The second suture is placed.

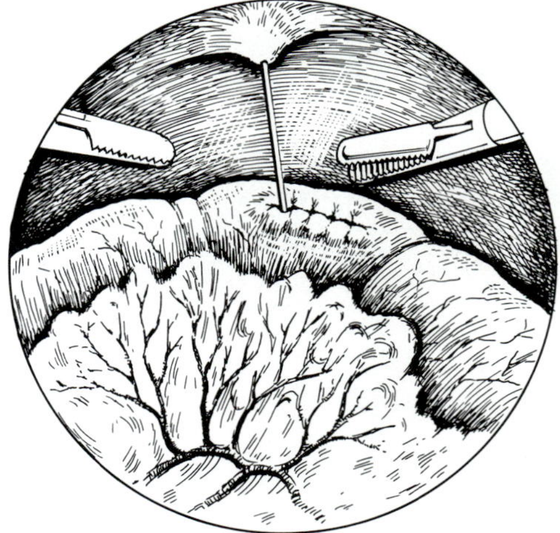

Reich—small bowel perforation
instilling sterile milk in
lumen before placing
last suture

FIGURE 12-10. Repair of small bowel laceration.

performed using 3-0 Vicryl, silk, PDS, or the stapler. Stay sutures are placed at the transverse angles of the defect and brought out through the lower quadrant port. The port is removed and then replaced through the same site, adjacent to the stay suture. After closure, Betadine solution can be injected into the rectum through a 26-French Foley catheter with a 30-mL balloon, and an underwater examination is conducted to check for any leaks, which if seen are reinforced with additional sutures.[8,9]

The decision to repair the unprepared bowel laparoscopically depends on the amount of fecal spillage present. Should a large amount of fecal contamination occur, laparotomy followed by repair should be considered. Laparoscopic suture closure, followed by copious irrigation until the effluent runs clear, may be satisfactory.[10,11] Generally, there is little indication for colostomy during the repair of bowel injuries noted during the course of a laparoscopic procedure.

The practice of performing a colostomy when treating a bowel injury began in 1944, after Ogilvie reported significant reduction in mortality after treatment of colon injuries during World War II.[12] Moreover, in 1943, the Surgeon General of the United States issued an order that all colon injuries sustained in battle should be treated by doing a colostomy.[13] In 1951, Woodhall and Ochsner reported their experience with primary repair without colostomy: their mortality rate fell from 23% to 9% with primary repair.[14] In 1979, Stone and Fabian reported the first well-controlled prospective randomized study on primary closure of traumatic colon perforations.[15] Morbidity for the randomized colostomy group was tenfold higher and the average hospital stay was 6 days longer than the primary closure group. Similar results were obtained by George and coworkers and Burch and coworkers.[16,17] Thus, there is little indication for colostomy during the repair of bowel injuries noted during a laparoscopic procedure.

Unrecognized or Delayed Perforation. Delayed bowel injury can result from traumatic perforation not recognized during the procedure (Veress needle or trocar puncture or laceration during adhesiolysis or excision) or from thermal damage from any source. Rarely, delayed injuries can occur from perforation of mechanically devascularized bowel or hemorrhagic ischemic necrosis after mesenteric venous thrombosis. Bowel perforation after thermal injury usually presents 4 to 10 days after the procedure. With traumatic perforation, symptoms of peritonitis usually occur within 24 to 48 hours, although their occurrence up to 11 days later has been reported.[18] The gross appearance of traumatic and electric injuries is similar: the perforation is usually surrounded by a white area of necrosis. Histologic examination should include a Mallory's trichrome stain that turns desiccated tissue blue. Microscopic examination of an electric burn lesion reveals the persistence of dead amorphous tissue without polymorphonuclear infiltration or capillary ingrowth. With puncture injuries, there is rapid and abundant capillary ingrowth, white cell infiltration, and fibrin deposition at the edge of the injury site.[19] Treatment is bowel resection.

Soderstrom reviewed 66 cases of legal action because of bowel perforation (personal communication). In 58 of these cases, the major reason for the lawsuit was a bowel burn. There was evidence of a thermal injury from electricity in only six cases. Of the 60 cases of bowel trauma, a disposable trocar was used in 12 and an open technique in three cases. The small bowel was involved in 53 cases and the large bowel in 13 (Richard Soderstrom, MD, personal communication, International Society of Gynecologic Endoscopists [ISGE], Washington DC, June 26, 1993).

BLADDER

Cystitis occurs rarely after laparoscopic surgery. Patients are encouraged to void before going to the operating room, and a catheter is not always inserted at the start of the procedure. Because of the large volume of fluid left in the peritoneal cavity, in most cases a Foley catheter is inserted before completion. If the procedure has lasted less than 2 hours, the Foley catheter is removed in the short-stay unit when the patient is alert and awake. At the same time, the patient may be given one tablet of trimethoprim-sulfamethoxazole (Septra DS) and 25 mg of bethanechol chloride (Urecholine). When surgery lasts more than 2 hours, the patient may require 2 g of either cefoxitin sodium (Mefoxin) or cefotaxime sodium (Claforan).

Bladder perforation may occur from supraperitoneal thrusting of the umbilical trocar. These injuries present with postoperative hematuria or leakage of urine from the umbilical incision. Treatment by catheter drainage for 7 days usually results in complete healing.

The bladder may also be injured during attempts to resect endometriosis from the vaginal cuff posthysterectomy. The endometriosis frequently invades the bladder and one or both ureters, making the bladder extremely adherent to the vaginal cuff. When noted, injury should be repaired, ideally laparoscopically, and an indwelling catheter left in place for 5 days.

The second-puncture trocar can perforate the bladder, especially in a patient who has had previous pelvic surgery. A reliable diagnostic sign of this event is the sudden appearance of gas in the Foley catheter drainage bag. Thus, when bladder identification cannot be made because no bladder distention occurs during the surgery, consideration should be given to inserting a Foley catheter to observe for gas.

The most important factor in treatment is early detec-

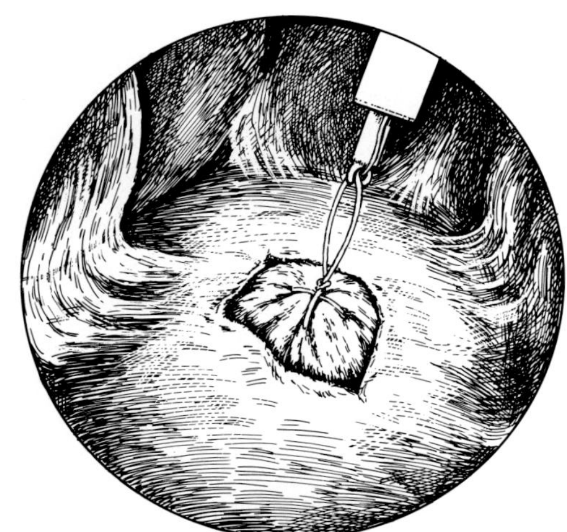

Bladder repair
Reich complications

FIGURE 12-11. Repair of bladder laceration.

tion. Treatment consists of the placement of an indwelling catheter for 7 to 10 days and prophylactic antibiotics. Should the defect be large from manipulation through the trocar sleeve during laparoscopic surgery, it should be closed with a figure-eight suture through the surrounding bladder muscularis and a second suture to close the overlying peritoneum (Fig. 12-11). A watertight seal should be documented by filling the bladder with blue dye solution and checking for leakage.[20]

Postoperative urinary retention may occur, especially with the use of large amounts of fluids for irrigation and hydroflotation. Urine can accumulate rapidly in the bladder in the drowsy patient recovering from anesthesia. The Foley catheter should not be removed at the end of operative procedures lasting more than 2 hours. Foley catheter removal should be delayed until the patient is awake in the short-stay unit and aware that the catheter is in place, usually 1 hour postoperatively. At this time, a useful protocol is to administer Urecholine (bethanechol chloride, MSD) 25 mg. Should spontaneous voiding not occur within 3 hours of catheter removal, straight catheterization is performed and the patient is given another 25 mg of Urecholine.

URETER

An intravenous pyelogram should be obtained if postoperative flank or pelvic pain presents after adnexal surgery. Thermal injury to a ureter results in ureteral narrowing and hydroureter formation. Treatment during the early phase is often possible by the placement of a ureteral stent for 3 to 6 weeks. Intraoperatively, ureteral integrity can be checked by injecting 5 mL of indigo carmine solution intravenously. Elimination of the dye begins soon after the injection, usually appearing in the urine within 5 to 10 minutes. Methylene blue should not be injected intravenously because it can result in methemoglobinemia.

References

1. Kadar N, Reich H, Liu CY, Manko GF, Gimpelson R: Incisional hernias after major laparoscopic gynecologic procedures. Am J Obstet Gynecol 1993;168:1493.
2. Morales J, Kibsey P, Thomas PD, Poznansky MJ, Hamilton SM: The effects of ischemia and ischemia-reperfusion on bacterial translocation, lipid peroxidation, and gut histology: studies on hemorrhagic shock in pigs. J Trauma 1992; 33:221.
3. Drouard F, Delamarre J, Capron JP: Cutaneous seeding of gallbladder cancer after laparoscopic cholecystectomy. N Engl J Med 1991;325:1316.
4. Yuzpe AA: Pneumoperitoneum needle and trocar injuries in laparoscopy. J Reprod Med 1990;35:485.
5. Zweigel D, Thiele H, Schworm HD: Die Verletzung grosser Gefasse durch Laparoskopie. (Injuries of the large vessels caused by laparoscopy.) Zentralbl Gynakol 1987; 109(10):673.
6. Reich H, McGlynn F, Budin R: Laparoscopic repair of full-thickness bowel injury. J Laparoendosc Surg 1991;1:119.
7. Reich H: Laparoscopic bowel injury. Surg Laparosc Endosc 1992;2:74.
8. Vilardell F, Seres I, Marti-Vicente A: Complications of peritoneoscopy. A survey of 1455 examinations. Gastrointest Endosc 1968;14:178.
9. Ruddock JC: Peritoneoscopy: a critical clinical review. Surg Clin North Am 1957;37:1249.
10. Hudspeth AS: Radical surgical debridement in the treatment of advanced generalized bacterial peritonitis. Arch Surg 1975;110:1233.
11. Reich H: Endoscopic management of tuboovarian abscess and pelvic inflammatory disease. In: Sanfilippo J, Levine R, eds. Operative gynecologic endoscopy. New York: Springer-Verlag, 1988:5.
12. Ogilvie WH: Abdominal wounds in the Western desert. Surg Gynecol Obstet 1944;78:225.
13. Office of the Surgeon General: Circulation letter, no. 178: October 23, 1943.
14. Woodhall JP, Ochsner A: The management of perforating injuries of the colon and rectum in civilian practice. Surgery 1951;29:305.
15. Stone HH, Fabian TC: Management of perforating colon trauma: randomization between primary closure and exteriorization. Ann Surg 1979;190:430.
16. George SM Jr, Fabian TC, Voeller GR, Kudsk KA, Mangiante EC, Britt LG: Primary repair of colon wounds. A prospective trial in nonselected patients. Ann Surg 1989; 209:728.
17. Burch JM, Brock JC, Gevirtzman L, et al: The injured colon. Ann Surg 1986;203:701.
18. Penfield AJ: How to prevent complications of open laparoscopy. J Reprod Med 1985;30:660.
19. Levy BS, Soderstrom RM, Dail DH: Bowel injuries during laparoscopy: gross anatomy and histology. J Reprod Med 1985;30:168.
20. Reich H, McGlynn F: Laparoscopic repair of bladder injury. Obstet Gynecol 1990;76:910.

Chapter 13

Laparoscopic Surgery: An Atlas for General Surgeons, edited by Gary C. Vitale, Joseph S. Sanfilippo, and Jacques Perissat. J. B. Lippincott Company, Philadelphia, © 1995.

Laparoscopic Common Bile Duct Exploration

Edward H. Phillips

The treatment of common bile duct calculi was relatively straightforward until the advent of laparoscopic cholecystectomy in 1989. Before the laparoscopic era, patients suspected of harboring common bile duct calculi underwent intraoperative cholangiography. If common bile duct calculi were found, the bile duct was opened and the stones retrieved. One had to decide which patients, too old or too ill for open surgery, would benefit from preoperative endoscopic sphincterotomy.

The introduction of therapeutic laparoscopy altered the surgical approach to patients undergoing cholecystectomy. Preoperative endoscopic retrograde cholangiopancreatography became the standard diagnostic procedure for patients suspected of having choledocholithiasis to avoid having to "open" patients found to have common bile duct stones. Postoperative endoscopic sphincterotomy became the preferred method for treating common bile duct calculi encountered at surgery or found after surgery. In the first few years of performing laparoscopic cholecystectomy, intraoperative cholangiography was performed infrequently, and preoperative endoscopic retrograde cholangiopancreatography was performed instead. New techniques (laparoscopic common bile duct exploration through the cystic duct or by choledochotomy) allow intraoperative removal of bile duct calculi, reducing the need for endoscopic sphincterotomy.

TRANSCYSTIC BILE DUCT EXPLORATION

Most transcystic techniques of common bile duct exploration involve the dilation of the cystic duct with balloon dilators or sequentially graduated bougies to gain access to the common bile duct. Flexible biliary endoscopy, balloon trolling of the common bile duct, fluoroscopically guided wire-basket stone retrieval, ampullary balloon dilation with lavage, and transcystic endoscopically assisted sphincterotomy are all techniques that can be performed laparoscopically through the cystic duct.

The most commonly employed technique is flexible biliary endoscopy with wire-basket retrieval of calculi. This appears to be the safest technique because stone capture and manipulation is performed under direct vision, without manipulation of the ampulla, and is feasible in 80% to 90% of cases.[1] One limitation is that only in about 10% of cases can the endoscope be passed into the proximal bile ducts.[2] Multiple stones; small, fragile cystic ducts; and stones proximal to the cystic duct–common duct junction usually must be dealt with by choledochotomy, endoscopic sphincterotomy, or ampullary balloon dilation.

Technique

After review of the intraoperative cholangiography, the treatment plan should consider the patient's age and physical condition. If the location of the stones and the patient's condition permit, the cystic duct should be bluntly and carefully dissected close to its junction with the common duct. It is often necessary to make an incision in the larger portion of the cystic duct, close to the common duct, so that less duct requires dilation. The location of the incision should allow for an adequate stump for closure with an Endoloop (Ethicon, Cincinnati, OH) at the end of the procedure, which increases its success. A Phantom 5 balloon dilating catheter (Microvasive, Boston, MA), which has a balloon 4 cm long and 6 mm in diameter, is preloaded with a .038″ 150 cm long hydrophilic guide wire. The assembly is inserted through a 5-mm trocar in the anterior axillary line, just under the right costal margin. Depending on the laparoscopic cholecystectomy technique employed, it may be necessary to add an additional 5-mm trocar in a better location to intubate the cystic duct.

After radiographic or fluoroscopic confirmation of the guide-wire location, the balloon dilating catheter or sequential bougies are inserted over it. Two thirds of the balloon should be inserted. It is then slowly inflated with a LeVeen syringe, which is attached to a pressure gauge. The balloon and cystic duct are observed laparoscopically on the monitor while the assistant or nurse slowly inflates the balloon as the pressures are read aloud. The balloon should be inflated to the insufflation pressure recommended by the manufacturer (usually 12 atm). If the cystic duct begins to tear, stop inflation and wait 3 minutes before resuming inflation. With patience, most cystic ducts can be dilated to 7 mm but they should never be dilated larger than the inner diameter of the common bile duct. When exploring a small common duct, care must be taken to use the proper diameter of dilating balloon, determined when performing the intraoperative cholangiography.

The cystic duct should be dilated to the size of the largest stone to prevent the stone entrapped in the wire basket from becoming impacted on removal. Stones larger than 1 cm have to be fragmented with a dye-pulse laser or electrohydraulic lithotripsy or they must be removed by choledochotomy. After the duct is dilated, the balloon catheter is deflated and withdrawn. The endoscope can be inserted over the guide wire if the wire is 150 cm long, or the endoscope can be inserted freehand or gently guided with an atraumatic grasping instrument. The working channel of some endoscopes are eccentric to their cross section, making insertion over the guide wire difficult.

The endoscope should have bidirectional deflection and a working channel of at least 1.2 mm. An outer diameter of 2.7 to 3.2 mm is ideal. Smaller endoscopes compromise the working channel, and larger ones are more difficult to pass. A camera should be attached and the image should be projected on a TV monitor with an A-V (audio-visual) mixer (picture in picture) or it should be projected on its own monitor. It is convenient to set up a mobile cart with a monitor, light source, camera box, video recorder, endoscopes, wire baskets, balloon dilating catheters, and other instruments needed for a laparoscopic common bile duct exploration. This cart can also function as an emergency cart or a backup cart for other laparoscopic procedures. Having all the required instruments in one place decreases the frustration and delays when common duct calculi are encountered.

Once the endoscope is in the cystic duct, irrigation with warm normal saline should be initiated. Attention must be paid to the temperature of the irrigation fluid because it is not uncommon to have instilled 3 to 6 L by the end of the procedure. The operating surgeon manipulates the endoscope, inserting and torquing with the left hand and deflecting the end of the endoscope with the right hand on the deflecting lever. Grasping the endoscope with a grasper can damage it.

Once a stone is identified, it should be removed. Always entrap the stone closest to the endoscope and do not bypass any because they can be irrigated upward into the liver. A straight four-wire basket (2.4 French) is preferable. The closed basket should be advanced beyond the stone, opened, and then pulled back to entrap it. The basket should be closed gently, and the basket and stone should be pulled up against the end of the endoscope so that they can be withdrawn in unison (Fig. 13-1). This process is repeated until all the stones are removed. A completion cholangiogram is essential.

At this point, a decision regarding cystic duct drain-

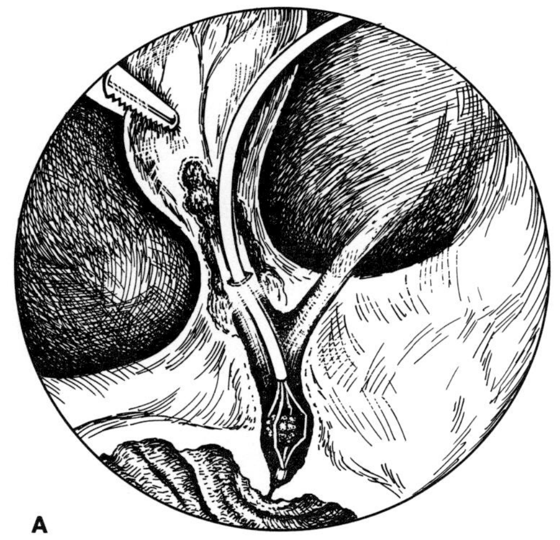

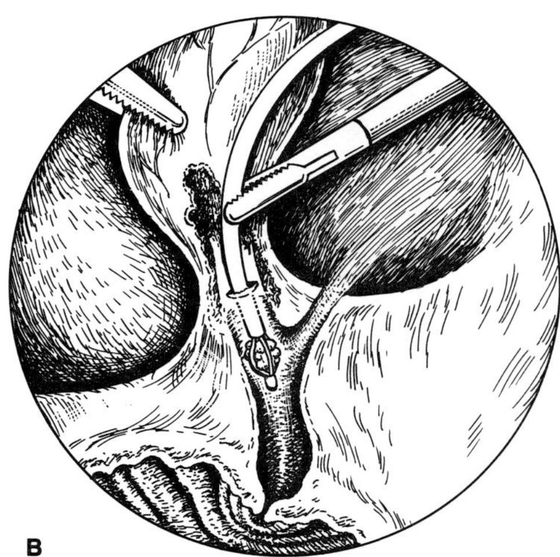

FIGURE 13-1. Technique of endoscopic-guided transcystic basket retrieval of common bile duct stones.

age must be made. Older or immunosuppressed patients with cholangitis should have a latex (not silicone) tube placed for postoperative decompression of their biliary system. Patients who may be harboring a retained stone should have a drainage tube placed in anticipation of postoperative cholangiography and if necessary, percutaneous tube tract stone extraction. If the preexploration intraoperative cholangiography shows a different number of common duct stones than was found on endoscopy, a tube should also be placed.[3]

FLUOROSCOPIC WIRE-BASKET STONE RETRIEVAL

Fluoroscopic wire-basket stone retrieval is feasible if fluoroscopy is available. Special spiral wire baskets with flexible leaders must be used to avoid injuring the common bile duct. The basket is inserted into the common bile duct through the cystic duct and with the aid of fluoroscopy, it is advanced into the lower portion of the common bile duct or duodenum and then opened.[4] Then it is pulled back until the stone is captured. The advantage of not having to dilate the cystic duct is offset by the problem of extracting the wire basket with the captured stone through the nondilated cystic duct. In our experience, this technique is not as successful as other transcystic duct techniques; it can lead to an impacted stone-containing basket, requiring choledochotomy for its removal.

BILIARY BALLOON CATHETER STONE RETRIEVAL

This technique is occasionally helpful, especially when the cystic duct is dilated. A biliary balloon catheter can be passed blindly or under fluoroscopic control through the cystic duct into the duodenum, where the balloon is inflated. The catheter is then gently withdrawn, modulating the pressure on the balloon. This procedure is often successful using choledochotomy but when used through the cystic duct, it has the potential to pull the stone into the common hepatic duct, out of reach of an endoscope.

AMPULLARY BALLOON DILATION

This controversial technique can be employed when the cystic duct is extremely small, so that an endoscope cannot be inserted. One milligram of glucagon is administered intravenously. A specifically sized balloon dilating catheter is chosen that is appropriate for the inner diameter of the common duct. A hydrophilic guide wire is inserted into the catheter lumen. The assemblage is inserted through the subcostal trocar and the guide wire is advanced into the duodenum through the cystic duct. The balloon catheter is advanced under fluoroscopic guidance so that the balloon's radiographic markers span Oddi's sphincter. The balloon is inflated to the manufacturer's recommended pressure, with a LeVeen syringe attached to a pressure gauge (Fig. 13-2). Hypaque 25% is used to inflate the balloon, so that it is visible on fluoroscopy. The balloon is left inflated for 3 minutes and is then deflated and withdrawn. A large-bore catheter or the dilating balloon catheter is placed in the cystic duct and using a pump or high-flow irrigators, warmed normal saline is used to forcibly flush the common duct. A cholangiogram is mandatory on completion of the procedure.

Carroll and Phillips report that small common bile duct stones and stone debris were successfully lavaged into the duodenum in 17 of 20 cases (85%) using this method.[5] Postoperative hyperamylasemia was noted in four patients. Mild clinical pancreatitis was observed in

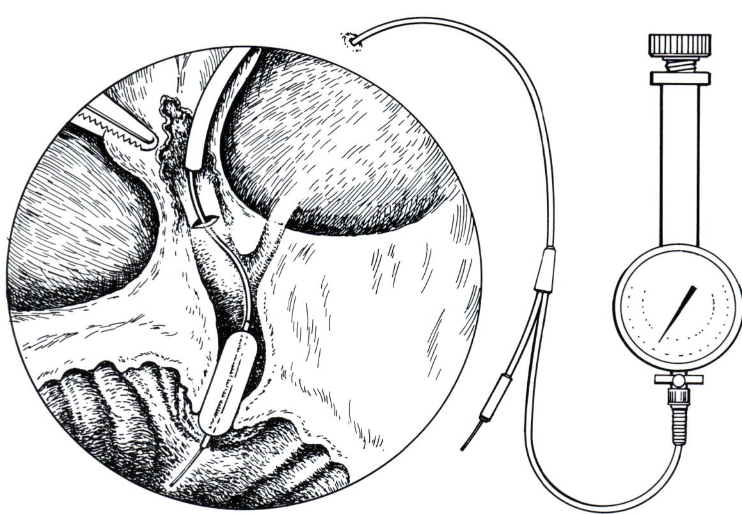

FIGURE 13-2. Technique of fluoroscopically guided transcystic duct ampullary balloon dilation.

three patients (15%). Appel reports 16 cases without complications.[6] This technique, however, should be attempted only when the alternative is endoscopic sphincterotomy or choledochotomy (in a small common duct).

LAPAROSCOPIC CHOLEDOCHOTOMY

Laparoscopic choledochotomy is an excellent choice for patients with a dilated common duct, stones 1 cm or larger, multiple stones, or when lithotripsy is required for impacted stones. It is contraindicated when the ducts are small because of the risk of stricture. The advantage of choledochotomy is that stones can be easily irrigated out of the common duct, and an endoscope can be inserted into the intrahepatic ducts. A large diameter (8 mm) choledochoscope can be used, with better optics and a larger working channel that can accommodate larger and less delicate wire baskets. Another advantage of the technique is that a T-tube is placed in the common bile duct, which decompresses the duct and provides access for later cholangiography and stone retrieval. The disadvantage of choledochotomy is that a T-tube is required, and considerable laparoscopic suturing skill is needed to close the choledochotomy.

Technique

The procedure is performed before the gallbladder is removed, so that it can be used to elevate the liver, applying tension to the cystic duct. The anterior wall of the common bile duct is bluntly dissected. Occasionally, it is necessary to aspirate bile to confirm the identity of the structure thought to be the common duct. Two stay sutures should be placed in the common bile duct and its anterior wall tented before an incision is made with a microscissor. The choledochotomy should only be made as long as the circumference of the largest stone to minimize the amount of suturing required for closure. The most efficient technique is to insert a choledochoscope into the duct and irrigate with warm normal saline. A biliary balloon catheter or wire baskets can be used to remove the calculi in most cases. Occasionally, a three-pronged grasper or biliary lithotripsy is necessary to remove an impacted stone.

Dye-pulse laser energy is the safest form of lithotripsy but electrohydraulic lithotripsy can be used safely if it is performed carefully, under direct vision.[7] If a larger endoscope is used, baskets with a central lumen for the probe can be employed with increased safety. Because lithotripsy is usually performed when the stone is impacted, most of the time the basket cannot encircle the stone.

After the common bile duct is cleared, a decision must be made regarding the need for a drainage procedure. This decision can be made laparoscopically by performing a choledochoduodenostomy, Roux-en-Y choledochojejunostomy, or a postoperative or intraoperative facilitated endoscopic sphincterotomy. If a drainage procedure is not needed, a latex T-tube must be inserted entirely intracorporeally to avoid carbon dioxide (CO_2) loss and to allow easier manipulation of the T-tube. The "T" end should be inserted into the common bile duct as close to the duodenum as possible and a suture placed there to keep it in place. The next suture should be placed in the most proximal end of the choledochotomy and the two sutures lifted to facilitate the closure of the choledochotomy. The author's preference is to close the choledochotomy with interrupted sutures of Vicryl (Ethicon, Summerville, NJ) lubricated with mineral oil. The long end of the T-tube is then brought through the abdominal wall, and a cholangiogram is performed.

Results with this technique have been excellent. Franklin and coworkers have performed 80 procedures, leaving two retained calculi, and Berci and Cuschieri have performed 43 procedures, leaving one retained calculus.[8–11] The morbidity rate has been 5% and 7% and the mortality rate 1% and 2%, respectively (Table 13-1). Those who perform transcystic common bile duct exploration as the first technique in the treatment of common bile duct sphincterotomy (Arregui, Hunter, Petelin, DePaula, Phillips; Table 13-2) perform laparoscopic choledochotomy only in the most challenging cases of choledocholithiasis (10%).[4,7,12–14] This explains why the incidence of complications of laparoscopy choledochotomy (11%

TABLE 13-1
Laparoscopic Choledochotomy

Author	*Cases (n)*	*Morbidity (%)*	*Retained Stones (%)*	*Mortality (%)*
PRIMARY METHOD OF COMMON BILE DUCT EXPLORATION				
Franklin, et al[8–10]	80	5	2.5	1
Berci and Cuschieri[11]	43	7	2.3	2
SECONDARY METHOD OF COMMON BILE DUCT EXPLORATION				
De Paula, et al[13]	12	17	8.3	8
Phillips, et al[14]	9	11	22	0

TABLE 13-2
Laparoscopic Transcystic Duct

	Common Bile Duct Exploration			
Study	*TCD # (# endoscoped)*	*Failed (%)*	*Complications*	*Deaths*
Berci and Cuschieri[11]	20	—	—	
Petelin[12]	80 (48)	3 (4)	5 (6)	1
DePaula,[13] et al	99 (37)	10 (10)	5 (5)	0
Phillips, et al[14]	97 (87)	7 (7)	5 (5)	1

to 17%) and retained stones (8% to 22%) is higher for these surgeons than if laparoscopic choledochotomy or even "open" common bile duct exploration is the primary method of stone removal (see Table 13-1).[8–11] Biliary drainage procedures should be performed in many of these difficult cases to reduce the incidence of retained stones. Endoscopic sphincterotomy or choledochoduodenostomy can be performed laparoscopically but because cases that require drainage procedures involve only 1% of all cases undergoing laparoscopic cholecystectomy, converting these cases to "open" surgery seems appropriate, except in the hands of experienced laparoscopic surgical teams.

References

1. Carroll BJ, Phillips EH, Daykhovsky L, et al: Laparoscopic choledochoscopy: an effective approach to the common duct. J Laparoendosc Surg 1992;2(1):15.
2. Phillips EH, Carroll BJ: New techniques for the treatment of common bile duct calculi encountered during laparoscopic cholecystectomy. Probl Gen Surg 1991;8(3):387.
3. Shimi S, Banting S, Cuschieri A: Transcystic drainage after laparoscopic exploration of common bile duct. Minimally Invasive Therapy 1992;1:273.
4. Hunter JG, Soper NJ: Laparoscopic management of bile duct stones. Surg Clin North Am 1992;72(5):1077.
5. Carroll BJ, Phillips EH: Laparoscopic transcystic duct balloon dilatation of the sphincter of Oddi. Surg Endosc 1993;7:514.
6. Appel SD: Wire guided cholangiography and transcystic common duct exploration. Third World Congress of Endoscopic Surgery. Bordeaux, France, June 1992, Session CLII. Abstract #123.
7. Arregui ME, Davis CJ, Arkush AM, Nagan RF: Laparoscopic cholecystectomy combined with endoscopic sphincterotomy and stone extraction or laparoscopic choledochoscopy and electrohydraulic lithotripsy for management of cholelithiasis with choledocholithiasis. Surg Endosc 1992;6:10.
8. Franklin ME: Laparoscopic choledochotomy for management of common bile duct stones and other common bile duct diseases. In: Arregui ME, ed. Principles of laparoscopic surgery. New York: Springer-Verlag, 1994.
9. Franklin ME, Dorman JP: Laparoscopic common bile duct exploration. In: Braverman M, ed. Surgical technology international. Vol 2. San Francisco: Surgical Technology International, 1993.
10. Franklin ME, Pharand D, Rosenthal D: Laparoscopic common bile duct exploration. In: Zucker KA, ed. Surgical laparoscopy and endoscopy. New York: Raven Press, 1994.
11. Berci G, Cuschieri A: Practical laparoscopy. London: Bailliere Tindall, 1986.
12. Petelin JB: Laparoscopic approach to common duct pathology. Am J Surg 1993;165:487.
13. DePaula AL, Hashiba K, Bafutto M, Zago R: Laparoscopic management of choledocholithiasis. Surg Endosc. In press.
14. Phillips EH, Carroll JB, Pearlstein AR, Daykhovsky L, Fallas MJ: Laparoscopic choledochoscopy and extraction of common bile duct stones. World J Surg 1993;17:22.

Chapter 14

Laparoscopic Surgery: An Atlas for General Surgeons, edited by Gary C. Vitale, Joseph S. Sanfilippo, and Jacques Perissat. J. B. Lippincott Company, Philadelphia, © 1995.

Management of Biliary Complications After Laparoscopic Cholecystectomy

Claude Liguory
Gary C. Vitale

Laparoscopic cholecystectomy has greatly simplified the surgical process for many patients having symptomatic gallstones. For others, however, an associated intraoperative bile duct injury has greatly complicated their course, leading to long hospitalization, multiple operations, or even death. Appropriate initial recognition of the injury to the bile duct, accurate diagnosis of the postinjury ductal anatomy, and prompt treatment are essential to good outcome.[1–7] Use of interventional endoscopic techniques to definitively treat selected bile duct injuries is an acceptable alternative to standard open surgical repair, and this topic forms the basis of this chapter.[8]

Endoscopic retrograde cholangiopancreatography (ERCP) with stone extraction has been well accepted by surgeons but therapeutic measures such as endoscopic sphincterotomy for bile leaks or stenting for benign bile duct strictures are more controversial.[9–11] Endoscopic retrograde cholangiopancreatography is the procedure of choice for investigating the possibility of postoperative bile duct injury after cholecystectomy. Although computed tomography (CT) scanning or ultrasound may have a role in diagnosing a subhepatic bile collection or dilation of the biliary tree, ERCP definitively demonstrates the exact nature of the ductal injury. Management can be determined with full knowledge of the extent of injury; a therapeutic endoscopic intervention can be proposed at the time of diagnosis, if appropriate. The complexity of the injury, the patient's age, and medical risks help to determine whether an operative or endoscopic approach should be used.

Percutaneous transhepatic cholangiography (PTC) has been suggested as the best procedure for diagnosis in cases of severe bile duct injury because it can delineate proximal anatomy when the bile duct has been completely transected. Although this is true, opacification of the bile ducts may be difficult because the ducts are rarely dilated early, particularly when there is a leak to decompress the biliary system. At a later time for patients presenting with ductal obstruction and jaundice, PTC may be easier to perform and may yield more information than ERCP. Transhepatic routes for stricture dilation and stenting require hepatic tract dilation, and risk of infection or bleeding is high, approaching 20% to 30% in complex cases. Thus, we reserve PTC for selected indications, such as preoperative internal external drain placement to assist with intraoperative identification and anastomosis of ductal tissue in high bilateral duct excisions.

Injuries to the extrahepatic biliary system during cholecystectomy commonly present with abdominal pain, fever, or abdominal distention. If a drain was placed at operation, copious drainage may be present; if no drain was used, bile may leak through one of the abdominal wall puncture sites. Biochemical profile usually demonstrates mildly elevated liver functions; the white blood count may be elevated. Jaundice and cholangitis occur next and are clear indicators of bile duct injury. Some patients present with sepsis of unclear etiology. A CT scan may be obtained and may show bile ascites, subhepatic abscess, or simple dilation of the biliary system. Ultrasound may be performed but CT scan is more complete in demonstrating loculated fluid collections or interloop abscesses that may occur from a bile leak. A hepatobiliary scan may demonstrate extravasation of bile from the biliary system (in case of leak) or obstruction to flow (in case of a stenosis or clip across the duct). An abnormality

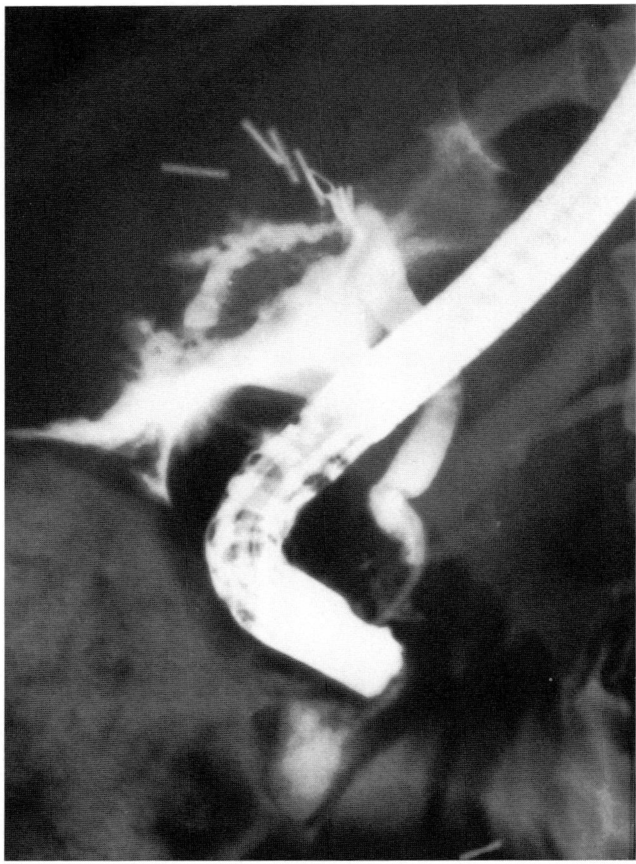

FIGURE 14-1. Common bile duct, obstructed by transversely placed metallic clips. When associated with contrast leak (as pictured here), one must be concerned about excisional loss of common duct tissue above clips.

in any of the aforementioned studies should prompt performance of an ERCP to more accurately assess ductal anatomy. If a patient is not doing well, particularly if septic complications are present, an ERCP should be performed even if the CT, ultrasound, and hepatobiliary scans are normal. Clipping of the bile duct can be partial or complete. Endoscopic retrograde cholangiopancreatography demonstrates complete or partial obstruction of the bile duct at the level of a metallic clip seen fluoroscopically (Fig. 14-1). The image must be confirmed in two views to ascertain clip location in relation to intraductal contrast. Surgical removal of the clip is the best treatment in all cases of clipping of the common duct. In cases of complete obstruction one must be concerned about a transection of the common duct above the clip. Access to the proximal biliary system is impossible endoscopically, and surgical exploration is warranted for clip removal and examination of the common duct. This may be done laparoscopically and converted to laparotomy if concomitant ductal injury is present. If the clip is only tangentially applied to the common duct, endoscopic balloon dilation may push the clip laterally enough to create

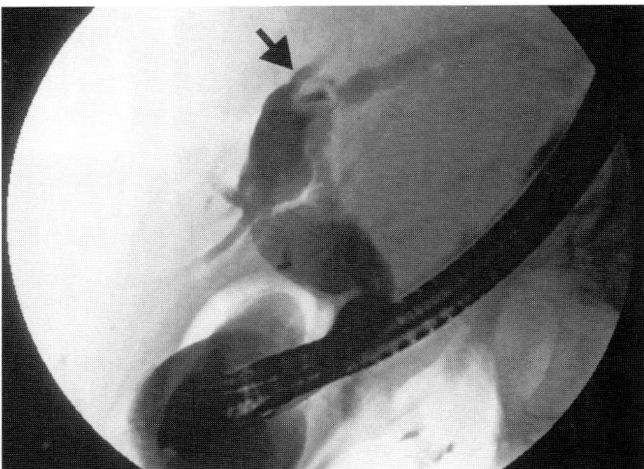

FIGURE 14-2. Common bile duct stone associated with metallic clips. The clips moved with the stone when the stone was retrieved.

a normal-appearing lumen to the bile duct by cholangiogram but the clip is most likely still applied to the biliary tissue. Laparoscopic or open operative removal of the clip is still the best treatment because this reduces the possibility of stricture or late migration of the clip into the bile duct (Figs. 14-2 and 14-3).

Simple cystic duct stump leak can usually be treated by sphincterotomy alone or with stent placement. The decompression of the biliary system afforded by sphincterotomy or stenting usually allows spontaneous closure of the leak. If there is an adjacent subhepatic fluid collection, percutaneous drainage should be performed. Leak-

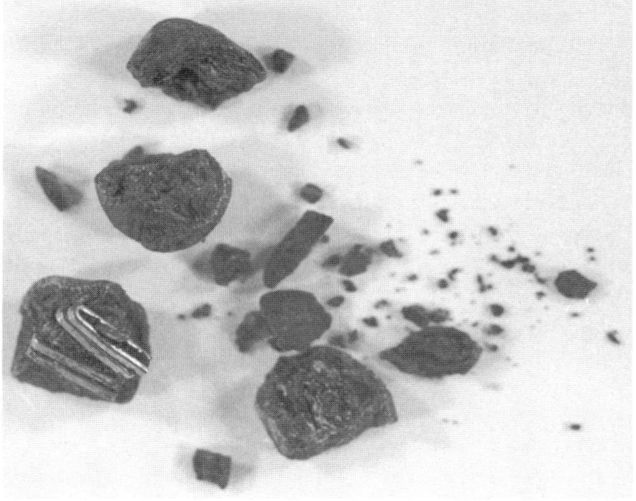

FIGURE 14-3. Common bile duct stone pictured in Figure 14-2. Fracture of stone revealed metallic clips inside. The stone had formed around these clips when they migrated into the common bile duct after being placed at the cystic duct–common bile duct junction years earlier during cholecystectomy.

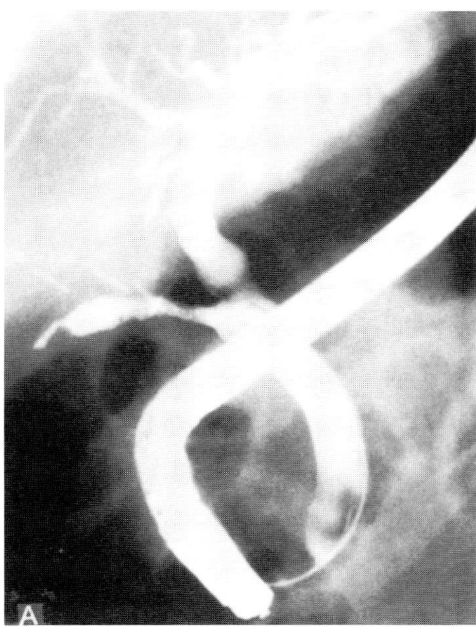

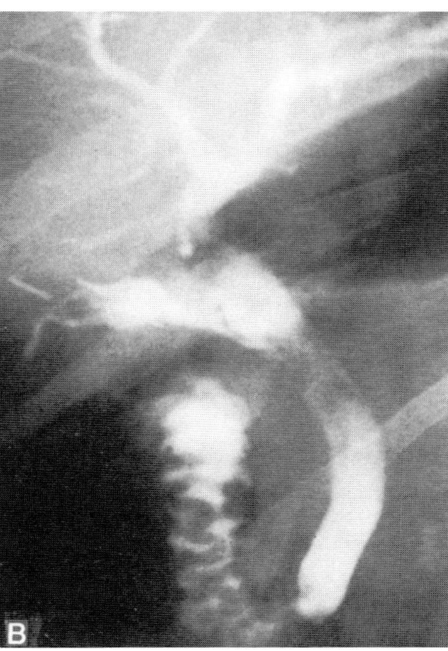

FIGURE 14-4. (**A**) Cystic duct stump leak, with unexpected distal common bile duct stone identified by ERCP. (**B**) Sphincterotomy and stone retrieval was sufficient to treat the cystic duct leak in this case.

age from the undersurface of the liver in the dissected bed of the gallbladder can be treated in a similar fashion. A small leak from an accessory duct in the right hepatic ductal system is often the culprit and responds well to sphincterotomy alone. Larger leaks should be stented.[12] Percutaneous subhepatic drainage may be necessary unless these leaks are identified early. In some of these cases, ERCP reveals distal obstruction from a previously unsuspected common duct stone or ampullary stenosis that has precipitated the leak by increasing intrabiliary pressure (Figs. 14-4 and 14-5).

A tangential or partial transection of the common duct, if identified at the time of the initial surgery, should be repaired by an open operation. Repair over a T-tube may be possible but the surgeon should be aware that the incidence of stricture post–T-tube removal is high. This may be because of the extensive circumferential dissection that occurs if the bile duct is mistakenly thought to be cystic duct or even gallbladder during the early part of the laparoscopic procedure (Figs. 14-6 and 14-7). Electrocautery injury may also play a role. Consideration should be given to endoscopic placement of a

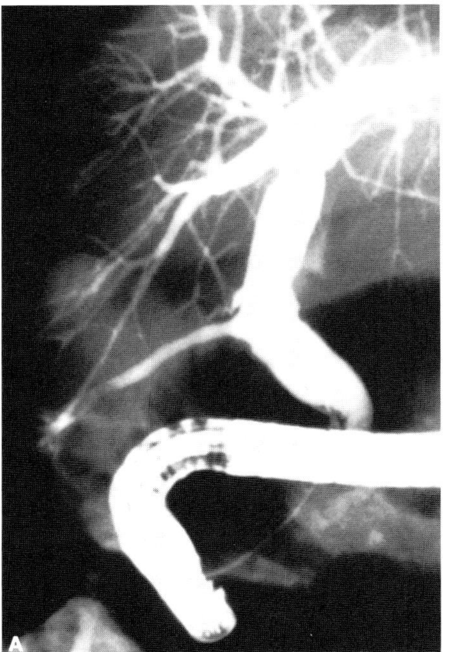

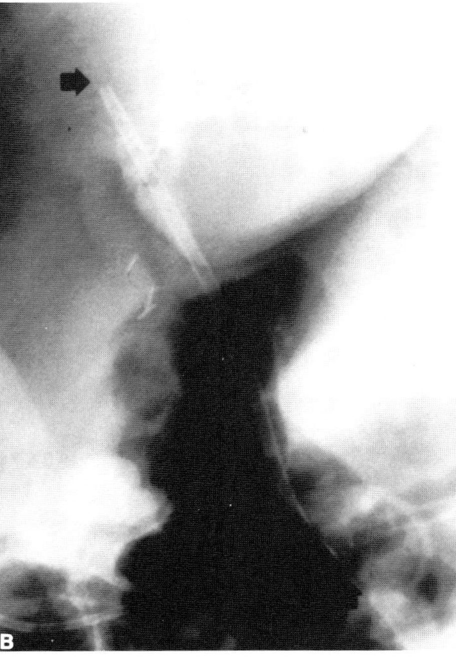

FIGURE 14-5. Common bile duct fistula after T-tube removal. (**A**) Fistula closed after sphincterotomy and stent placement (*arrow* indicates top of 10-French stent). (**B**) In this case, ampullary stenosis kept the fistula open by increasing intrabiliary pressure.

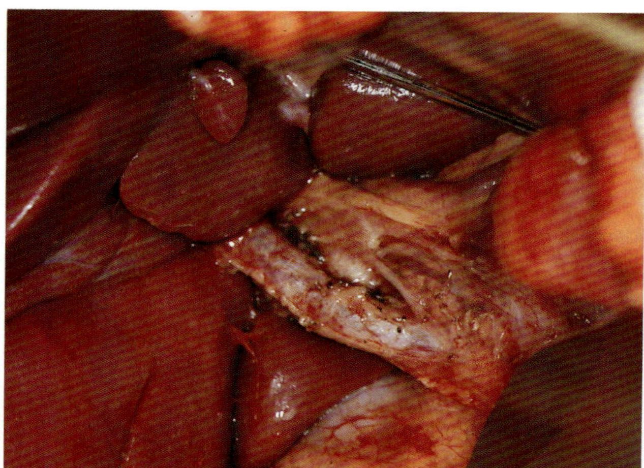

FIGURE 14-6. Unusual case in which ultrasound showed a contracted, scarred gallbladder. Extensive laparoscopic dissection revealed that what was first thought to be gallbladder was actually a mildly dilated common bile duct. The common bile duct after dissection is shown.

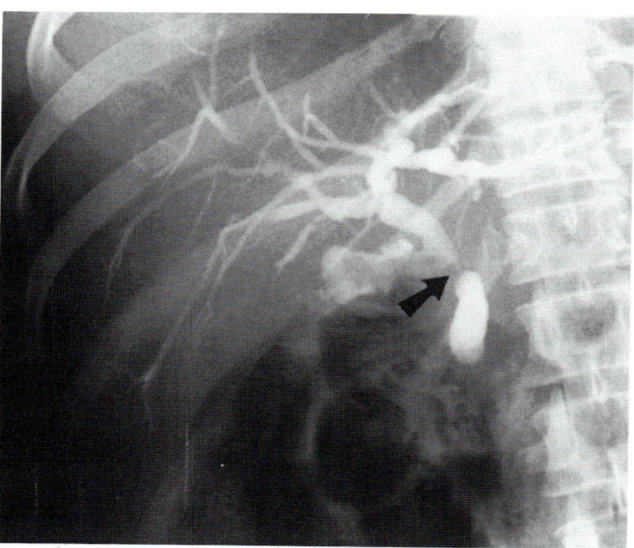

FIGURE 14-8. Stricture of common bile duct after repair of a tangential common bile duct injury over a T tube. *Arrow* indicates stricture, as it appeared 2 months after T-tube removal.

large stent (10 or 11.5 French) at the time of T-tube removal, particularly in cases with any tangential loss of ductal tissue or for injuries involving more than 50% of the ductal diameter. These injuries are at high risk for stricture, and stenting early may decrease the incidence of subsequent stricture formation. The ability to maintain ductal caliber during the healing process is certainly preferable to dilating the stricture after the scarring process and stricture formation has taken place. Endoscopic stenting should last from 6 months to 1 year, depending on the nature of the injury and presence of stricture. The stent is changed every 3 months and should be accompanied by endoscopic balloon dilation if ERCP demonstrates any narrowing at the site of the injury (Figs. 14-8 through 14-10).

If partial transection is not identified at the initial surgery, it presents as abscess, fistula, or stricture. The combination of fistula and stricture is common (Figs. 14-11 through 14-14). Endoscopic stenting is clearly an option in these cases, as long as infection can be controlled. If sepsis remains a problem after initial stenting, open operation is indicated. At operation, debridement of infected tissue and adequate drainage are necessary in addition to definitive repair (Fig. 14-15). In most cases with extensive infection, a repair over a T-tube is unlikely

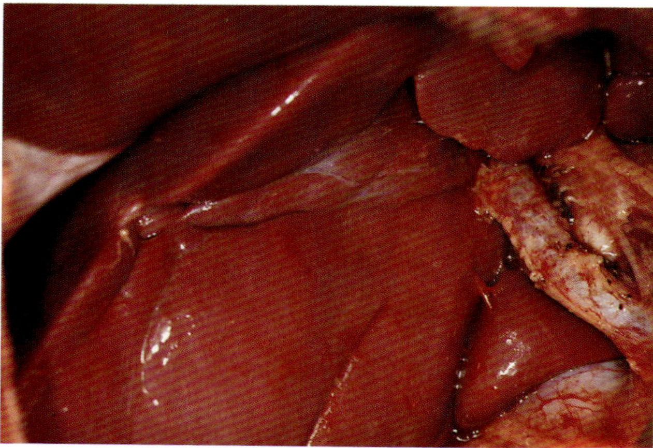

FIGURE 14-7. When a gallbladder could not be found laparoscopically in the patient described in Figure 14-6, open operation revealed that the patient had congenital absence of the gallbladder. The empty gallbladder fossa in the liver is shown. Although the common bile duct had been initially misidentified as a contracted gallbladder and was extensively dissected, no ductal injury occurred at operation and 3-year follow-up documents no late occurrence of stricture.

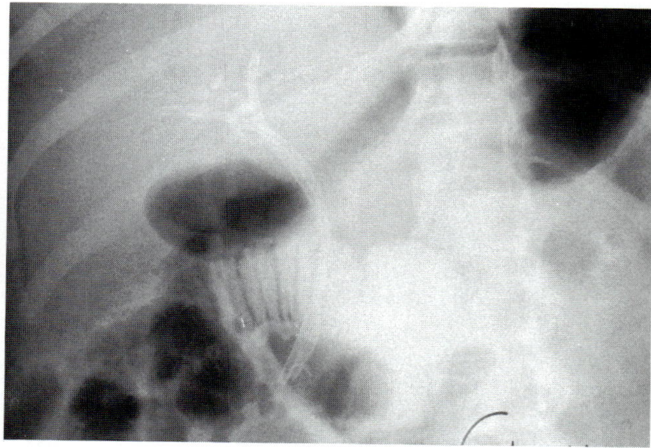

FIGURE 14-9. Insertion of two 10-French stents side-by-side into bile duct after dilation of the common bile duct stricture shown in Figure 14-8.

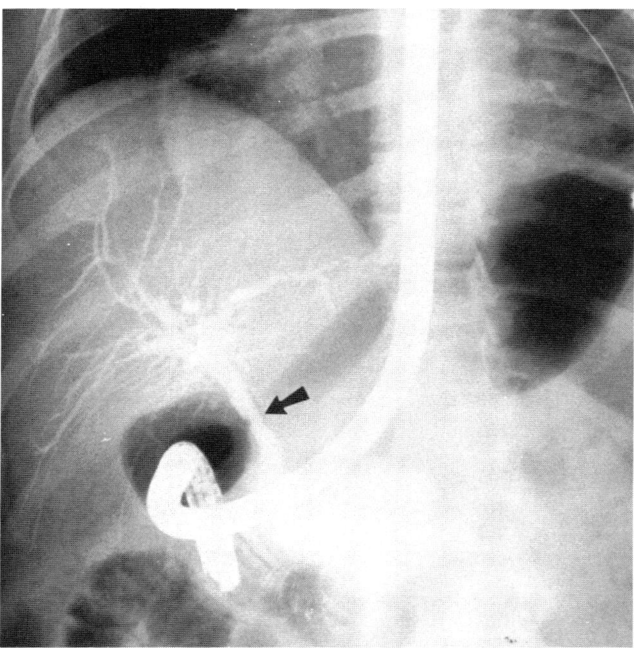

FIGURE 14-10. Common bile duct after 1 year of stenting. *Arrow* indicates the level of previous stricture. This patient is now 3 years post–common bile duct injury, with no clinical evidence of recurrent stricture.

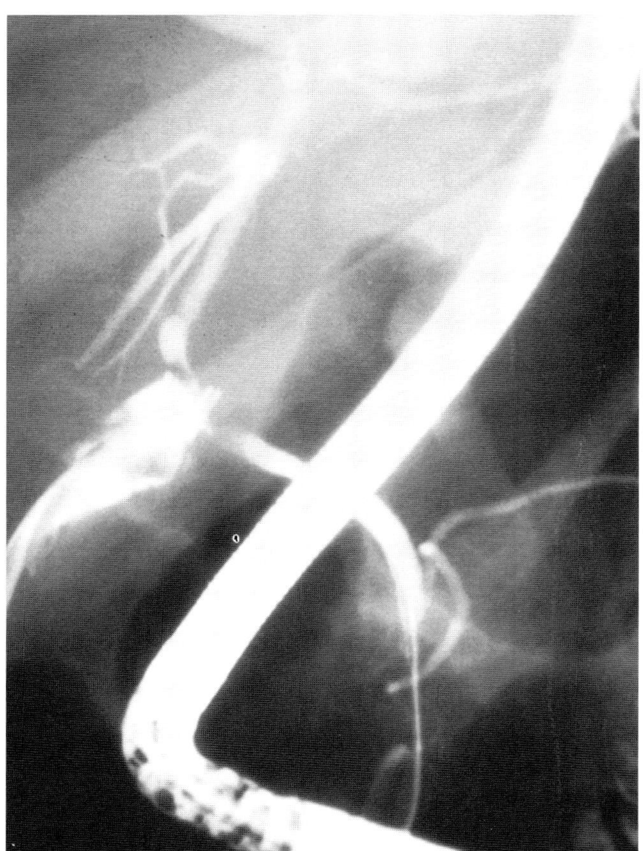

FIGURE 14-11. Common hepatic duct stricture and associated fistula after laparoscopic cholecystectomy.

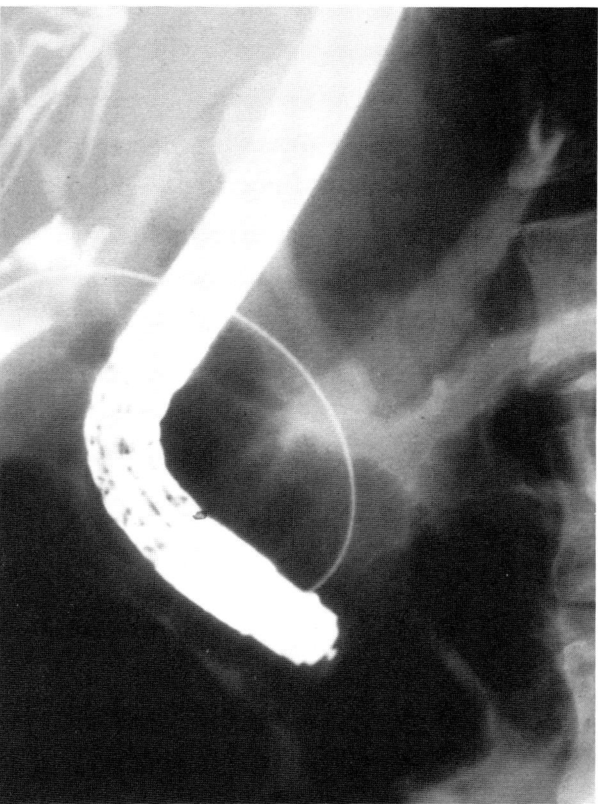

FIGURE 14-12. Guide wire is passed through the area of injury (same patient as in Fig. 14-11), which is just above the level of the cystic duct clips.

to be successful long term, and excision of the injury site with the use of a Roux-en-Y choledochojejunal anastomosis is recommended (Fig. 14-16). Frequently, the injuries are at or below the level of insertion of the cystic duct. In these cases, the duct should be excised to just below the level of the junction of right and left hepatic ducts. Failure to do this may increase chances of anastomotic stenosis due to poor choledochal blood supply at the distal end of the common duct where the anastomosis is being performed. If it occurs, anastomotic stricture may be treated with anastomotic dilation, with or without stenting by the percutaneous transhepatic route. If a choledochoduodenal anastomosis or a non–Roux-en-Y jejunal loop has been used in the repair, an endoscopic approach is possible and should be attempted first (Figs. 14-17 through 14-19). The ease of internal stent exchanges by the endoscopic route and risk of hemorrhage or problems due to infection with external percutaneous drains are reasons to proceed endoscopically first, if possible.

Endoscopic stenting of strictures and fistulas resulting from partial transection or electrocautery burn of the common bile duct, common hepatic duct, or right or left hepatic ducts is an acceptable treatment option,

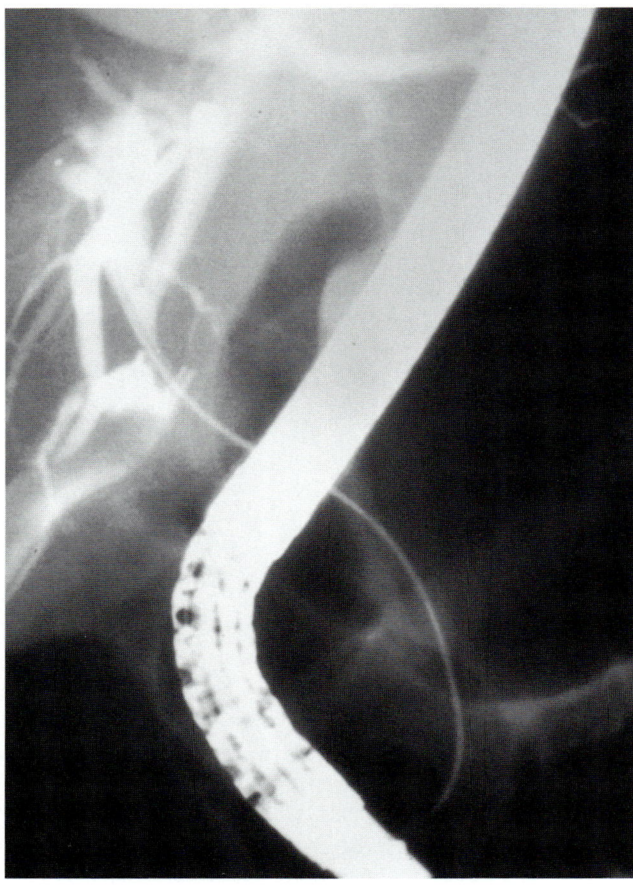

FIGURE 14-13. Guide wire is repositioned across the stricture and area of injury to allow dilation and stenting (same patient as in Fig. 14-11).

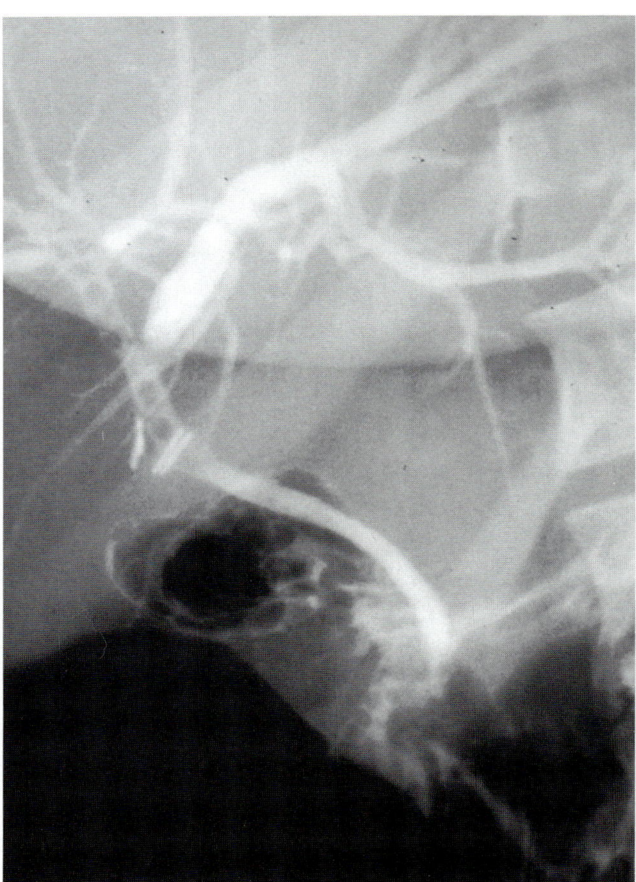

FIGURE 14-14. Common bile duct at 6 months after injury, demonstrating normal caliber and good drainage of contrast through area of prior stricture.

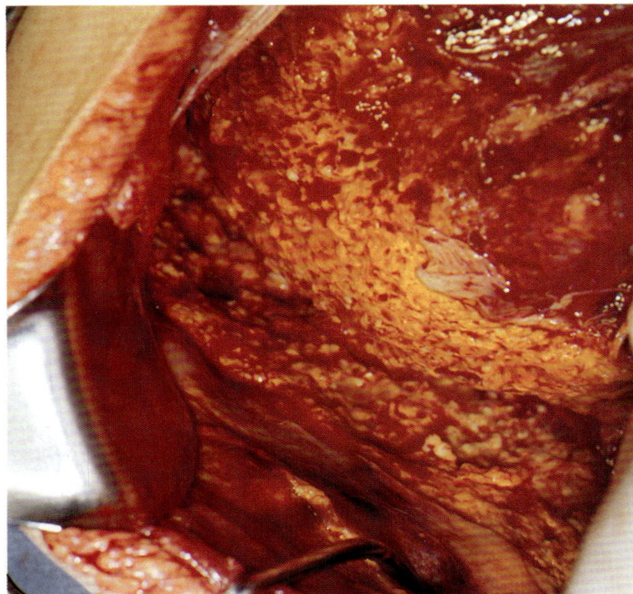

FIGURE 14-15. Severely inflamed dome of liver and peritoneum of right upper quadrant in young woman with a bile duct injury, which went unrecognized for 6 weeks. The severity of inflammation and presence of abscess limit application of interventional endoscopic techniques.

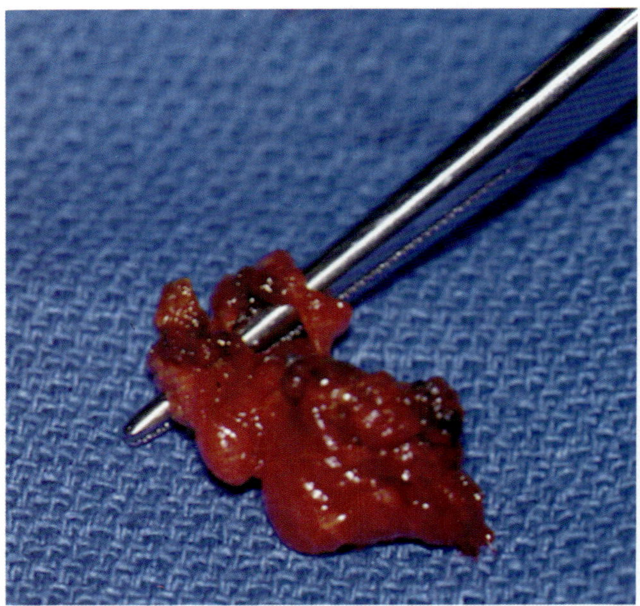

FIGURE 14-16. Segment of bile duct excised in same patient as in Figure 14-15. Forceps through lumen of bile duct show tangential injury to the wall of the bile duct, with loss of some tissue. This injury was repaired with a Roux-en-Y choledochojejunostomy, and the patient is doing well 2 years postinjury.

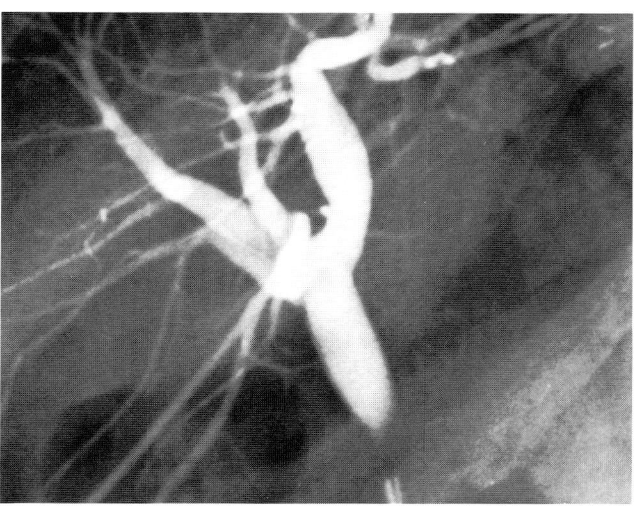

FIGURE 14-17. Stricture of choledochoduodenal anastomosis after repair of complete common bile duct transection.

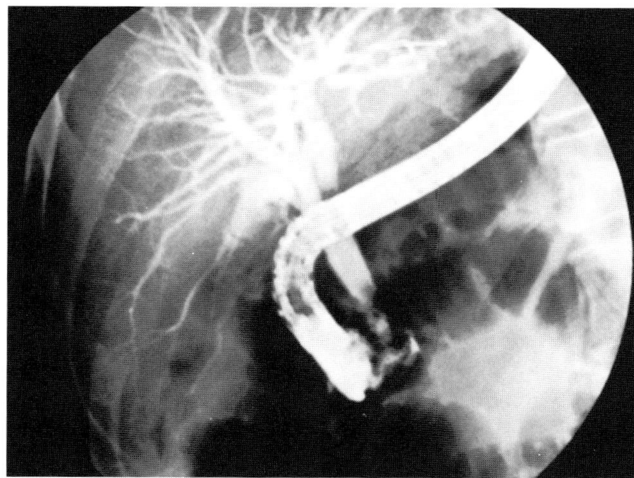

FIGURE 14-19. Anastomosis after 3 months of stenting (same patient as in Fig. 14-17).

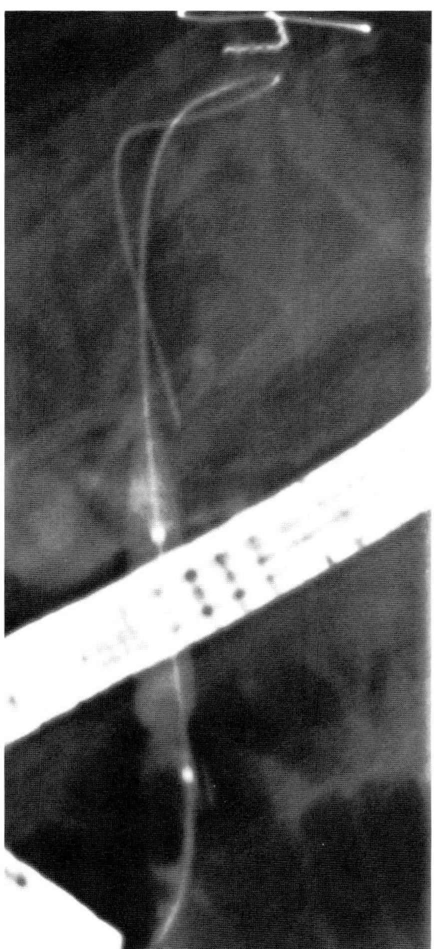

FIGURE 14-18. Endoscopic balloon dilation of anastomosis shown in Figure 14-17. Anastomosis was subsequently stented with two 10-French stents.

with good outcome documented in 80% of cases. These results are not significantly different from long-term results reported after operative treatment.[13–16] Best results are obtained in cases with shorter strictures occurring in larger ducts but all strictures that can be traversed with a guide wire and dilation catheters or balloon are amenable to an endoscopic approach. The endoscopic approach should clearly be used for higher-level strictures and fistulas because operation for these frequently nondilated smaller ducts may have a higher incidence of postoperative stricture. Also, older patients, with their attendant higher operative risk and shorter remaining lifespan, are more ideal candidates for an endoscopic approach. The endoscopic technique consists of passing a guide wire across the stricture, performance of a small sphincterotomy, and passing of a 10-French or 11.5-French polyethylene stent across the stricture. Dilation is often required, and axial balloon dilators or sequential passage dilators may be passed over guide wires before stenting. Stents are changed routinely on a 3- to 4-month basis; one should avoid leaving the stents unchanged for longer periods because obstruction and cholangitis occur and may produce inflammation and edema, which promote scar formation.

The length of time required for treatment of complex strictures is a year or more of intermittent balloon dilation and stenting, progressing from single 10-French stents potentially to double (side by side) 11.5-French stents (Figs. 14-20 through 14-25). Consideration should be given to operative repair for longer or more complex strictures in younger patients. If the stricture is located in a position of easy surgical access (i.e., the common bile duct or common hepatic duct) and the patient is young, without high surgical risk, a single definitive operative intervention may be preferable to the endoscopic approach. One factor that is not clear from reported se-

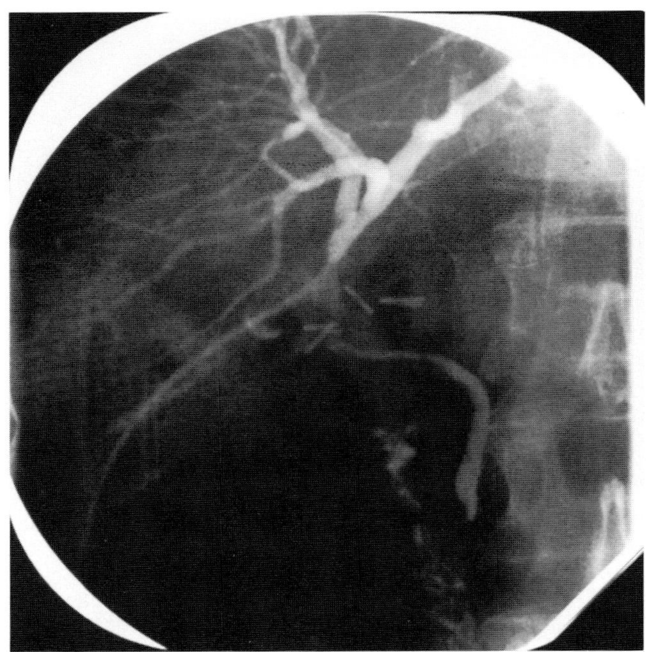

FIGURE 14-20. Severe stricture of common hepatic duct at presentation, shortly after laparoscopic cholecystectomy. A 7-French stent was placed through the stricture at this time.

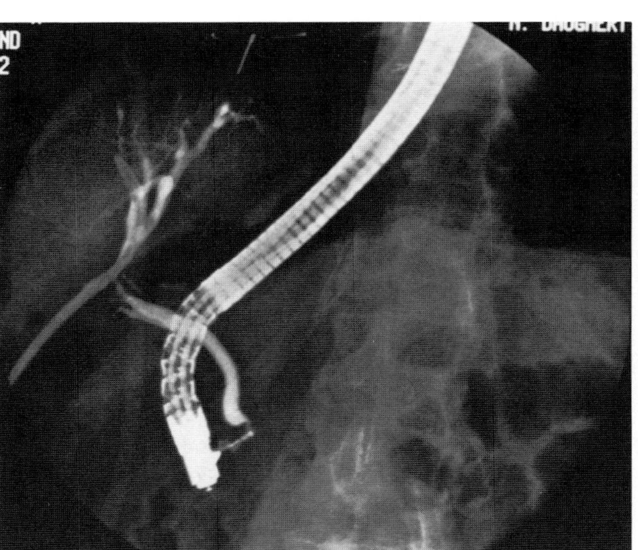

FIGURE 14-21. Stricture after removal of 7-French stent 2 months later (same patient as in Fig. 14-20).

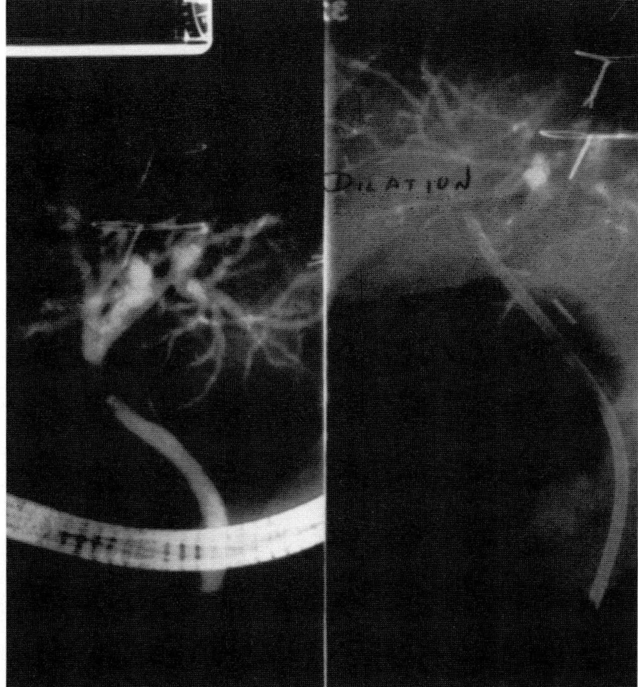

FIGURE 14-22. Stricture after balloon dilation and placement of a 10-French stent 5 months after injury (same patient as in Fig. 14-20).

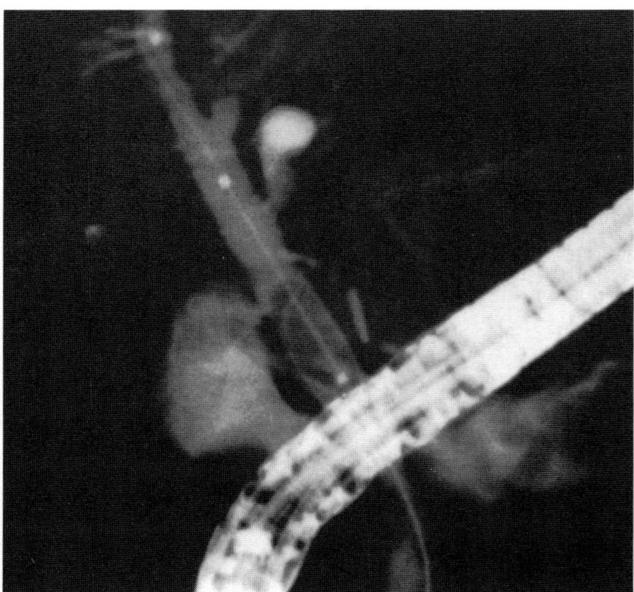

FIGURE 14-23. Endoscopic balloon dilation of stricture, using an 8-mm diameter balloon dilator. Balloon is seen in place across stricture in this radiograph (same patient as in Fig. 14-20).

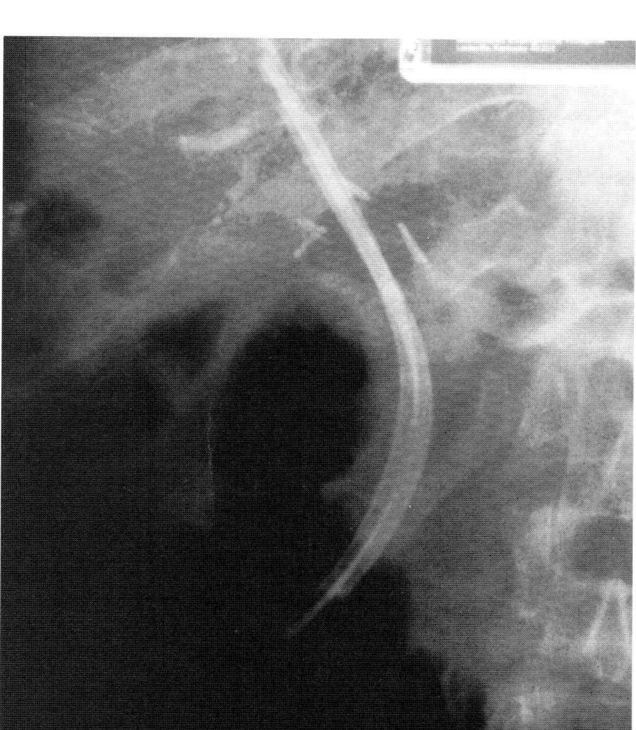

FIGURE 14-24. Nine months after injury, two 10-French stents are placed across the stricture after balloon dilation seen in Figure 14-23.

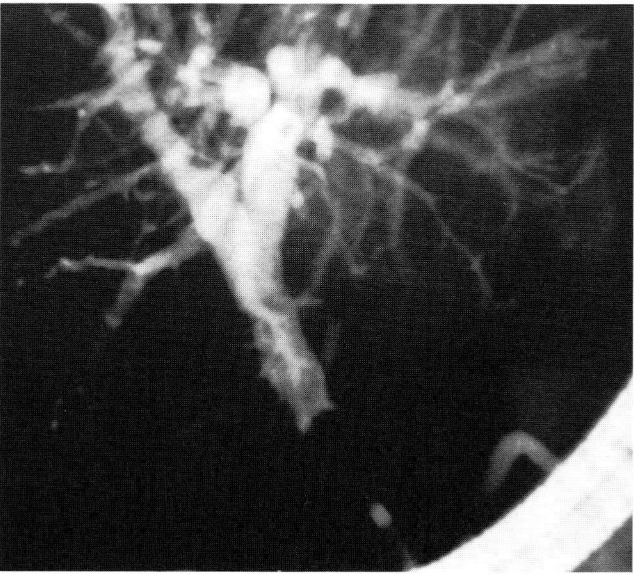

FIGURE 14-25. Bile duct opacification at 1 year after injury reveals a normal caliber bile duct, with good intrahepatic drainage through the area of previous stricture (same patient as Fig. 14-20). The reverse meniscus is a balloon-tipped catheter used to fill the bile duct. The patient is 2 years postinjury and 1 year post–stent removal, with normal liver functions.

ries of bile duct injuries treated by stenting is whether there is a significant incidence of late stricture recurrence. Thus, these patients require careful lifelong follow-up to avoid the possibility of partial bile duct obstruction, leading to chronic hepatic injury and biliary cirrhosis. The time frame of surgical anastomotic stenosis has been documented and if it is going to occur, it usually occurs within the first year after operation. Although there is an incidence of late anastomotic stricturing, operation may still be the best choice for younger patients, who for whatever reason may be difficult cases, to be sure of long-term careful follow-up. Failure of an initial endoscopic approach with recurrent stenosis after stent removal can be treated operatively without untoward effects.

Complete transection of the common bile duct, with or without excision of ductal tissue, is best treated by open repair, using a Roux-en-Y limb of jejunum (Fig. 14-26). These injuries are usually discovered at surgery

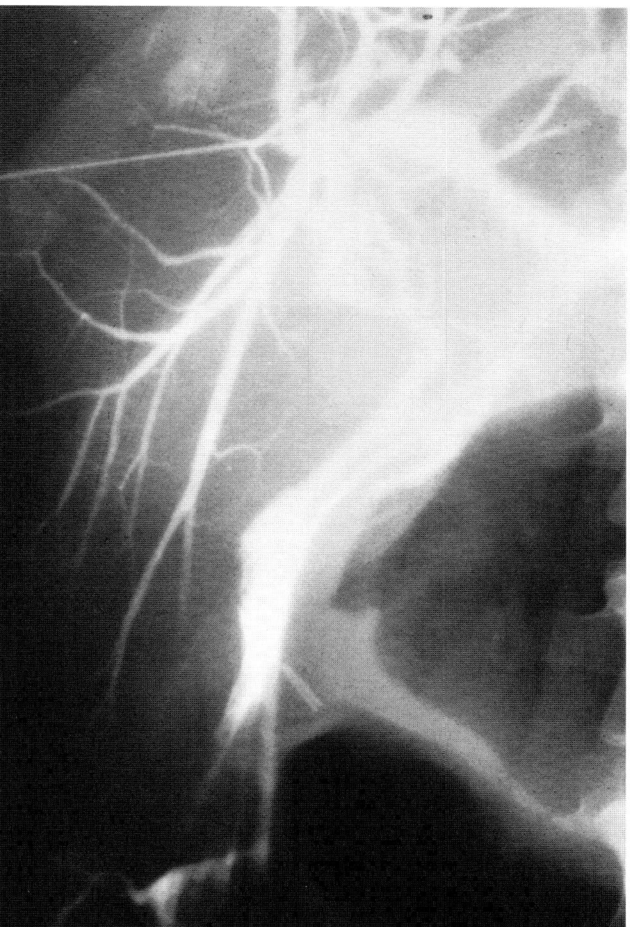

FIGURE 14-26. Percutaneous transhepatic cholangiogram in patient with laparoscopic excision of a segment of common duct. Cholangiogram reveals loss of duct and extravasation of contrast.

or early postoperatively and should be operated on as soon as possible; in occasional cases, patients may be mistakenly treated with antibiotics and external drainage for long periods before being referred for definitive repair. Late operation is fraught with difficulty due to severe cholangitis. In these cases, instead of dilating, the ductal tissue becomes severely edematous, with almost no lumen available for anastomosis, even in the intrahepatic ducts. The lack of continuity of proximal and distal bile duct makes an endoscopic approach impossible, but a transhepatic catheter greatly assists the operative approach if the catheter can be passed to the level of the common hepatic duct or to the porta hepatis in cases of ductal excision. The use of endoscopic stenting for stricture resulting from initial operative repair of a complete transection is possible but the possibility of recurrent stenosis would have to be considered high.

All patients who have undergone repair of a bile duct injury should have lifetime follow-up consisting of liver enzyme determination, including alkaline phosphatase and bilirubin on a yearly basis. Those who have had endoscopic dilation and stenting of complex bile duct injury should have an ERCP early after stent removal, at 3 to 6 months, and again at 1 year to 18 months post–stent removal to document biliary anatomy and evaluate for progressive stricture recurrence.

In summary, ERCP has an important role, both diagnostically and therapeutically, after laparoscopic cholecystectomy. Its ability to clearly define ductal anatomy is critical to subsequent plans for treatment; unexpected pathology such as ampullary stenosis or distal common duct stones may be found to be contributing to the problem.[17] Finally, interventional techniques of sphincterotomy and stenting may have a definitive management role in selected cases.[18]

References

1. Deyo GA: Complications of laparoscopic cholecystectomy. Surg Laparosc Endosc 1992;2:41.
2. Peters JH, Gibbons GD, Innes JT, et al: Complications of laparoscopic cholecystectomy. Surgery 1991;110:769.
3. Moossa AR, Easter EW, VanSonnenberg E, Casola G, D'Agostino H: Laparoscopic injuries to the bile duct. Ann Surg 1992;215:203.
4. Ferguson CM, Rattner DW, Warshaw AL: Bile duct injury in laparoscopic cholecystectomy. Surg Laparosc Endosc 1992;2:1.
5. Soper NJ, Brunt LM, Sicard GA, Edmundowicz SA: Diagnosis and management of biliary complications of laparoscopic cholecystectomy. Am J Surg 1993;165:663.
6. Davidoff AM, Pappas TN, Murray EA, et al: Mechanisms of major biliary injury during laparoscopic cholecystectomy. Ann Surg 1992;215:196.
7. Larson GM, Vitale GC, Casey J, et al: Multipractice analysis of laparoscopic cholecystectomy in 1,983 patients. Am J Surg 1991;163:221.
8. Vitale GC, Stephens G, Wieman TJ, Larson GM: Use of endoscopic retrograde cholangiopancreatography in the management of biliary complications after laparoscopic cholecystectomy. Surgery 1993;114:806.
9. Liguory C, Lefebvre JF, Bonnel D, Vitale GC: Crushing stones: mechanical, intracorporeal and extracorporeal lithotripsy in the clearance of common bile duct lithiasis. Can J Gastroenterol 1991;4:564.
10. Vitale GC: Interventional endoscopic retrograde cholangiopancreatography: state of the art. Part I. J R Coll Surg Edinb 1992;37:389.
11. Vitale GC: Interventional endoscopic retrograde cholangiopancreatography: state of the art. Part II. J R Coll Surg Edinb 1992;37:357.
12. Liguory C, Vitale GC, Lefebvre JF, Bonnel D, Cornud F: Endoscopic treatment of postoperative biliary fistulas. Surgery 1991;110:779.
13. Lillemoe KD, Pitt HA, Cameron JL: Postoperative bile duct strictures. Surg Clin North Am 1990;70:1355.
14. Pitt HA, Kaufman SL, Coleman J, et al: Benign postoperative biliary strictures: operate or dilate? Ann Surg 1989; 210:417.
15. Berkelhammer C, Kortan P, Haber GB: Endoscopic biliary prostheses as treatment for benign postoperative bile duct strictures. Gastrointest Endosc 1989;35:95.
16. Davids PHP, Rauws EAJ, Coene PPLO, Tygat GNJ, Huibregtse K: Endoscopic stenting for post-operative biliary strictures. Gastrointest Endosc 1992;38:12.
17. Cotton P: Endoscopic retrograde cholangiopancreatography and laparoscopic cholecystectomy. Am J Surg 1993; 165:474.
18. Traverso LW, Kozarek RA, Ball TJ, et al: Endoscopic retrograde cholangiopancreatography after laparoscopic cholecystectomy. Am J Surg 1993;165:581.

Chapter 15

Laparoscopic Surgery: An Atlas for General Surgeons, edited by
Gary C. Vitale, Joseph S. Sanfilippo, and Jacques Perissat.
J. B. Lippincott Company, Philadelphia, © 1995.

Laparoscopic Appendectomy

Michael Edye
Denis Collet
Jacques Perissat

Conventional appendectomy through a short muscle–splitting incision is rapidly performed and returns good results, but laparoscopic access allows superior visualization and lavage of the peritoneal cavity. Additionally, irrespective of the site of the appendix or its pathology, it can usually be removed laparoscopically.[1]

INDICATIONS

Indications for laparoscopic appendectomy are not different from those of the open procedure. The surgical procedure is particularly useful in young women because it allows excellent simultaneous evaluation of the reproductive organs.

PRECAUTIONS

Preexisting cardiac or respiratory disease that may complicate general anesthesia is a point of concern. In small children, specially adapted instrumentation is advised.[2]

Instrumentation

The following instruments are necessary for the performance of laparoscopic appendectomy:

- Laparoscope (0°), light source, insufflator, video monitor, and camera
- Two or three 10-mm ports; one 5-mm port
- Mono- or bipolar diathermy
- Laparoscopic scissors, hook dissector, grasper, and Babcock forceps
- Irrigation–suction cannula, connected to physiologic saline at 37°C
- Absorbable ligature material (eg, braided 0-polyglycolic acid) that will allow a slip knot to be placed
- Disposable loop and slip knot (Endoloop, Ethicon-Endosurgery, Cincinnati, OH) or knot pusher

Preparation

A single dose of a broad-spectrum antibiotic that includes anaerobic coverage is administered preoperatively. A urinary catheter and a gastric tube are inserted. The patient is in a supine position. For female patients, it may be advantageous to have vaginal access, should there be gynecologic disease.

The surgeon stands on the patient's left side, with the camera operator to the surgeon's right. The video monitor is placed on the patient's right, facing the surgeon (Fig. 15-1).

TECHNIQUE

A left hypochondral puncture for insufflation is recommended, although it is distant from the operative site. Close to the costal margin, the abdominal wall is more fixed, permitting easier penetration with the Veress needle. Adhesions are rare in this area and there is little risk of injury to an organ or major vessel. Insufflation proceeds to 10 TORR. The table is placed in a 10° to 15° Trendelenburg's position and tilted toward the operator.[3]

Because of the absence of a three-dimensional view, laparoscopic techniques are facilitated by (1) having instruments meet at the operative site, roughly at right angles; and (2) avoiding cannula sites, which orient the instruments too close to the optical axis.

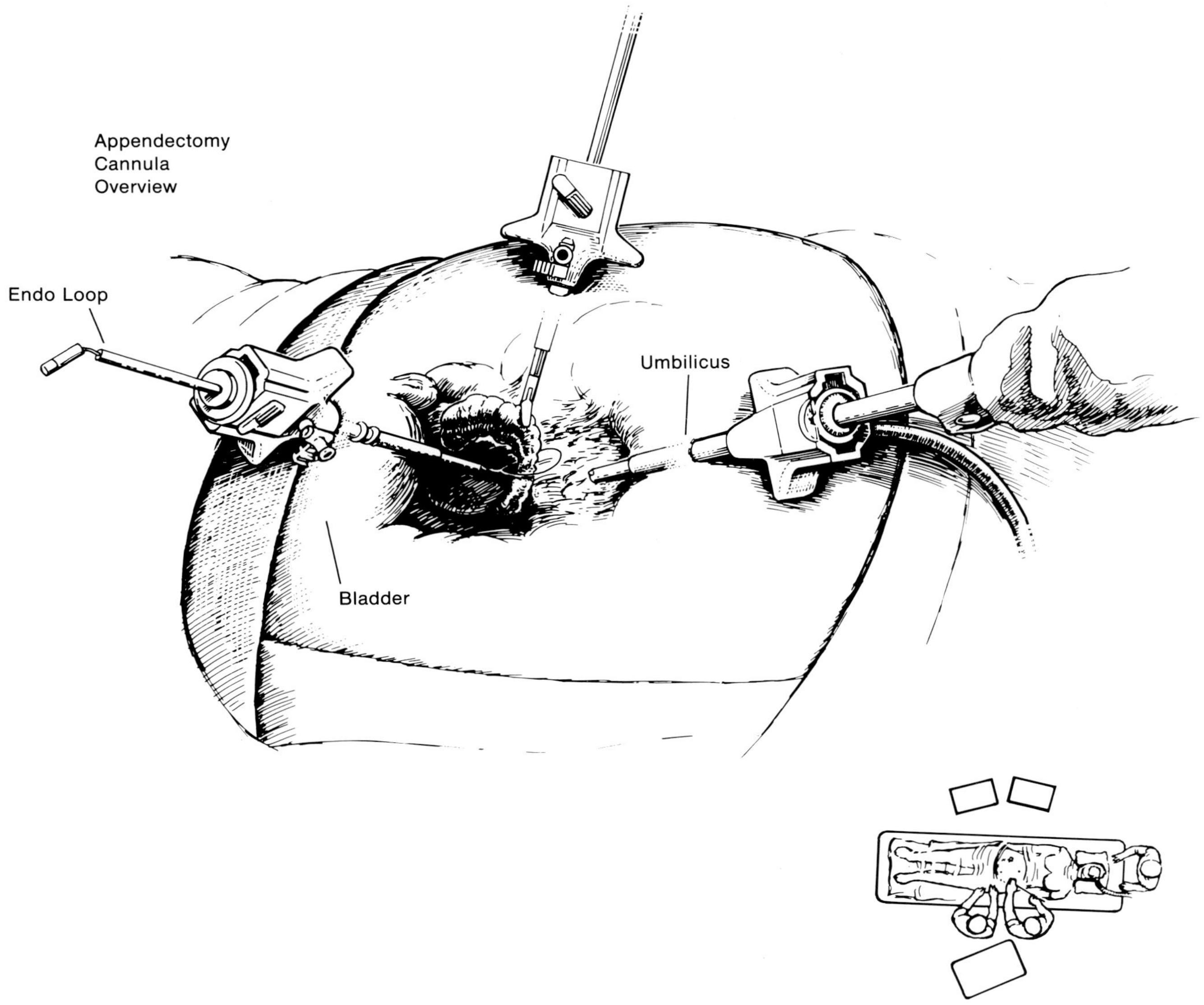

FIGURE 15-1. Positioning of trocars and surgeon.

Placing the cannulas at the corners of a broad-based isosceles triangle with the laparoscope at the apex usually achieves these goals.

A 10-mm trocar (port 1) for the 0° laparoscope is inserted through the umbilicus and directed toward the pelvis. If there is a lower abdominal scar, an 8-mm trocar should first be inserted in the left flank to inspect the umbilicus for adhesions. Alternatively, an open-insertion technique with a Hasson cannula can be used.

A 5-mm trocar (port 2) is inserted in or slightly left of the midline, just below the pubic hairline. The trocar must be sharp because the peritoneum is lax in this region and tents on the point. Transillumination of the inferior mesenteric vessels is helpful to avoid injury by a trocar. A blunt palpator or forceps is used to expose accessible structures, including the appendix.

Once the surgeon has decided to proceed with appendectomy, a 10-mm trocar (port 3) is inserted through the abdominal wall, directly over the appendix base or lower for cosmetic considerations.

A diagnostic laparoscopy is performed to permit inspection of the cecum, terminal ileum, and pelvic viscera in the female patient. If the appendix is not visibly inflamed, the small bowel is methodically inspected for the presence of a Meckel's diverticulum, and the mesentery is checked for inflamed or enlarged lymph nodes.

It may be necessary to mobilize the cecum to expose the appendix base (Fig. 15-2). Gentle application of the laparoscopic Babcock forceps to the teniae coli helps with retraction.

If accessible, the appendix is seized with the Babcock forceps through port 3 and pulled gently in the axis of

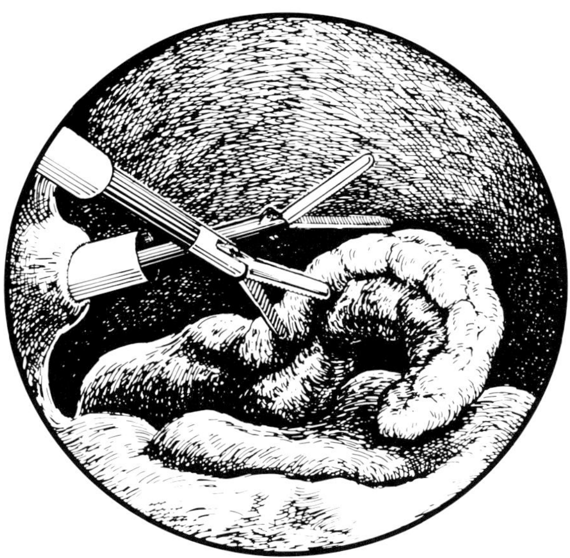

FIGURE 15-2. Appendix is dissected free from inflammatory attachments to the surrounding bowel.

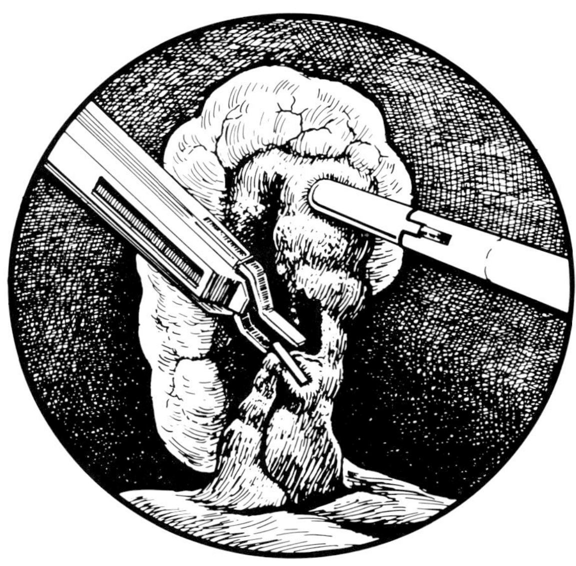

FIGURE 15-4. Arteries in the mesoappendix are divided between the clips.

the trocar port. The forceps handle can often be left to dangle, thus applying traction to the appendix and freeing a hand.

There are two ways to deal with the mesoappendix:

1. Coagulation of the mesentery close to the appendix, from the tip to the base, which seals the vessels where they are branched and small[4]
2. Placement of a ligature and extra- or intracorporeal knot or ligaclips around the mesoappendix after creation of a window adjacent to the base (Figs. 15-3 through 15-6)

It is unusual for ligation material to slip easily through a loaded trocar, and therefore it must be pulled firmly. If using an extracorporeal knot, a length of thread equal to more than twice the distance from cannula head to pedicle is fed through the cannula into the abdomen. The end is passed through the window and around the mesoappendix, withdrawn without tension to avoid "sawing the pedicle," and tied using a Roeder slip knot or knot pusher. If the mesoappendix is bulky, it may be safer to divide it into two or more stages.

In each case, the mesentery is divided close to the appendix to reduce its bulk and facilitate extraction. The

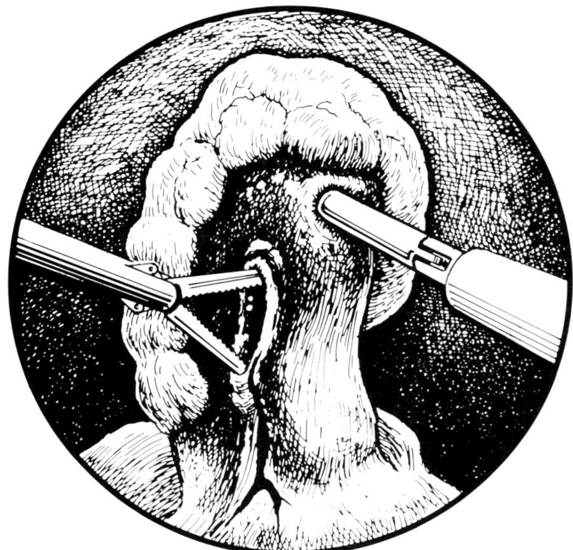

FIGURE 15-3. The mesoappendix is opened and the vessels are isolated.

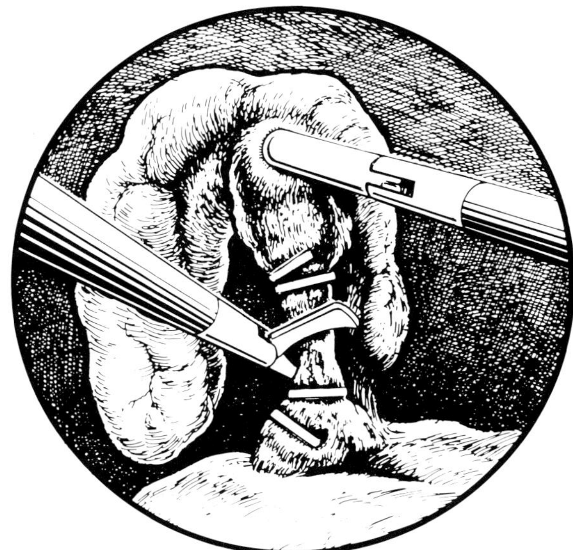

FIGURE 15-5. Arteries in the mesoappendix are clipped.

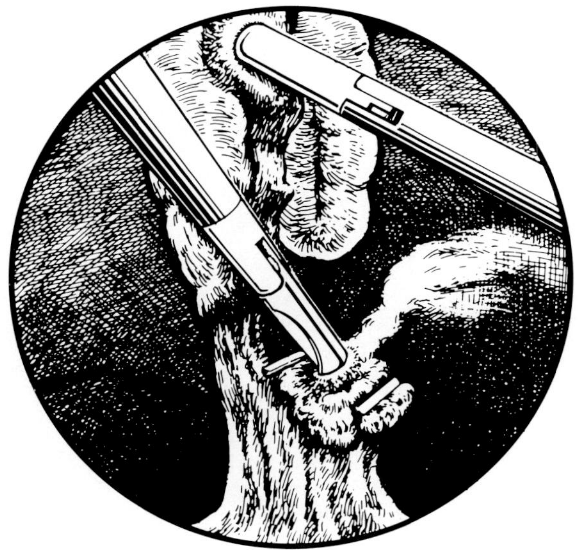

FIGURE 15-6. Cautery is applied to small vessels in mesoappendix.

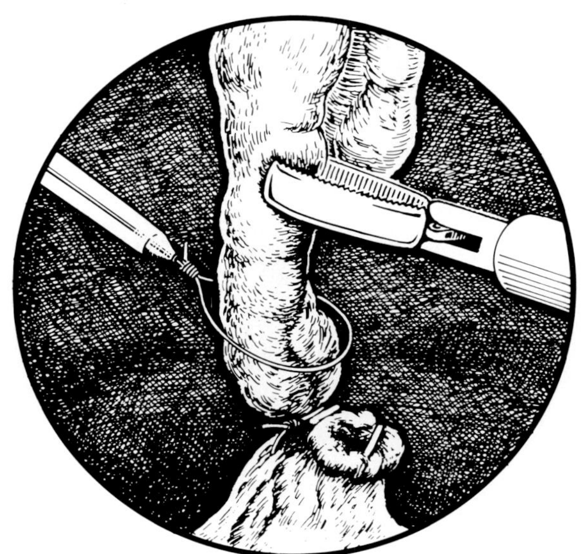

FIGURE 15-8. A second Endoloop is placed around the base of the appendix.

base is tied flush with two Endoloop sutures and divided (Figs. 15-7 through 15-9).

The pouch of Douglas is checked for exudate and irrigated and aspirated along with the operative field if necessary. If generalized peritonitis is present, careful lavage of the entire peritoneal cavity using copious volumes (2 to 3 L) of warm normal saline is necessary. Collections of loculated exudate are sought between the loops of small bowel, taking care to handle the inflamed, fragile structures gently.

Poking and firm grasping of inflamed bowel with narrow laparoscopic instruments is likely to perforate its wall. The subdiaphragmatic spaces are checked, and if necessary, a fourth trocar is inserted subcostally, so that the irrigation—aspiration cannula can reach them. It is usually necessary to tilt the table in several directions to achieve a thorough cleansing without being hindered by loops of bowel. Membranous exudate is peeled away where practicable.

If the diameter of the appendix permits, it is drawn into the port (3) and its base is divided flush with the cannula tube to reduce the chance of spillage (Fig. 15-10). The trocar containing the appendix is withdrawn; a finger is placed over the incision, controlling escape of

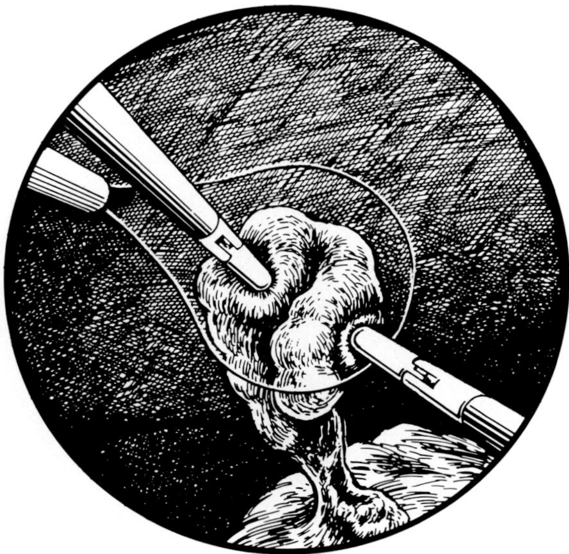

FIGURE 15-7. An Endoloop chronic suture is passed into the trocar port and placed around the appendix.

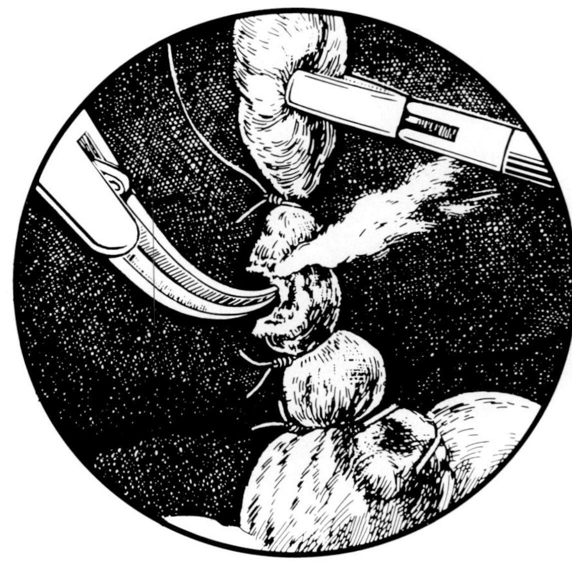

FIGURE 15-9. The appendix is divided near its junction with the cecum; two Endoloop ties secure the appendiceal stump.

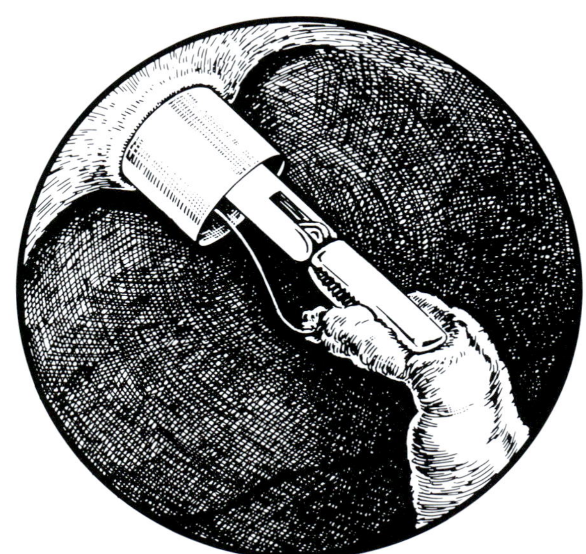

FIGURE 15-10. The appendix is removed through the trocar sleeve. If the appendix is large and fleshy, it should first be placed in a specimen bag.

gas; and a clean, nondisposable 10-mm cannula is reinserted. The mucosa of the stump is gently coagulated. No pursestring suture is necessary.

If the appendix is too thickened, it can be placed in a bag and extracted by slight dilation of the incision where trocar 3 was previously placed.

If the cecum is mobile and the abdominal wall thin, the abdomen is deflated and the appendix is drawn through the wound and divided after ligature, terminating the operation.

If indicated, a suction drain is placed in the pouch of Douglas through port 3. The puncture sites are inspected internally for bleeding before removal of the laparoscope.

The abdominal cavity is deflated, taking care to evacuate all CO_2; the fascial layer of the trocar sites are closed with absorbable sutures; and the skin is reapproximated with subcuticular sutures and adhesive strips.

AFTERCARE

Although laparoscopic removal of the appendix is performed in the same fashion as with an open procedure, it is usual to observe earlier return of intestinal transit. Patients can normally take fluids after 6 to 12 hours and solids when transit is established. Healthcare providers commonly underestimate the discomfort the patient has at the trocar sites. Although analgesic requirements may be reduced, one or two parenteral doses are often needed. A patient treated for a perforated appendix with local or general peritonitis should be expected to be more uncomfortable, with more delayed transit, when compared with less complicated pathology.

References

1. Nouaille JM: Techniques, resultats et limites de l'appendicectomie par voie coelioscopique. A propos de 360 malades. Chirurgie 1990;116:834.
2. Gans SL, Berci J: Peritoneoscopy in infants and children. J Pediatr Surg 1973;8:399.
3. Semm K: Endoscopic appendectomy. Endoscopy 1983;15:59.
4. Mouret P: L'abord coelioscopique de l'appendice. In: Testas P, Delaitre B, eds. Chirurgie digestive par voie coelioscopique. Paris: Maloine Ed, 1991:150.

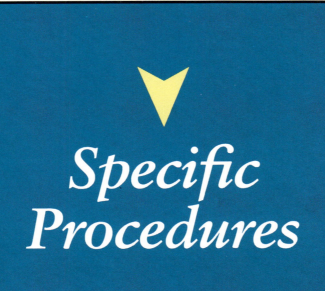

Specific Procedures

Chapter 16

Laparoscopic Surgery: An Atlas for General Surgeons, edited by Gary C. Vitale, Joseph S. Sanfilippo, and Jacques Perissat. J. B. Lippincott Company, Philadelphia, © 1995.

Laparoscopic Cholecystectomy: The French Experience

Jacques Perissat

In the history of surgery, few procedures have so rapidly changed the surgeon's custom of thinking and acting as has laparoscopic cholecystectomy. It has been the true detonator of the laparoscopic revolution in digestive surgery.

Laparoscopic cholecystectomy was developed in Lyon, France, in March 1987 by Mouret, a general surgeon who was highly skilled in gynecologic surgery and in the use of laparoscopy.[1] In 1988 in Paris, Dubois and coworkers—firm proponents of minilaparotomy for cholecystectomy—tried the laparoscopic method.[2] Rapidly, he improved his technique and began using it routinely. During the same year, the technique of internal lithotripsy for removing gallstones using a laparoscopic access was developed by the author. The gallbladder, once cleared of its stone contents, could easily pass through a 10-mm port after being dissected free from its duct, vessels, and peritoneal attachment.

First publications in 1989 about the technique of laparoscopic cholecystectomy and its results were received with skepticism and even criticism, mainly from academic circles.[3,4] In contrast, other physicians were enthusiastic. For the first time in the United States, a videotape of laparoscopic cholecystectomy using intracorporeal lithotripsy techniques was presented at the annual meeting of the Society of American Gastrointestinal Endoscopic Surgeons in Louisville, Kentucky, in April 1989.

By this time, Reddick and coworkers had already embarked on this technique, using laser surgery.[5] Thus began the revolution that would change the routine practice of all surgeons. As early as 1992, laparoscopic cholecystectomy had become the procedure of choice to remove the gallbladder with calculi for two main reasons: constant improvement of results and simplification of technique.

TECHNIQUE

Instruments

The basic instruments required for most laparoscopic surgical procedures are listed below (see Chap. 6 for details).

- A 10-mm direct laparoscope; an additional 10-mm scope with a 30° view may be useful under certain circumstances (e.g., obese patients, patients with hepatomegaly)
- Two 5-mm and two 10-mm trocars
- Two 5-mm forceps: one grasping forceps with teeth and one with nontraumatizing jaws and a sharp tip
- One 10-mm grasping "crocodile" forceps
- One forceps for cystic duct catheterization, for the intraoperative cholangiography
- One 10-mm curved dissector
- One 5-mm irrigation–suction cannula
- One bipolar electrocautery forceps
- One dissecting hook that can be connected to monopolar electrocautery
- One smooth spatula that can be connected to monopolar electrocautery
- One 10-mm clip applier

This equipment must also be available:

- A needle holder and 3-0 absorbable sutures set on 3/8″ 17-mm needles

- A Roeder loop ligature
- An adjustable camera holder
- An internal lithotriptor, either ultrasonic, or mechanical (laparolith)

Preparation of Patient and the Surgical Team

The patient, ideally wearing antithrombosis stockings, is placed in the supine position, with legs apart. The patient is firmly strapped on the table to permit rotation of the table. The surgeon stands or sits between the patient's legs. The first assistant is on the patient's left, the scrub nurse is on the patient's right, with the instrument table. A rack containing monitor, insufflator, light source, camera, and recording system is at the patient's head on the right side. An electrosurgical unit and a mobile radiograph machine are on the patient's left side. The table is rotated in proclive (reverse Trendelenberg) position (20° to 25°), with several degrees tilt into the left lateral decubitus position.

Procedure

INSUFFLATION AND PLACEMENT OF INSTRUMENTS

Insufflation is achieved with the Veress needle, which is introduced at the anterior mid-axillary line in the left hypochondrium, 3 cm below the costal margin. The abdomen is then progressively inflated and the pressure maintained at 10 mm.

A 10-mm trocar (for the laparoscope), inserted through the umbilicus, is directed toward the liver. Once the laparoscope is placed, the surgeon must check the intra-abdominal position of the tip of the Veress needle in the left hypochondrium and inspect the entire abdominal cavity.

A second trocar (port 1; Fig. 16-1) is placed 1 cm

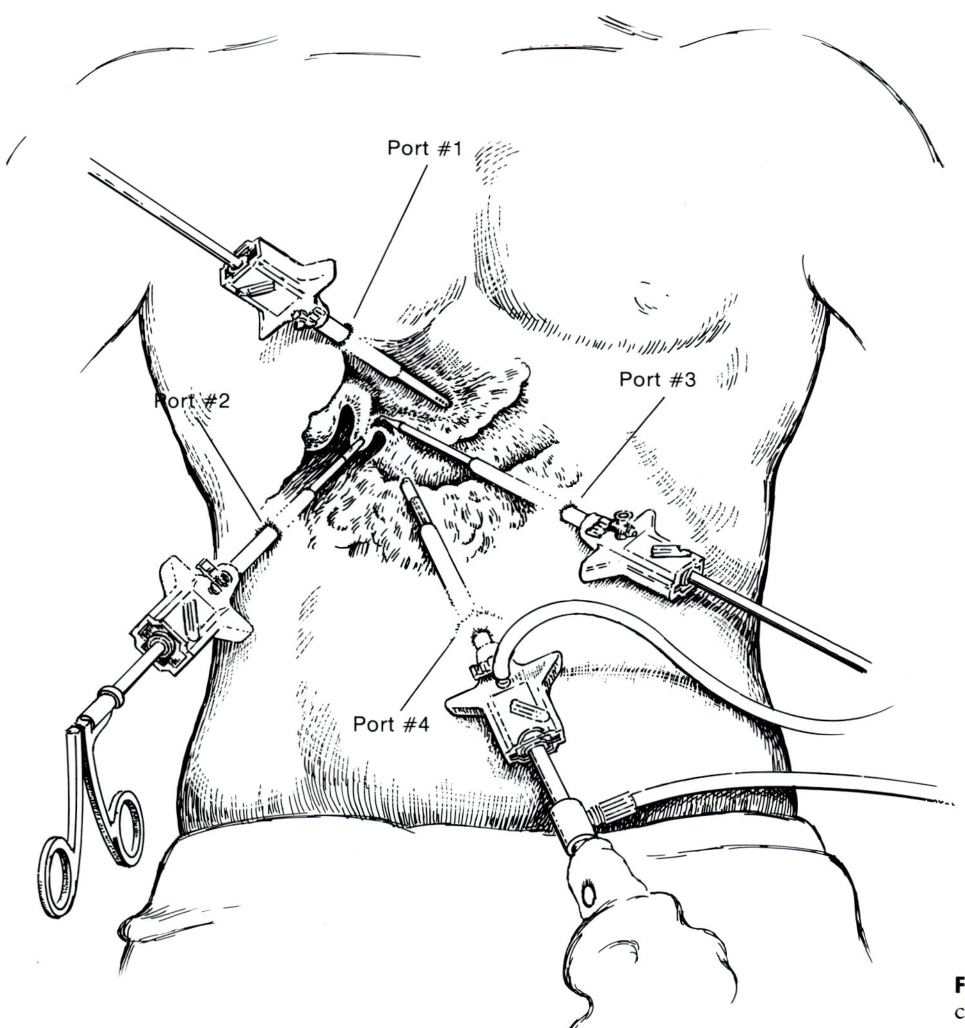

FIGURE 16-1. Positioning of trocars for French technique of laparoscopic cholecystectomy.

below the right costal margin, vertical to the fundus of the gallbladder. It is 5 mm in diameter and permits the introduction of the irrigation–suction cannula.

The next trocar, 5 mm in diameter (port 2), is inserted into the patient's right flank on the anterior axillary line, facing the fundus of the gallbladder. The exact point is determined by pressing the finger on the abdominal wall until this pressure brings the parietal peritoneum in contact with the fundus of the gallbladder. The light of the laparoscope transilluminates the abdominal wall, enabling the operator to avoid injuring the wall vessels. To grasp the neck of the gallbladder, a 5-mm grasping forceps is inserted through this port.

The fourth trocar (port 3) is placed in the left hypochondrium at the site where the Veress needle has been withdrawn. This 10-mm port is for passage of the dissector, scissors, electrocautery hook or forceps, and the clip applier (see Fig. 16-1).

Trocars must be placed according to a general principle of laparoscopic surgery (i.e., introduction of the two most important instruments perpendicular to the view axis). In such a manner, the surgeon works with both hands—one holding the structure to be dissected and the other maneuvering the instruments for dissection and suction hemostasis.

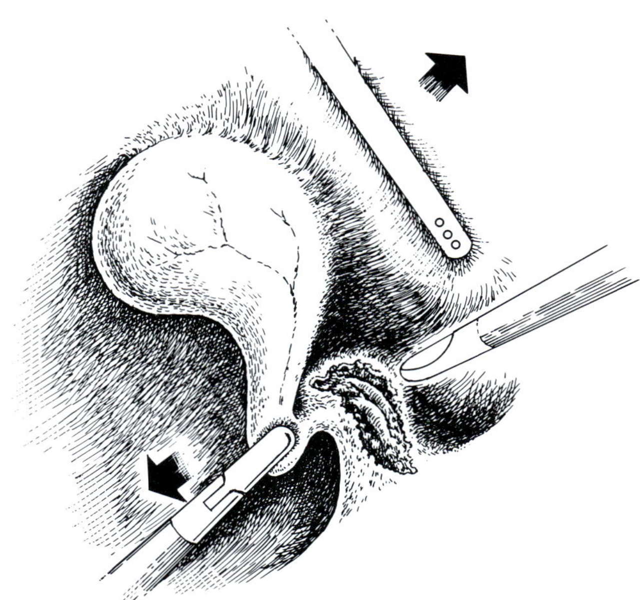

FIGURE 16-2. The neck of gallbladder is pulled inferiorly while undersurface of right lobe of the liver is pushed superiorly.

DISSECTION OF CALOT'S TRIANGLE

The patient's liver is lifted up with the irrigation–suction cannula, allowing access to the anterior aspect of the neck of the gallbladder and to the liver pedicle and Calot's triangle. The grasping forceps, inserted through port 2, is used to grasp and pull the neck of the gallbladder downward to the right (Figs. 16-2 and 16-3). This maneuver opens Calot's triangle like a fan. Scissors are passed through port 3 to open the anterior layer of the visceral peritoneum of Hartmann's pouch. One can dissect the connective tissue, either with the scissors or bluntly with the dissector, going from the gallbladder's neck to the site of the cystic duct–common duct junction. Adhesions exist frequently between the hepatic flexure of the colon, the duodenum, and the gallbladder. They must be divided, either with the scissors or with bipolar electrocautery and scissors, if they contain vessels. Dissection of Calot's triangle should always progress from the gallbladder neck toward the common bile duct. The usual instruments for this purpose must be either scissors or a dissector. Monopolar electrocautery should never be used near the common bile duct.

Maneuvering the grasping forceps inserted in port 2 permits the surgeon to change the orientation of the neck of the gallbladder and expose alternatively the anterior and posterior aspects of Calot's triangle, thus surrounding the cystic duct. A free space between the cystic artery and the cystic duct must then be identified (Figs. 16-4 and 16-5). Mascagni's lymph node, situated on the neck of the gallbladder at the point where the cystic artery or its branches reach the gallbladder, serves as a landmark.

The three components of Calot's triangle must be clearly delineated: (1) the cystic duct and the cystic duct–common duct junction below it, (2) the right aspect of the hepatic duct, and (3) the cystic artery. Clips can be applied only after this anatomic configuration is accurately identified; this is the key aspect of the cholecystectomy (Fig. 16-6). The clip applier is passed through port 3. One must put two clips proximal and one distal on

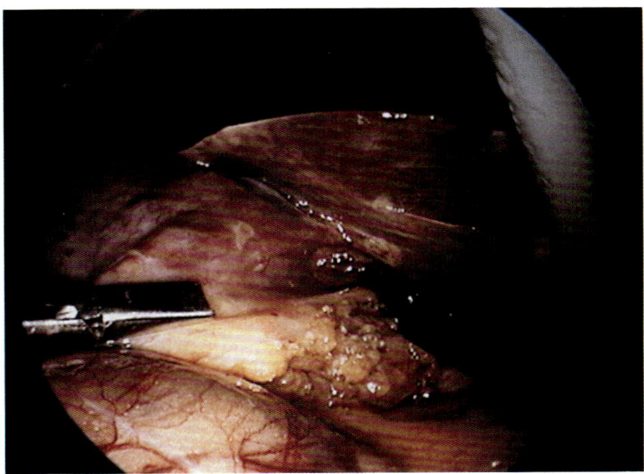

FIGURE 16-3. Neck of gallbladder is pulled inferiorly and peritoneum is opened over cystic duct and artery.

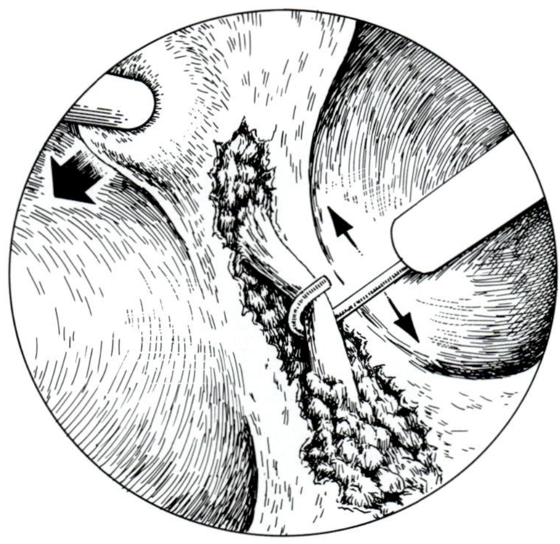

FIGURE 16-4. Cystic duct is dissected free from surrounding fat tissue. *Arrows* indicate motion of hook dissector.

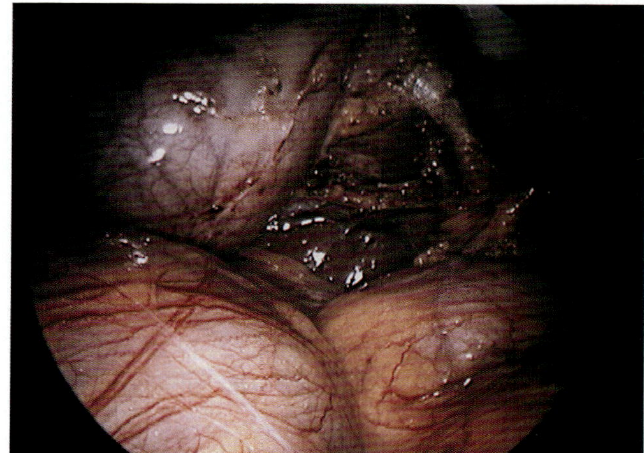

FIGURE 16-6. Triangle of Calot is dissected clear.

the cystic artery, which is then divided. The distal part of the cystic duct is then clipped and its anterior aspect is opened proximally, with the scissors inserted through port 3 (Figs. 16-7 through 16-9).

INTRAOPERATIVE CHOLANGIOGRAPHY

The nontraumatizing 5-mm forceps is passed through port 3 and used to gently and progressively squeeze the cystic duct, from the cystic duct–common duct junction to the incision on its anterior aspect (previously performed). The cystic duct can then be demonstrated to be free of stones; often, this maneuver brings out small calculi that otherwise may have been pushed into the common bile duct by the catheter used for the cholangiography. If there are no calculi, this maneuver delivers only bile. The 5-mm forceps holds and orients the cystic duct for cannulation. The irrigation–suction cannula is removed from port 1 and is replaced by the cholangiography forceps. It contains ureteral catheter 3, 4, or 5, according to the diameter of the cystic duct. After the cystic duct is cannulated, the cholangiography forceps is secured to the duct to prevent any leak of contrast material between the catheter and the duct. The insufflator is then switched off, the instruments are withdrawn, and the trocars are withdrawn to the level of the peritoneum. As the common bile duct is progressively filled with 50% diluted contrast material, the progression is followed with fluoroscopy. A first radiograph is taken when the lower part of the common bile duct becomes opaque. Further contrast material is injected until it reaches the first duodenal passage, when another radiograph is taken. The entire common bile duct must then be filled with contrast material until the upper part above the cystic duct–common duct junction becomes opaque, yielding an image of the hepatic duct, the biliary convergence, and the intrahepatic ducts. If there is no abnor-

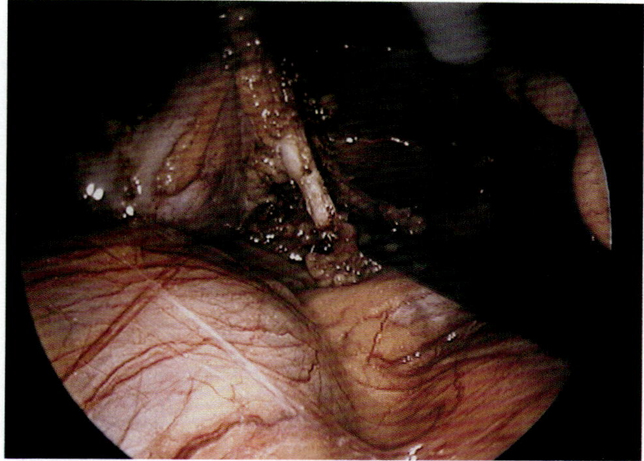

FIGURE 16-5. Cystic duct is dissected free from surrounding tissue.

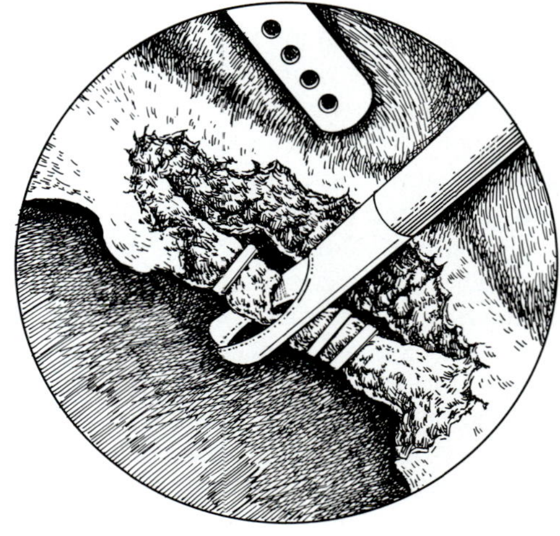

FIGURE 16-7. Cystic duct is doubly clipped and divided.

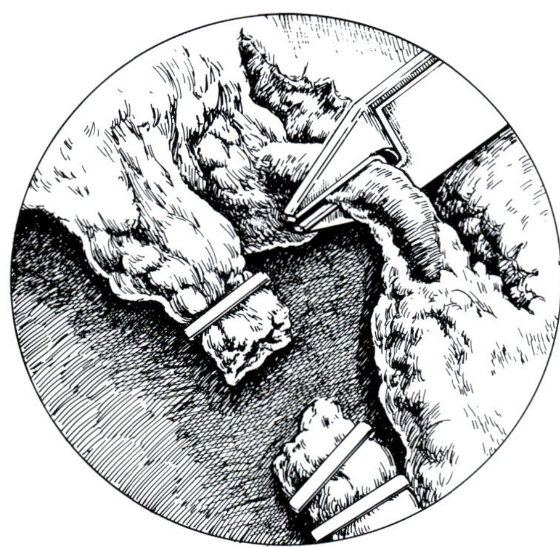

FIGURE 16-8. Cystic artery is clipped and subsequently divided.

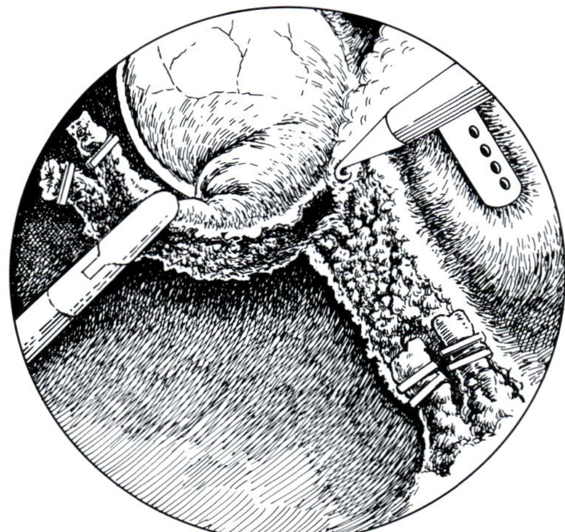

FIGURE 16-10. Gallbladder is dissected free from the liver bed using hook dissector and electrocautery.

mality or calculi in the common bile duct, insufflation is resumed and the cholangiography catheter is removed by opening the jaws of the cholangiography forceps. The clip applier is inserted into port 3 and the cystic duct can be clipped proximally, against the cystic duct–common duct junction. A second clip must be applied more distally for security; the duct can then be divided. At this point, the gallbladder is held only by its liver attachments.

SEVERING THE LIVER ATTACHMENTS OF THE GALLBLADDER

The liver is progressively liberated with either the scissors, the spatula, or the hook connected to a monopolar cautery (Figs. 16-10 and 16-11). The grasping forceps inserted through port 2 is applied to the neck of the gallbladder, pulling it up and to the right, exposing the division between the gallbladder and the liver parenchyma. Hydrodissection is useful at this point. If some injury of the liver parenchyma occurs, hemostasis must be achieved with either the spatula or the hook connected to a monopolar cautery and passed through port 3. When only the fundus remains attached, the grasping forceps in port 2 is elevated, widely opening the liver bed. Hemostasis is completed and the last attachments of the gallbladder are divided.

EXTRACTION OF THE GALLBLADDER

According to the pathologic status of the gallbladder, several technical methods can be used to extract the gallbladder. These are categorized as follows:

Simple. If the gallbladder wall is solid, supple, not damaged by the dissection, if the stones are few and

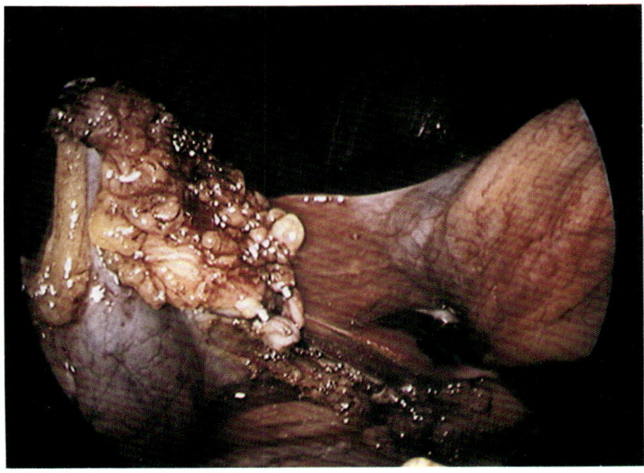

FIGURE 16-9. Cystic duct is divided between clips.

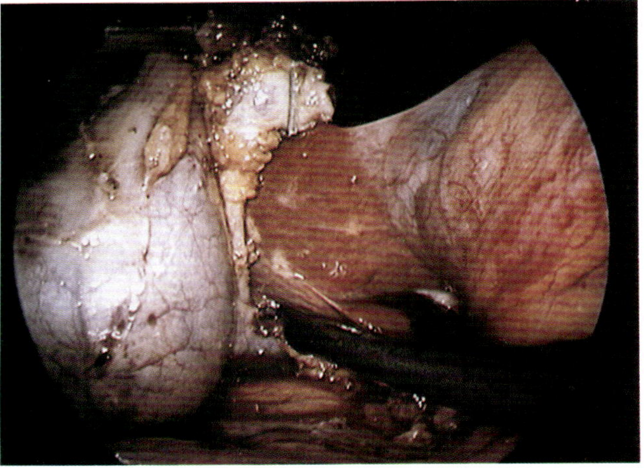

FIGURE 16-11. Gallbladder is dissected off of the liver using electrocautery.

smaller than 5 mm, and the bile is liquid, the gallbladder can be extracted through port 3 in the left hypochondrium. A crocodile forceps passed through this port is used to grasp the neck of the gallbladder and the cystic stump with its clip and to remove them from the abdominal cavity. The exposed part of the gallbladder is then incised and its contents aspirated with the irrigation–suction cannula. The emptied gallbladder can then pass easily through the 10-mm port or an incision in the right hypochondrium.

Complex. When the above-mentioned conditions are not present, it is better to extract the gallbladder through the umbilicus because it is the point where the abdominal wall is less thick. The laparoscope must be moved to the 10-mm trocar (port 3) in the left hypochondrium and the crocodile forceps inserted into the 10-mm umbilical trocar (Fig. 16-12).

If the gallbladder has a supple wall, if it is not damaged by the dissection, if the calculi are larger than 10 mm or numerous, if the bile is fluid and there is a long gallbladder neck, Hartmann's pouch is directly exteriorized with the crocodile forceps. When the gallbladder is opened, the bile is aspirated. Calculi that cannot pass through must be fragmented, either crushed with a Kocher forceps or powdered with an ultrasonic lithotriptor. The gallbladder can then pass easily through the umbilical orifice after the calculi debris has been aspirated.

Conversely, if the gallbladder wall is infected, thickened, or damaged by the dissection, if the bile is thick, or if there is an empyema or a gangrenous gallbladder, the "bag extractor" technique should be used. A plastic bag, packed in a special sheath, is introduced through the transumbilical port, unfolded, and opened in the abdomen. The gallbladder is placed in this bag. A suture is applied to the cystic stump, its tail left long (5 cm), and it is pulled out of the bag. The gallbladder is then widely opened inside the bag and the bile is aspirated while the stones remain in the bag. The bag is then brought outside of the abdominal cavity, still opened. The gallbladder, previously opened and emptied, can be easily pulled outside the abdomen by the suture tail. The bag's content can be cleared with the irrigation–suction cannula and the stones identified. They are then fragmented with one of the techniques mentioned above, and the bag is withdrawn. This technique, which prevents any spillage into the abdominal cavity, must be used when the gallbladder is gangrenous or if it has been opened during the dissection. Under these circumstances, the stones are immediately placed in the bag that has just been introduced. If the gallbladder is inflamed, its anterior aspect must be incised. This allows evacuation of the stone contents and partial resection to be performed, leaving the hepatic aspect intact (the mucosa having been eliminated by electrocautery).

END OF THE OPERATION

A peritoneal lavage is then performed. The laparoscope is placed again through the umbilical port, a 10-mm forceps is inserted in port 3, and the irrigation–suction cannula is placed in port 1. The subhepatic and subdiaphragmatic spaces are washed with an abundance of warm saline. The table is rotated into the Trendelenburg's position and to the right to collect all the fluids in the patient's right hypochondrium. In this position, the laparoscope can be turned to check the right gutter and the pouch of Douglas. The lavage is continued until it runs clear (Fig. 16-13).

The last steps are:

1. Return the table to the flat position.
2. Discontinue the insufflation.
3. Remove the instruments and the laparoscope.
4. Close the fascia with an absorbable suture.
5. Close the skin incisions.

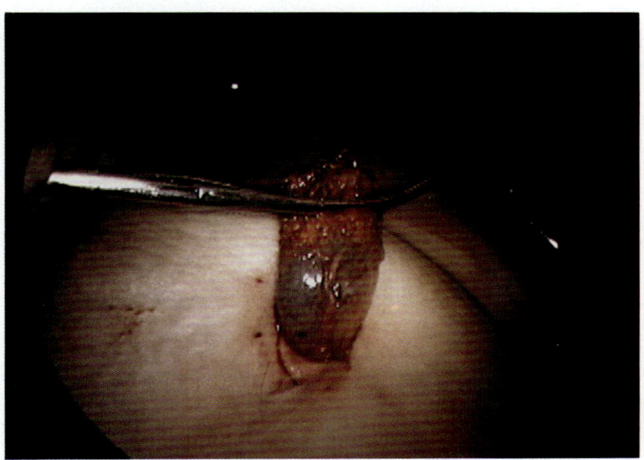

FIGURE 16-12. Gallbladder is extracted through the umbilical incision.

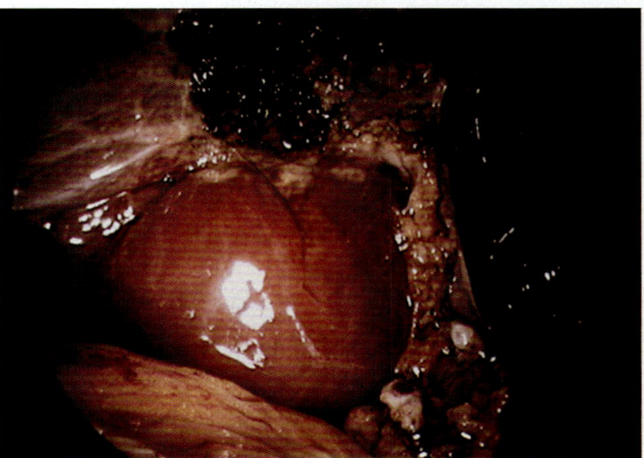

FIGURE 16-13. Completed dissection, showing cystic duct and artery stumps with dry liver bed.

Variation of Technique

SUBHEPATIC DRAINAGE

A suction drain can be inserted through either port 1 or 2 and placed in the gallbladder bed at the end of the procedure. I recommend placing a drain in those patients who have an infected or inflamed gallbladder. In such patients, the cystic stump is fragile and there is a high risk of postoperative leakage. Moreover, drainage is recommended when the liver parenchyma has been entered several times during the dissection. Any bleeding must be stopped rapidly. Drainage permits the exterior diversion of an early bile leak, transforming it into a biliary fistula, which spontaneously resolves in some patients, avoiding a biliary peritonitis and its sequelae.

LAPAROSCOPIC ACCESS TO THE COMMON BILE DUCT DURING LAPAROSCOPIC CHOLECYSTECTOMY

Two situations can lead to laparoscopic procedures on the common bile duct: the presence of a silent stone, discovered by intraoperative cholangiography, or a common bile duct injury, intraoperatively diagnosed.

The Silent Stone. For transcystic access to the common bile duct, the cystic duct must be more than 4 mm in diameter; otherwise, it must be dilated with a coronary artery angioplasty balloon catheter. All the instruments that are to be brought into the cystic duct are inserted through port 1 or 2, according to the duct orientation. They are guided by an atraumatic forceps, which is inserted in port 3.

The calculi can be removed from the common bile duct with a Dormia basket. This is a blind maneuver that requires intraoperative fluoroscopy control. It is preferable to perform a transcystic choledochoscopy, using a flexible fiberscope ranging from 1.8 to 3.2 mm. This procedure allows the surgeon to see the calculi, pass a Dormia basket through the operating channel, and capture the stones under a controlled view.

If the common bile duct is too narrow to admit the above-mentioned fiberscope, an ultrathin fiberscope with an operating channel that admits a laser fiber (300 μm/m) can be used. The tip of this fiber is brought in contact with the stones, which are then powdered by the pulsed laser. The fragments are washed out by continuous lavage, allowing it to pass through the papilla. Should these maneuvers fail, one should not persist if the common bile duct is narrow. A transient biliary drainage must be installed: either a classic transcystic biliary drain or a transcystic–transpapillary drain that drains into the duodenum. This type of drainage can be helpful for the postoperative endoscopic sphincterotomy, which is always difficult in the narrow common bile duct. Finally, one can perform a transcystic balloon dilation of the papilla. It may permit the stones to pass out of the common bile duct with pressurized irrigation.

In patients with a narrow common bile duct, stones ranging from 2 to 3 mm pass through the papilla spontaneously.

Only the transcystic route to the common bile duct can be used during laparoscopic surgery when the diameter of the main duct is less than 6 mm. In contrast, if this diameter is more than 8 mm, the duct can be approached laparoscopically.

Direct laparoscopic approach of the common bile duct requires an additional 10-mm port in the right hypochondrium, vertical to the medial part of the common bile duct and placed so that the surgeon can orient this port and introduce instruments toward either the upper or the lower part of the duct. A knife with a retractable blade is inserted to open the anterior aspect of the duct at the level of the cystic duct–common duct junction. An attempt is then made to clear the common bile duct of stones by passage of a Dormia basket under fluoroscopic control. A choledochoscope is introduced through the 10-mm port. A supple trocar sleeve is used to avoid damage to the sheath of the laparoscope. Choledochoscopy facilitates identification of stones, dislodging them with a Dormia basket and determining the vacuity of the upper as well as of the lower part of the duct. The opening of the duct is closed and the laparoscope is removed. One can either leave in a T-tube drain (through port 2) or close the duct with a running suture and install a transcystic drain.

We recommend introducing a bag into the abdominal cavity before opening the duct to collect the stones as soon as they are removed.

After peritoneal lavage is performed, a suction drain is systematically placed in the subhepatic space.

These maneuvers are described because they are occasionally necessary during laparoscopic cholecystectomy since calculi in a dilated duct are rarely silent. Usually, large stones are diagnosed before the intraoperative cholangiogram is performed. In these cases, an endoscopic sphincterotomy is recommended before laparoscopic cholecystectomy. Indeed, the deliberate laparoscopic approach to the common bile duct should be performed only in specialized centers because this procedure has not been proven to be superior to endoscopic sphincterotomy.

Recognizing Common Bile Duct Injuries. Injuries that can occur during laparoscopic cholecystectomy include transection of the common bile duct, either partially or totally, and narrowing or obstruction of the duct caused by the inadvertent placement of a clip.

Partial or total transection of the common bile duct can occur during a difficult dissection of the neck of the gallbladder when it is attached by dense and inflamed adhesions. This injury can be prevented by good exposure of Calot's triangle and by initiating the dissection from the inferior edge of the neck of the gallbladder toward the hepatic pedicle. The second cause of transection is excessive pulling upward on the gallbladder, creating a curve in the common bile duct. Transection may also occur when the biliary anatomy is not adequately understood, given the natural variance of anatomy in this area.

A punctiform lateral opening can be repaired by inserting a T-tube in the breach if the diameter of the main duct is more than 6 mm. Otherwise, the surgeon can attempt to suture the traumatized duct, provided there is allowance for a transcystic biliary drainage. Direct repair of small wounds to the common bile duct can be performed if transcystic biliary drainage can be accomplished. These repairs have a high incidence of stricture and should be performed by laparotomy. Total transection of the common bile duct cannot be repaired laparoscopically, and a laparotomy is required.

Narrowing by a clip or a suture can occur under two circumstances. There may be confusion regarding the configuration of the biliary anatomy before the operative cholangiogram. A clip can be applied to the common bile duct instead of the cystic duct while the common bile duct is opened to perform the cholangiography. This situation becomes apparent when the upper common bile duct cannot be filled with the contrast medium, which is stopped by the clip. Because the clips are minimally traumatic, one can attempt to remove them and close the lateral opening, provided that transient biliary drainage is possible through the cystic duct.

It may be difficult to achieve hemostasis of the cystic artery. The arterial stump can retract into the hepatic pedicle and if the artery is not individually identified, a clip can be applied to both the artery and the common bile duct. This complication is diagnosed by intraoperative cholangiography, which must always be performed after the artery has been controlled and divided. If the upper common bile duct is poorly filled or not filled with the contrast medium, it may be partially or completely clipped. After the hepatic artery is clamped with a nontraumatic forceps, the clip can be removed. The arterial cystic stump must be identified to apply (electively) a clip on it. The clamp on the hepatic artery can then be released.

Whenever a common bile duct injury is recognized intraoperatively, the surgeon must consider that the safe limits of laparoscopic surgery may have been reached. If the situation cannot be easily controlled with the simple maneuvers described above, an open procedure should be performed.

CONVERSION TO LAPAROTOMY

Laparoscopic surgery can be performed only in an operating room that is set up for the possibility of converting the procedure to a laparotomy. Instruments for open surgery must always be available. Conversion does not require major changes, either in patient positioning or in the anesthetic protocol. The route is a subcostal laparotomy, a standardized procedure routinely performed by all surgeons.

The indications for conversion fall into two categories: conversion for necessity and conversion for prudence.

Conversion for Necessity. A complication may occur at any step of the laparoscopic cholecystectomy. The bowel can be damaged, either during trocar insertion or during dissection of the hepatic flexure and the gallbladder–duodenal ligament. Perforations, hematomas, or electric burns can occur. The omentum and small and large vessels such as the vena cava or porta vena can be traumatized. Hemorrhage can occur from the liver after the gallbladder is removed or from the liver pedicle, especially in the presence of unexpected portal hypertension. All of these complications can be repaired laparoscopically if they are minor—the best example being the bowel injury that can be repaired through the laparoscope. If the complication is major, however, an open procedure must rapidly follow.

Conversion for Prudence. Any event that turns the laparoscopic procedure into one that may compromise the patient's security requires conversion to laparotomy. Any mechanical or instrument failure is a reason for conversion. Particular dangers are poor lighting, bad image transmission, difficulty with intra-abdominal pressure due to a defective insufflator, a malfunctioning electrocautery system, and insulation instrument defects. The importance of a well-coordinated surgical nursing team cannot be overemphasized.

Other reasons for conversion arise from disease related to the gallbladder and the surgeon's experience. These two reasons are closely entwined. Gallbladders of patients who have had multiple acute attacks of chronic cholecystitis and who have been medically treated are the most difficult to remove. We recommend that surgeons who are beginning to use laparoscopic cholecystectomy select patients carefully.

Severe inflammation makes the identification of the biliary and vascular anatomy more difficult than congenital anatomic variations. If the surgeon, after his laparoscopic dissection, cannot accurately identify the vascular and biliary components of Calot's triangle, a clip should not be applied and no strictures should be divided, even partially. In these instances, the above-described intraoperative cholangiography cannot be used to look for common bile duct calculi. Under these circumstances, intraoperative cholangiography must be performed through a puncture of the gallbladder. One must use a large needle to extract a certain amount of bile and to inject the 50% diluted contrast medium. Opacification of the cystic duct is followed by fluoroscopy, which identifies the cystic duct–common duct junction. Stones frequently obstruct the cystic duct (in 30% to 40% of patients) and the transvesicular cholangiography does not produce information with respect to biliary anatomy. One must puncture the main duct directly with a fine needle to obtain a map of the biliary tree. The intraoperative cholangiography may be helpful in identifying the biliary components of Calot's triangle but it cannot totally replace knowledge of anatomy or experience in difficult biliary dissections. Laparoscopic cholecystectomy is a safe procedure only when performed by a surgeon experienced in open biliary procedures.

CARE

Intraoperative

Candidates for laparoscopic cholecystectomy should have the following preoperative tests: ultrasound scan of the liver and biliary tree and liver function tests, particularly alkaline phosphatase, glutamyl transferase, and glutamyl transaminase. Preoperative medical evaluation before general anesthesia is important. These are usually outpatient procedures.

The operation is performed under general anesthesia, according to a protocol standardized for laparoscopic surgery (see Chap. 7).

Postoperative Follow-Up

The postoperative routine is similar to that of open gallbladder surgery. As soon as the patient awakens in the recovery room, the endotracheal tube, the nasogastric tube, and the Foley catheter are removed. Intravenous fluids are continued until oral fluids are tolerated. The patient may require analgesics; antiemetics or antispasmodics may be necessary during the first 24 hours. Intravenous fluids are discontinued one day postoperatively, and diet is advanced, as is physical activity. If there is appropriate surveillance at home, the patient is discharged on the evening of the first postoperative day.

References

1. Cuschieri A, Dubois F, Mouiel J, et al: The European experience with laparoscopic cholecystectomy. Am J Surg 1991; 161:385.
2. Dubois F, Icard P, Berthelot G, Levard H: Coelioscopic cholecystectomy: a preliminary report of 36 cases. Ann Surg 1990;211:60.
3. Perissat J, Collet D, Belliard R. Gallstones: laparoscopic treatment, intracorporeal lithotripsy followed by cholecystostomy or cholecystectomy. A personal technique. Endoscopy 1989;21:373.
4. Perissat J, Collet D, Belliard R: Gallstones: laparoscopic treatment—cholecystectomy and lithotripsy. Our own technique. Surg Endosc 1990;4:15.
5. Reddick EJ, Olsen DO, Daniel JF, et al: Laparoscopic laser cholecystectomy. Laser Med Surg News 1989;7:38.

Chapter 17

Laparoscopic Surgery: An Atlas for General Surgeons, edited by Gary C. Vitale, Joseph S. Sanfilippo, and Jacques Perissat. J. B. Lippincott Company, Philadelphia, © 1995.

Cholecystectomy: The American Technique

William G. Cheadle
Gerald M. Larson

It has been more than 100 years since Carl Langenbuch performed the first cholecystectomy in 1882. This has become a standard procedure that is performed by virtually all general surgeons for the treatment of symptomatic cholelithiasis. Despite various other therapeutic attempts to prevent gallstones, to dissolve them, or to fragment them with lithotripsy, cholecystectomy remains the definitive treatment for gallstone disease.

Laparoscopic cholecystectomy is a new technique for removal of the gallbladder. The practice of laparoscopic cholecystectomy has literally exploded over the last 4 years. Originally performed in Lyon, France, by Mouret and described by French surgical teams headed by Dubois and coworkers and Perissat and coworkers, the technique was mastered early in the United States by Reddick and coworkers, among others.[1–4] Today, most American surgeons have learned the technique and thousands of patients have undergone the procedure. Although the literature states that laparoscopic cholecystectomy has a complication rate similar to that of open cholecystectomy, several major complications that are directly caused by the procedure have been reported.[5,6] Proper training during the residency period and training courses for the practicing surgeon are necessary if this procedure is to be performed with minimal risk to the patient.

Over 500,000 cholecystectomies are performed each year in the United States. After a transition period of less than 2 years, most of these operations are being performed laparoscopically rather than by the traditional open technique. Many university teaching programs first developed and learned the laparoscopic technique in a research laboratory. In this chapter, we describe the "American perspective" of laparoscopic cholecystectomy.

DESCRIPTION OF METHOD

Patients are generally admitted to the hospital on the day of surgery having been NPO for ≥8 hours and they have had nothing by mouth or have fasted for 8 hours. The patient is placed on the operating table in the supine position. After general anesthesia is induced, bladder catheterization is performed. Routine placement of a nasogastric tube is not done unless the stomach is dilated at exploration. A vertical stab incision is made (#11 blade) from the middle of the umbilicus to its lower border. A Veress needle is then inserted into the abdominal cavity. (The sterile drop technique is not used routinely because preperitoneal instillation has occurred despite the drop easily passing through the syringe.) If the patient has had a previous midline incision, the needle is inserted above the umbilicus or a separate puncture is made in the left upper quadrant.

We determine the adequacy of the insufflation by physical examination of the tenseness of the abdomen and set the desired end-point pressure, generally near 12 to 14 mmHg. The skin incision is then extended to permit placement of a 10-mm trocar through the umbilicus. The laparoscope with camera attached is then inserted into the port at the umbilicus for routine exploration of the abdominal cavity. Three additional trocars (one 10-mm and two 5-mm) are then placed as shown in Figure 17-1. The second trocar (10 mm) is inserted about a third of the distance from the xiphoid to the umbilicus in the midline. It is important to keep the distance between the two 10-mm trocars at least 10 cm apart so that there is no interaction between the dissecting instrument and the scope. The first of the two

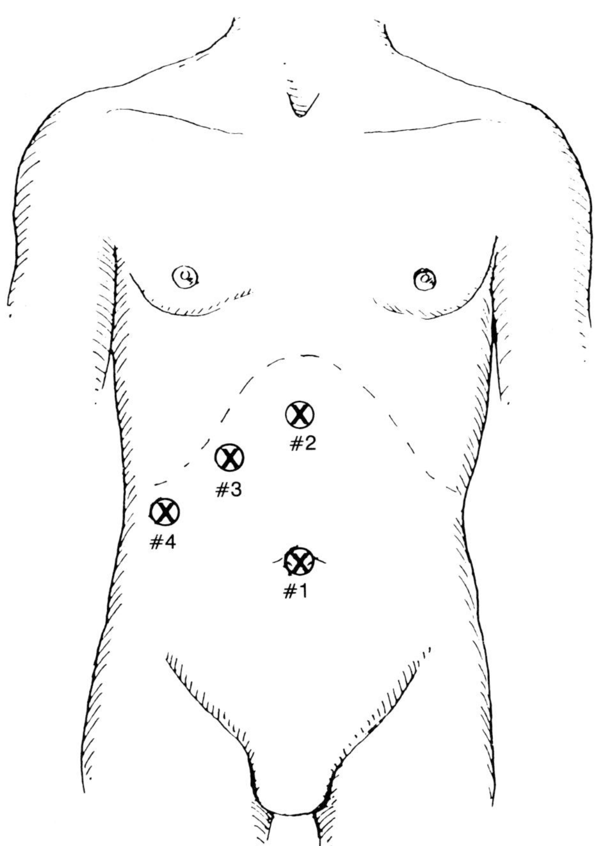

FIGURE 17-1. Proper placement of each trocar is shown. The two 10-mm ports are placed in the umbilicus and subxiphoid positions, and the two 5-mm ports are placed laterally.

5-mm trocars is inserted just underneath the right costal margin in the mid-clavicular line, and the other is placed as lateral as possible but anterior to the hepatic flexure of the colon (Fig. 17-2). An adaptor (4.5 or 5.5 mm) is placed into the superior 10-mm trocar to achieve a proper air seal for the dissecting instrument.

The surgeon stands on the left side of the patient and the first assistant is on the right side of the patient. The person operating the camera stands adjacent caudally to the surgeon. The patient is placed in reverse Trendelenburg's position, and the table is tilted toward the surgeon. This maneuver allows the upper abdominal hollow viscera to fall caudally while facilitating the exposure of the cystic structures and porta hepatis. Simultaneously, while the surgeon grasps the gallbladder with the dissecting forceps instrument, the first assistant grasps the gallbladder at its dome with a strong-grasping forceps (Fig. 17-3). The gallbladder is then directed anteriorly and superiorly, reflecting the liver with it, to reveal the porta hepatis and the peritoneum covering the cystic structures. To properly grasp the gallbladder in those patients with acute cholecystitis and hydrops, it is often helpful to decompress the gallbladder by aspiration with the percutaneous spinal needle. If the omentum and duodenum are adherent to the gallbladder, they are dissected free at this time (Fig. 17-4). If cautery is applied during this part of the dissection, one must be certain that the instrument is not in close proximity to the duodenum to avoid the chance of a burn injury. Once the cystic structures are evident, the first assistant grasps the infundibulum (Hartmann's pouch) of the gallbladder with the grasping forceps (the type with incisor teeth) and applies appropriate countertraction (Fig. 17-5).

At this point, the surgeon starts the dissection to display the cystic duct, cystic artery, and Calot's triangle. Countertraction during this part of the operation frequently stretches the cystic duct toward the gallbladder, so that the common duct can be tented into the area of dissection, particularly in those patients with a short cystic duct (Fig. 17-6). Therefore, it is just as important to stay as close as possible to the gallbladder in this operation as one would in the open operation. Generally, the surgeon identifies the cystic duct first and the duct is oriented in an oblique direction from left to right (Figs. 17-7 and 17-8). If a cholangiogram is to be done, it should be performed at this time. If the orientation and the exact identity of the structures are still unclear, we prefer to begin dissection of the gallbladder from its fossa just above the cystic duct. This creates an inferior window, in which one can be certain that there is not another ductal structure exiting into the distal gallbladder fossa from the gallbladder itself.

Ligation and division of the cystic duct is performed with clips, using a special clip applicator that is fitted through the subxiphoid 10-mm cannula (Fig. 17-9). The 4.5- or 5.5-mm adaptor is therefore removed. The clip applicator is used to place two clips on the remaining side of the cystic duct stump and one clip on the gallbladder side if a cholangiogram is not to be performed. The clips must be aligned so that they completely cross the cystic duct but do not overlap. If there is any doubt about the proper orientation of the clips, they are simply removed and reapplied. The cystic duct is cut and cauterized simultaneously. If a cholangiogram is to be performed, a single clip is placed on the cystic duct adjacent to the gallbladder. An incision is made with the scissors in the cystic duct and a cholangiocatheter of choice is inserted (Figs. 17-10 through 17-12). The cystic artery is then identified, clipped, and divided. Generally, the cystic duct is prominent and its division allows better access to the cystic artery. The cystic artery is isolated with the right angle or hook instrument and then doubly clipped proximally, singly clipped distally, and divided.

Further traction on the gallbladder brings into view the proper plane for dissection between the liver and the gallbladder. The gallbladder is then removed with an electrocautery instrument. One author (Cheadle) prefers to use the disposable scissors for dissection because it

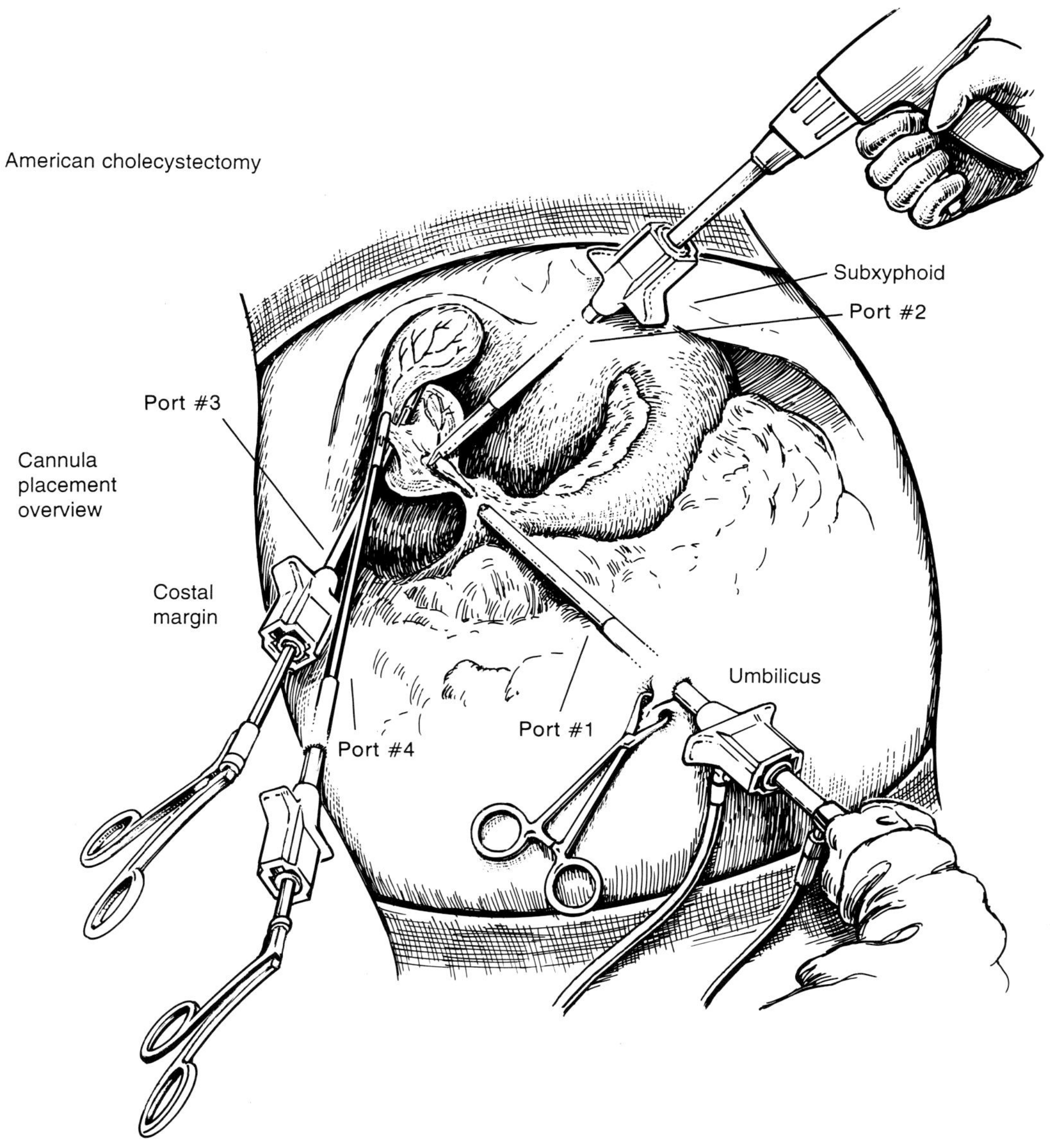

FIGURE 17-2. Overview of port and instrument placement for American technique.

has a slight curve and when closed, it has a narrow enough tip so that an electrocautery can be guided precisely. The other author (Larson) prefers to use the hook scissors and a dissecting hook for this part of the procedure. At times when electrocautery is difficult, the scissors can then be used for cutting the connective tissue (Fig. 17-13). This is often necessary during the last portion of the dissection, in which the fundus is freed from the liver, because the ability to apply traction and countertraction diminishes at this point. The grasping forceps on the neck of the gallbladder can be maneuvered into various positions, including clockwise and counterclockwise twists, to maintain proper countertraction and display the plane between the gallbladder and the liver (see Fig. 17-13). The gallbladder bed is best cauterized while the gallbladder is being removed and exposure of the area is optimal.

Once the gallbladder is freed from its fossa, it is directed over the dome of the liver with the grasping forceps and the lateral port. The 10-mm claw grasper is then placed through the upper midline 10-mm cannula and applied to the neck of the gallbladder (Fig. 17-14). It is important to grasp it at the neck because this is the easiest way to pull the gallbladder into the trocar. If the gallbladder is grasped in the middle, it bunches up and is difficult to pull through the abdominal wall. Once the gallbladder is firmly held by the claw grasper, the gallbladder is pulled into the trocar sleeve (Fig. 17-15). If

(text continues on page 163)

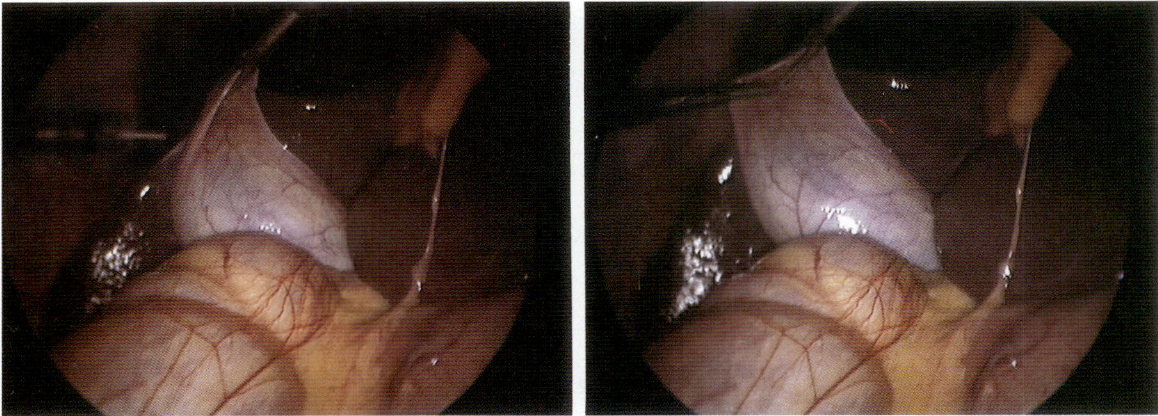

FIGURE 17-3. The surgeon grasps the gallbladder with a dissecting forceps instrument while the first assistant grasps the gallbladder at the dome.

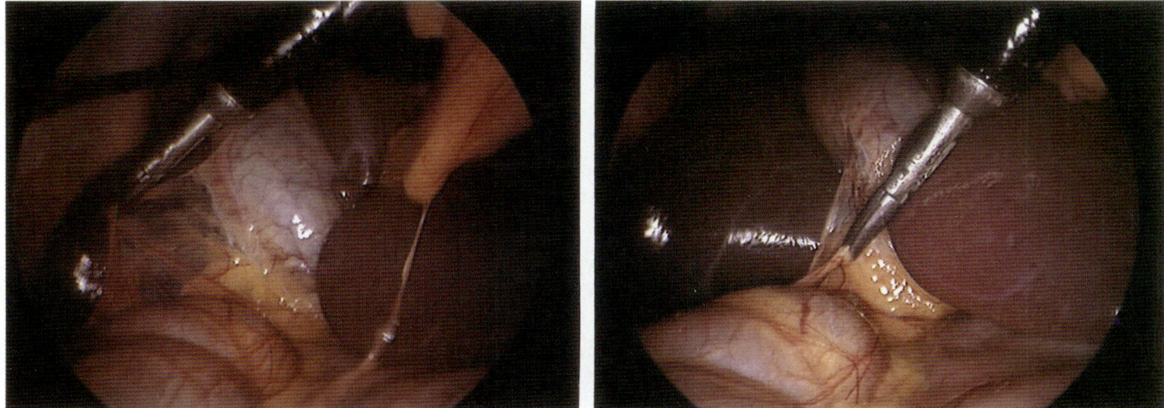

FIGURE 17-4. Omentum, colon or duodenum may be adherent to the gallbladder and are dissected free using a grasper.

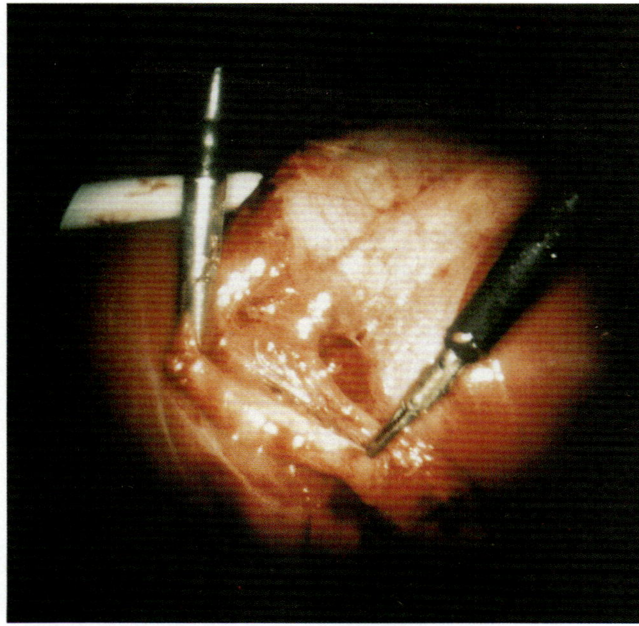

FIGURE 17-5. The first assistant is shown grasping the infundibulum (Hartmann's pouch) of the gallbladder with the grasping forceps with the incisor teeth and applying appropriate countertraction for the surgeon to begin dissection.

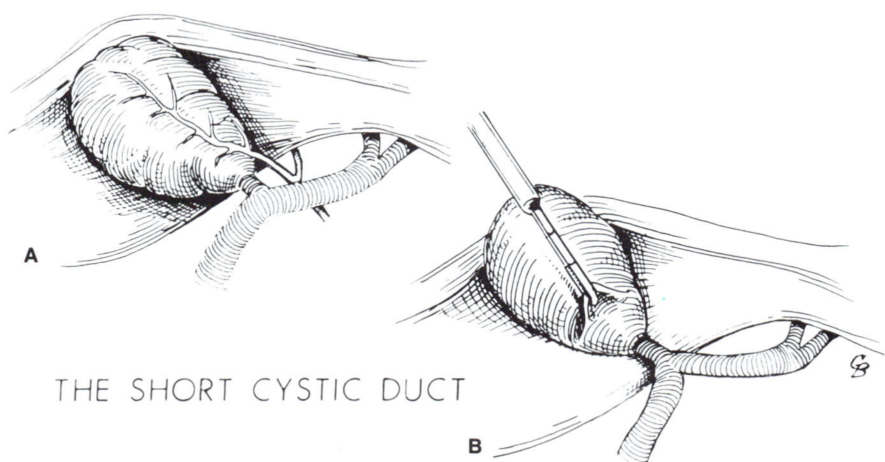

FIGURE 17-6. An example of a cystic duct stretched toward the gallbladder so that the common duct can be tented into the area of dissection.

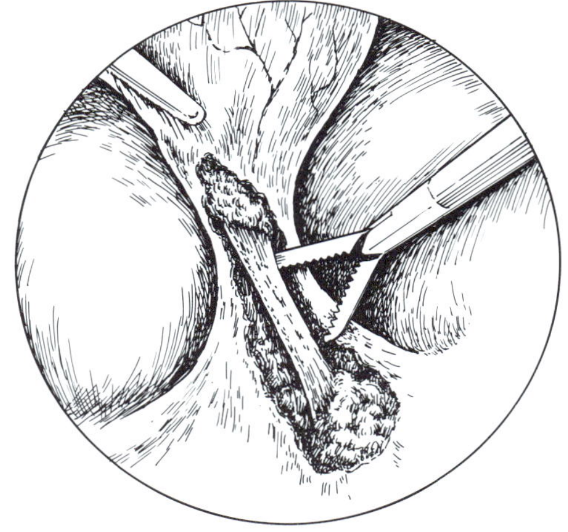

FIGURE 17-7. Cystic duct dissected free from surrounding tissue. Tension is placed by pushing gallbladder fundus superiorly over the liver edge and pulling the gallbladder neck laterally.

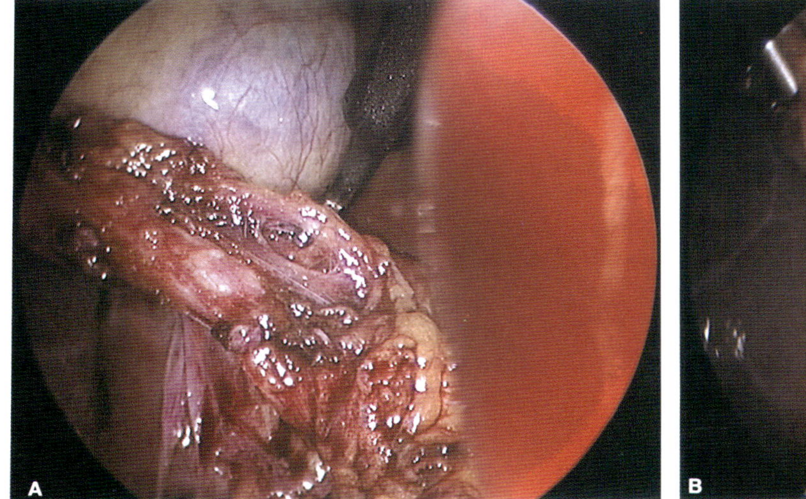

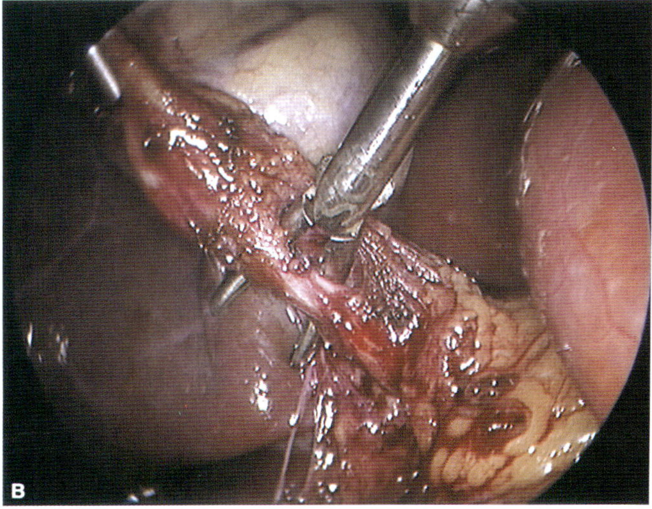

FIGURE 17-8. Dissection of cystic artery using hook dissector (A) and cystic duct using blunt dissector (B).

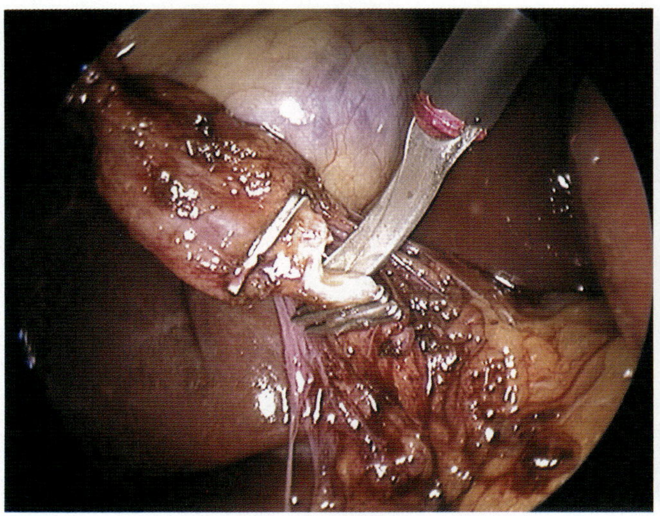

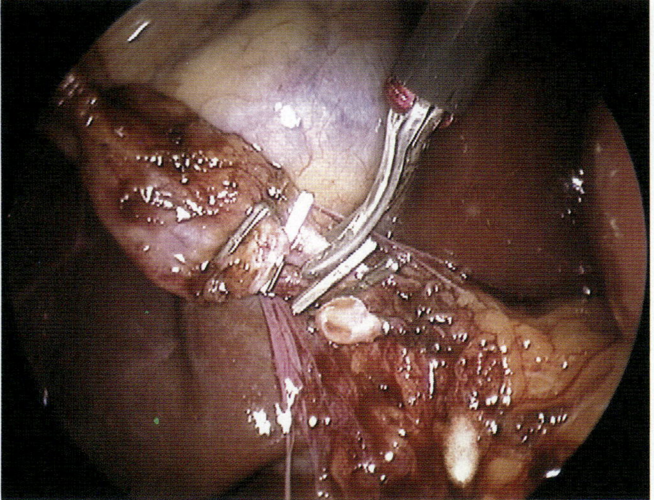

FIGURE 17-9. Division of cystic duct (**A**) and cystic artery (**B**) using scissors. Cautery is not applied due to risk of current being applied to the clips with necrosis of the tissue encompassed by the clips which could lead to late cystic artery bleeding or cystic duct stump bile leak.

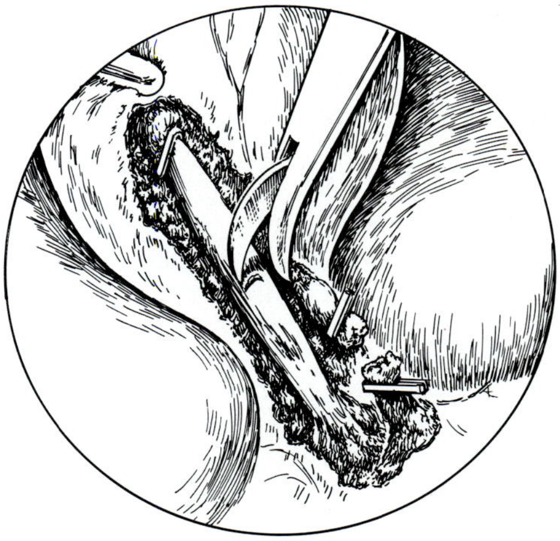

FIGURE 17-10. Incision of cystic duct to allow insertion of cholangiocatheter. Note the clip applied to the cystic duct at its junction with the gallbladder to prevent backflow of potentially infected bile.

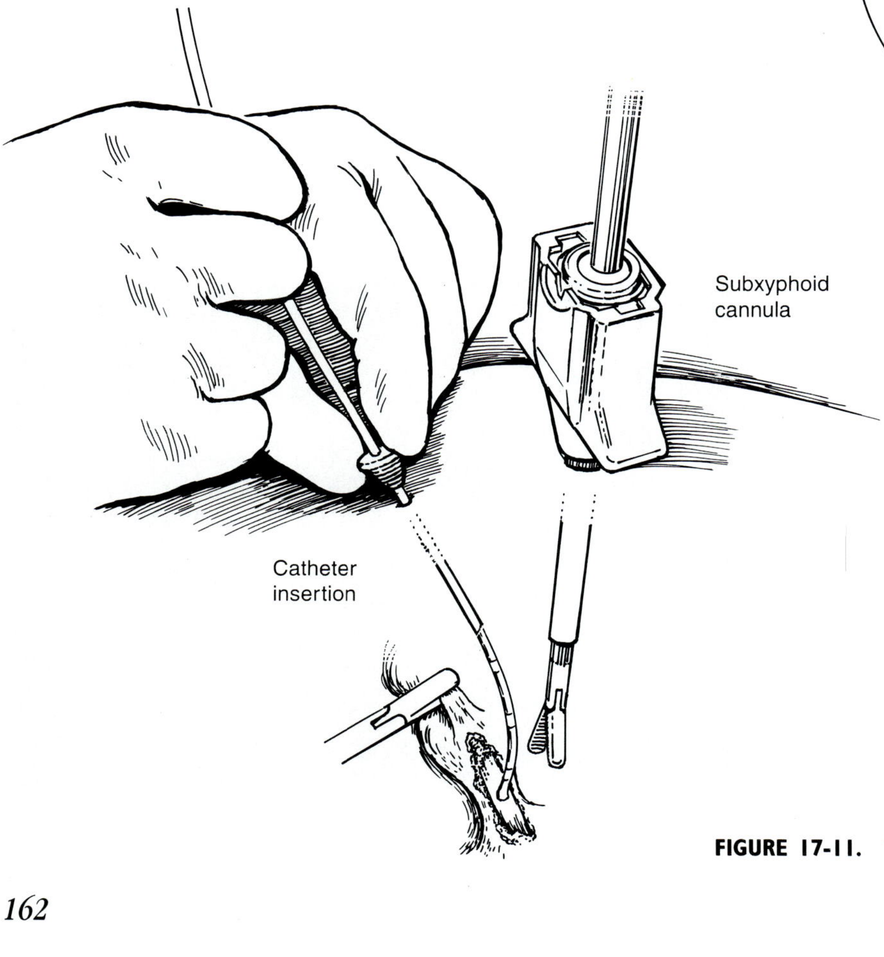

FIGURE 17-11. Technique of cholangiocatheter insertion.

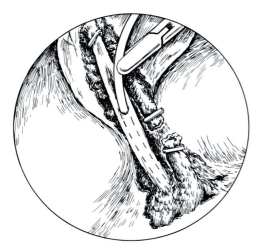

FIGURE 17-12. Insertion of catheter in cystic duct for cholangiogram.

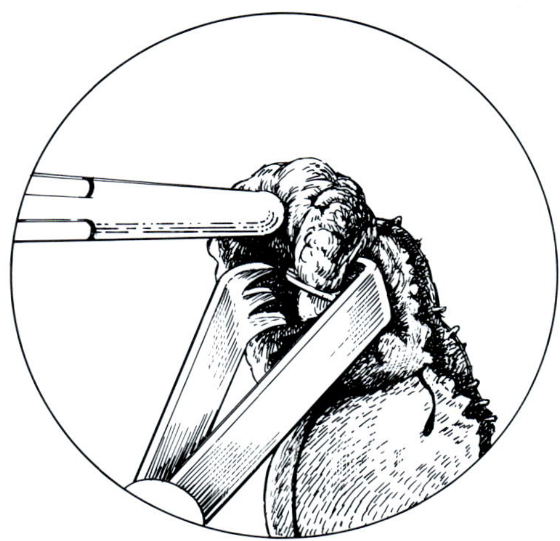

FIGURE 17-14. The gallbladder is grasped at the neck.

the gallbladder is small, it is simply removed through the trocar. More often, it is too large to be pulled all the way through the abdominal wall. In this case, the grasper and the trocar are simultaneously pulled out from the abdominal wall as far as possible and the trocar is then advanced along the grasper. This displays about 1 inch of the gallbladder, which is then grasped with a Kelly clamp. At this point, the gallbladder may be aspirated to remove excess bile. If there are multiple stones, creating a "beanbag" effect, the fascial defect created by the trocar is widened by spreading the fascia with a Kelly clamp or sharply with a scalpel. The gallbladder is then removed through the fascia. When the gallbladder is removed, the upper trocar is then replaced under direct vision. Sometimes the pneumoperitoneum is lost during this maneuver and a towel clip must be placed around the upper trocar to ensure adequate sealing of the skin around it. The assistant then uses the grasping forceps through a lateral port to elevate the liver and gallbladder bed, which is irrigated. The subhepatic and right subphrenic spaces are suctioned as dry as possible. The gallbladder fossa may be drained at this time by placing a medium round Silastic catheter through one of the 5-mm cannulas. Each trocar is removed within direct view while retaining the pneumoperitoneum. The camera is then removed. The abdomen is desufflated while the umbilical trocar is still within the abdomen. The anesthesiologist is then asked to perform a few Valsalva maneuvers with the ventilation bag. Because shoulder pain is due to residual CO_2 gas, as much CO_2 as possible is removed.

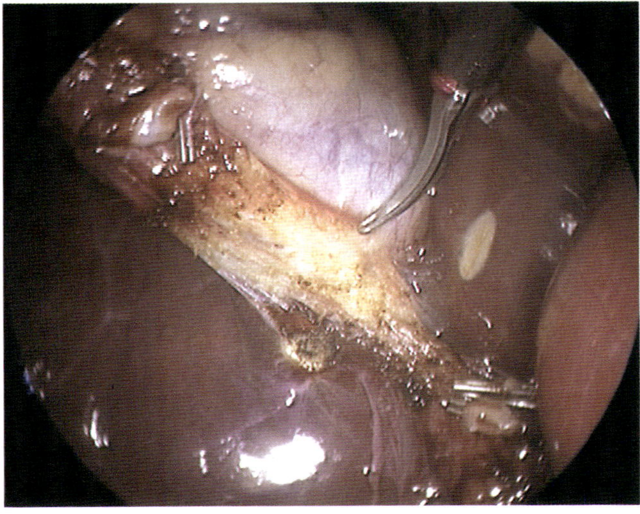

FIGURE 17-13. Gallbladder is dissected from liver bed using scissors and cautery.

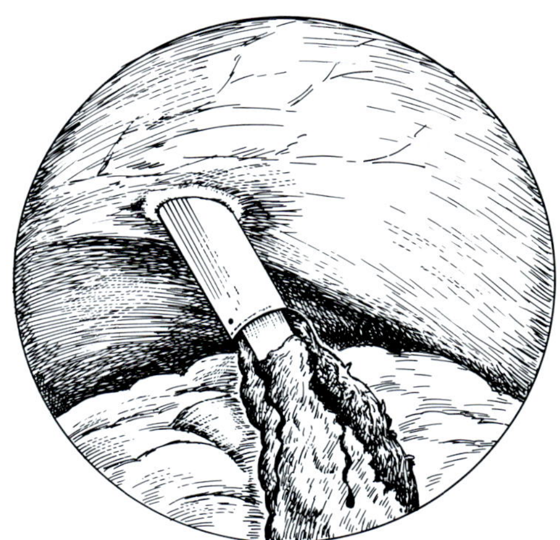

FIGURE 17-15. Removal of gallbladder through trocar sleeve, neck first.

If the fascial defect is larger than a fingertip, which occasionally occurs in the umbilical incision, it is repaired with a single 1-0 polyglycolic acid suture. All other skin wounds are closed with 4-0 polyglycolic acid subcuticular sutures; Steri-strips and protective dressings are then applied. A scopolamine patch is helpful preoperatively to prevent nausea, and all incisions are usually injected with a small amount of 0.5% Marcaine to minimize postoperative pain. The patient is kept from oral intake for the next several hours, started on clear liquids, and given a regular diet the following day. We do not discharge patients home the same day as the operation because of the risk of unobserved hemorrhage but most are discharged on postoperative day one.

References

1. Dubois F, Icard P, Berthelot G, Levard H: Coelioscopic cholecystectomy: preliminary report of 36 cases. Ann Surg 1990;211:60.
2. Perissat J, Collet D, Vitale G, Belliard R, Sosso M: Laparoscopic cholecystectomy using intracorporeal lithotripsy. Am J Surg 1991;161:371.
3. Reddick EJ, Olsen D, Daniell J, et al: Laparoscopic laser cholecystectomy. Laser Med Surg News 1989;7:38.
4. Zucker KA, Bailey RW, Gadacz TR, Imbembo AL: Laparoscopic guided cholecystectomy. Am J Surg 1991;161:36.
5. Graves HA Jr, Ballinger JF, Anderson WJ: Appraisal of laparoscopic cholecystectomy. Ann Surg 1991;213:655.
6. Schirmer BD, Edge SB, Dix J, Hyser MJ, Hanks JB, Jones RS: Laparoscopic cholecystectomy: treatment of choice for symptomatic cholelithiasis. Ann Surg 1991;213:665.

Chapter 18

Laparoscopic Surgery: An Atlas for General Surgeons, edited by Gary C. Vitale, Joseph S. Sanfilippo, and Jacques Perissat. J. B. Lippincott Company, Philadelphia, © 1995.

Laparoscopic-Assisted Colon and Rectal Surgery

E.L. Bokey
I.P. Davis
P. Hewitt

The success of laparoscopic cholecystectomy has compelled surgeons to define the role of laparoscopic colorectal surgery. A comparison of the two procedures emphasizes that laparoscopic resection of the colon is significantly more complex. Unlike the situation in laparoscopic cholecystectomy, the field of vision may be obscured by loops of bowel, intraoperative identification of any lesion may be difficult, and handling of the colon by instruments may result in serosal or full-thickness tears. In colon resection, several vessels of large caliber need to be ligated and divided, suitable anastomotic techniques need to be developed, and, if the colectomy is performed for malignancy, local recurrence and long-term survival must be considered.

INDICATIONS

Laparoscopic colon resection is a developing field. Precise indications still remain to be defined. Sound surgical principles must not be compromised by technical expedience. In carefully selected patients, it is possible to perform a laparoscopic procedure that has the same anatomic and functional outcome as the equivalent open procedure. If this cannot be accomplished, a traditional open procedure is mandatory.

Benign Tumors. Benign tumors not suitable for endoscopic resection are a common indication for laparoscopic resection.

Malignant Tumors. Patients with cancer should be selected with caution because there are insufficient prospective data on the outcome after laparoscopic surgery.

Inflammatory Bowel Disease. Patients requiring a limited resection for Crohn's disease and selected patients with ulcerative colitis requiring proctocolectomy, with or without J-pouch formation and ileoanal anastomosis, are good candidates for the laparoscopic approach.

Diverticular Disease. As with open surgery, laparoscopic colectomy for diverticular disease may be difficult. The bowel wall is thickened, the mesentery is shortened, adhesions to adjacent structures are common, and as a rule, mobilization needs to include the splenic flexure and upper third of the rectum. These conditions may lead to a difficult and hazardous laparoscopic dissection.

Stoma Formation. Laparoscopic techniques are well suited to the formation of both end and loop stomas.

Hartmann's Procedure. Laparoscopic restoration of intestinal continuity has been possible in some patients after Hartmann's procedure.

PREOPERATIVE ASSESSMENT

Evaluation of Lesion. Small tumors can be localized preoperatively by endoscopic injection of methylene blue within 24 hours of surgery. This enables the lesion to be readily identified laparoscopically (Fig. 18-1).

General Preparation. This includes orthograde bowel lavage, perioperative antimicrobial agents, anti-

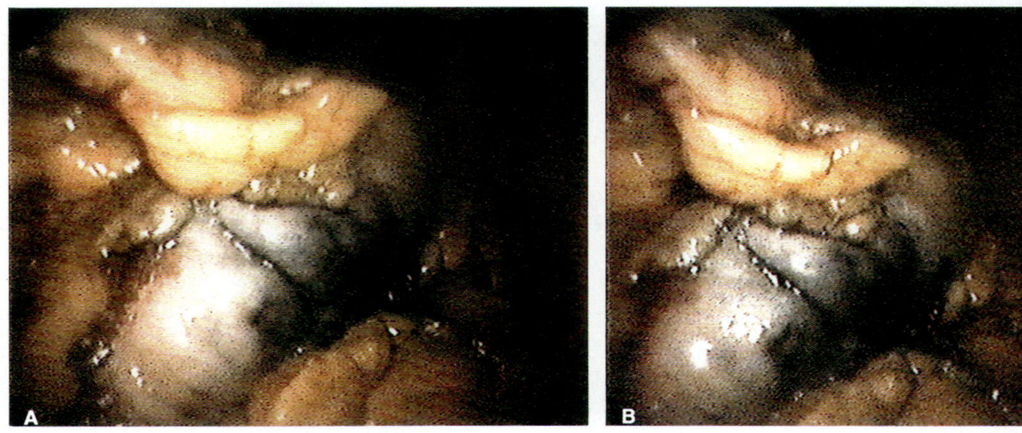

FIGURE 18-1. Tumor stained with methylene blue.

thrombotic prophylaxis, and appropriate stoma siting when indicated.

Anesthesia. A general anesthetic with endotracheal intubation and muscle relaxation is required. Insertion of a nasogastric tube and urinary catheter is essential.

Positioning. The patient is in the supine position, legs securely placed in stirrups (Fig. 18-2), with minimal flexion at the knees and hips. The patient's arms should be placed at his/her side to allow maximal access for the surgical team.

Pneumoperitoneum and Laparoscopy. Pneumoperitoneum is achieved through a Hasson trocar inserted under direct vision through a small paraumbilical incision. Laparoscopy is performed to assess the lesion, the liver, and other intraperitoneal organs. A 30° laparoscope is preferred during dissection.

Traction and Triangulation. Safe and gentle traction, countertraction, and triangulation are essential in laparoscopic surgery. Direct instrumentation of the colon is unavoidable and can lead to traction injury. The colon needs to be carefully inspected at the end of the procedure to ensure that no significant injury has occurred. Soft bowel clamps are preferred to Babcock forceps, which can cause significant trauma to the intestines.

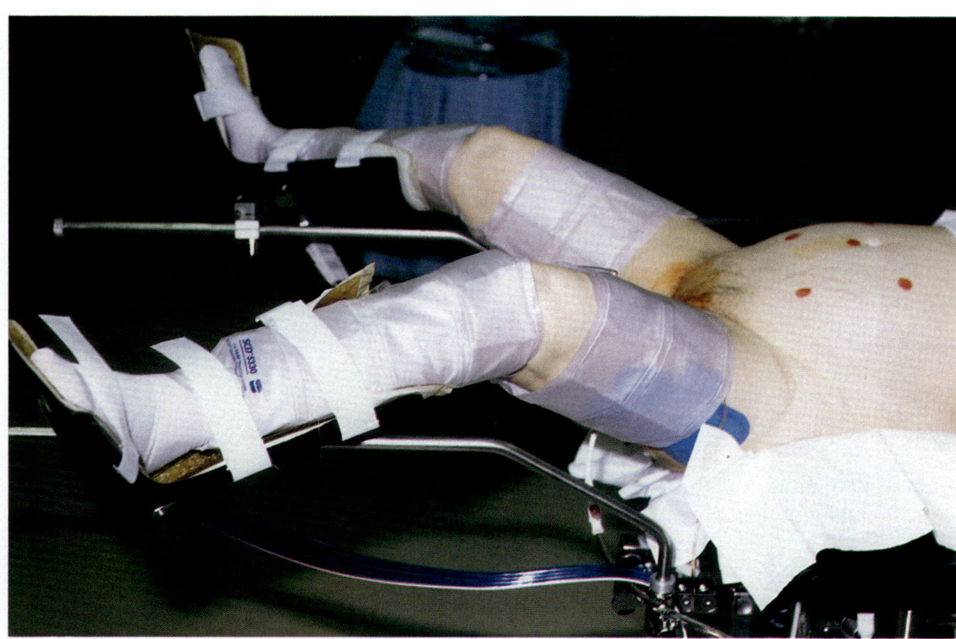

FIGURE 18-2. Patient is in the supine position with the legs securely placed in stirrups.

LAPAROSCOPIC-ASSISTED RIGHT HEMICOLECTOMY

Positions and Ports. The position of the surgeon, assistant, and the five sites for trocar placement are illustrated in Figure 18-3.

Mobilizing Cecum and Ascending Colon. The patient is placed in Trendelenburg's position and is tilted left side downward to improve exposure. Using soft bowel clamps inserted through port 2 or 3, the cecum is retracted medially (Fig. 18-4) to expose its peritoneal attachments to the posterior abdominal wall. An alternative to clamps is a blunt-tipped dissector, which is used to push the colon medially without grasping the serosa. Whenever grasping is necessary, one should try to grasp the edges of serosa or attached fat. One needs to avoid full-thickness injury to the bowel if it is a segment that will not be removed. These attachments are divided sharply with endoshears and electrocautery. The endoshears are placed through port 4 and the forceps through port 5. In this manner, the cecum and ascending colon are mobilized toward the midline. The remaining peritoneal attachments of the distal terminal ileum and cecum are then divided and the right ureter identified.

Mobilizing Hepatic Flexure. The table is tilted to the reverse Trendelenburg's position. The proximal transverse colon is retracted caudally while the greater omentum is elevated to display the line of separation between the two. This is accomplished with instruments inserted through ports 4 and 5. The omentum is dissected from the colon, using forceps and endoshears with electrocautery (ports 2 and 3) to expose the hepatic flexure (Fig. 18-5). The flexure is retracted caudally to expose the peritoneal attachments overlying the duodenum, which are often avascular. The attachments are appropriately divided, exposing the duodenum (Fig. 18-6). A hook dissector or endoshears inserted through port 2 or 3 is most useful for this. Depending on the anatomy, the camera and laparoscope may need to be moved to a port more distant from the operative site to complete this dissection (port 3, 4, or 5).

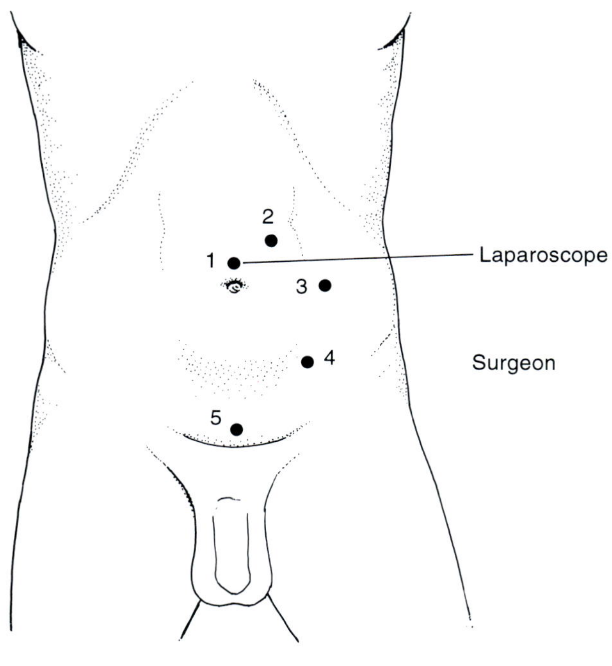

FIGURE 18-3. The position of the surgeon, assistant, and five port sites.

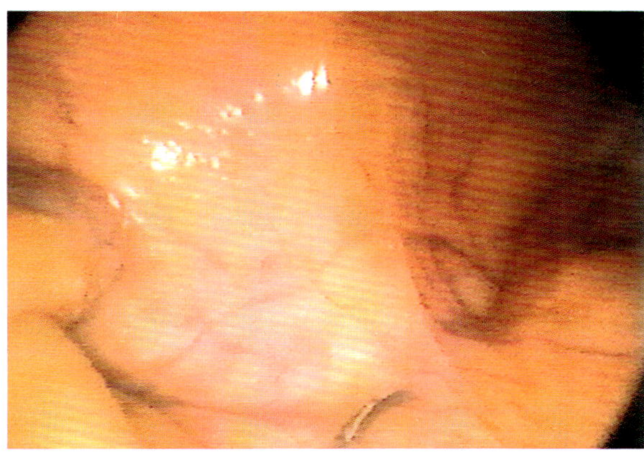

FIGURE 18-4. Lateral peritoneal attachment of cecum and ascending colon.

Division of Ileocolic Vessels. The mobilized right colon is held up between grasping forceps to demonstrate the peritoneal fold over the ileocolic vessels (Fig.

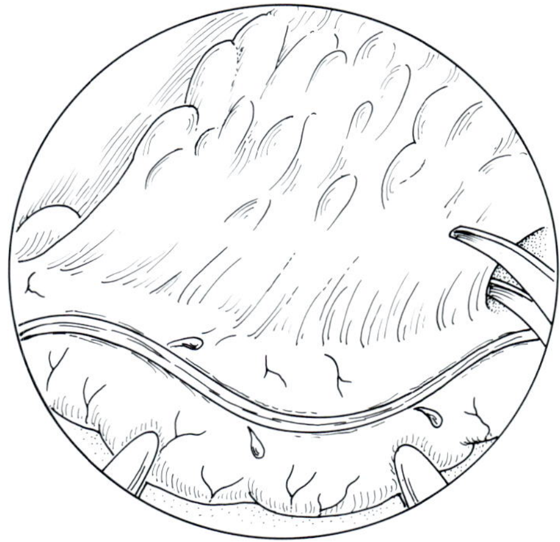

FIGURE 18-5. Hepatic flexure is exposed by dissecting the omentum from the colon.

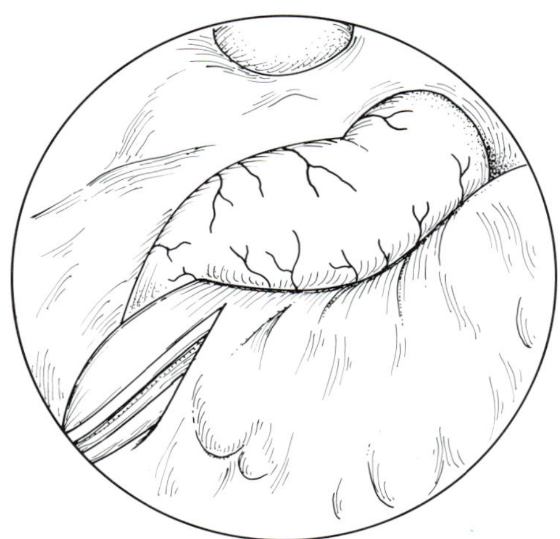

FIGURE 18-6. Duodenum exposed.

18-7). Scissors and forceps through ports 4 and 5 are used to develop a window in the mesentery on either side of the vascular pedicle and to divide the peritoneum over the ileocolic vessels (Fig. 18-8). The appropriate vascular Endo-GIA (U.S. Surgical, Norwalk, CT) instrument is used through port 5 to staple and divide the ileocolic vessels (Fig. 18-9).

Division of Right Colic Vessels. The colon is retracted medially with instruments placed through ports 3 and 5, and the right colic vessels are identified and dissected clear of the adjacent mesentery (Fig. 18-10). The vessels are ligated and divided, using an Endo-GIA vascular stapler placed through port 4 (Fig. 18-11).

Division of Ileal Mesentery. The ileal mesentery is triangulated. The overlying peritoneum is divided, and the mesenteric vessels are individually ligated and divided, using an Endo-Clip (Fig. 18-12).

Exteriorization of Specimen, Resection, and Anastomotic Technique. The specimen is exteriorized either through a small transverse muscle splitting incision or preferably by extending the midline paraumbilical incision through which the laparoscope was introduced (Fig. 18-13). The right branch of the middle colic and marginal vessels are ligated and divided extracorporeally. The transverse colon and terminal ileum are divided and an anastomosis performed, using the surgeon's preferred technique. The mesenteric defect is then closed and the bowel returned to the abdominal cavity. The wounds are closed in layers. Figure 18-14 is that of the abdomen of a 21-year-old patient, 3 weeks after a laparoscopic-assisted right hemicolectomy for Crohn's disease.

LAPAROSCOPIC-ASSISTED LEFT HEMICOLECTOMY

The preparation and positioning are essentially the same as for right hemicolectomy. The table is tilted right side downward to facilitate exposure of the left colon. Trocar placement and positions of surgeon and assistant are indicated in Figure 18-15.

Mobilizing Splenic Flexure. Mobilizing the splenic flexure is necessary to ensure a tension-free anastomosis in most left-sided colectomies, including sigmoid and anterior resections. This technically demanding step may be the limiting factor to a successful laparoscopic resection of the left colon. We recommend that this be the first step; if it is not possible to complete laparoscopically, the procedure is converted to an open one.

The patient is placed in a reverse Trendelenburg's position. The distal transverse colon is grasped through

(text continues on page 171)

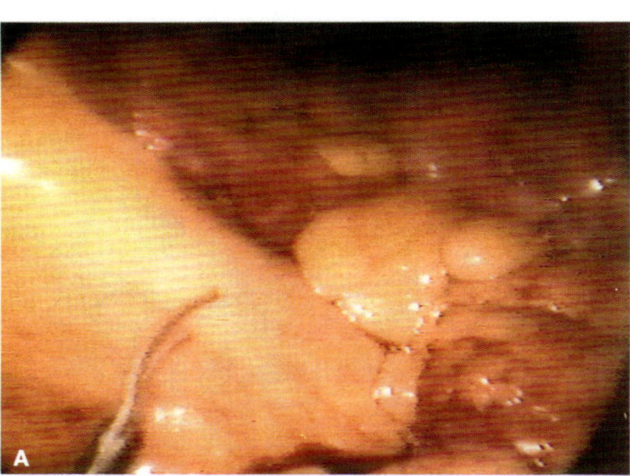

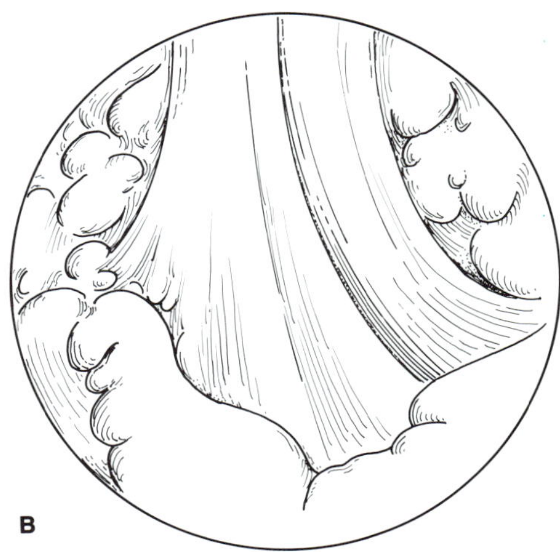

FIGURE 18-7. (**A**) Peritoneal fold over the ileocolic vessels. (**B**) Peritoneal fold.

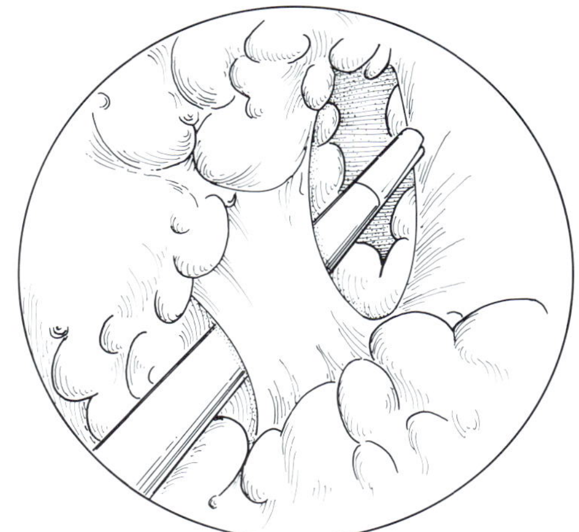

FIGURE 18-8. Ileocolic vessels.

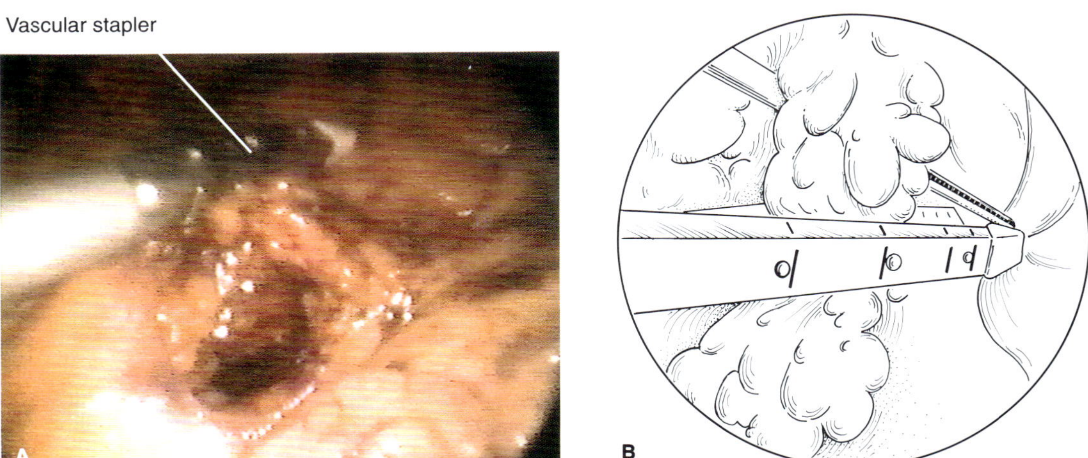

FIGURE 18-9. (**A**) Photograph of a vascular stapler. (**B**) Drawing of a vascular stapler.

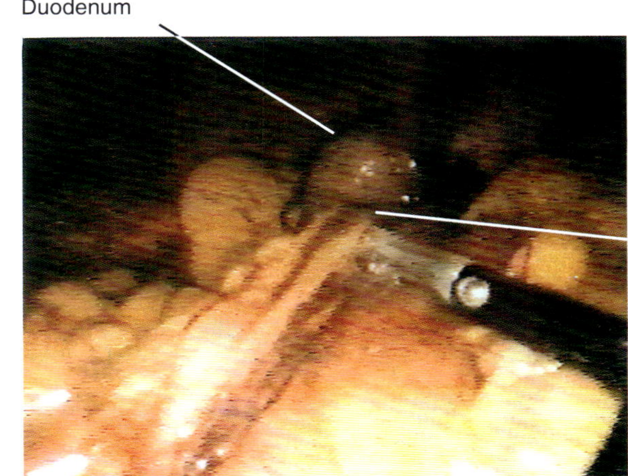

FIGURE 18-10. Identification of right colic vessels.

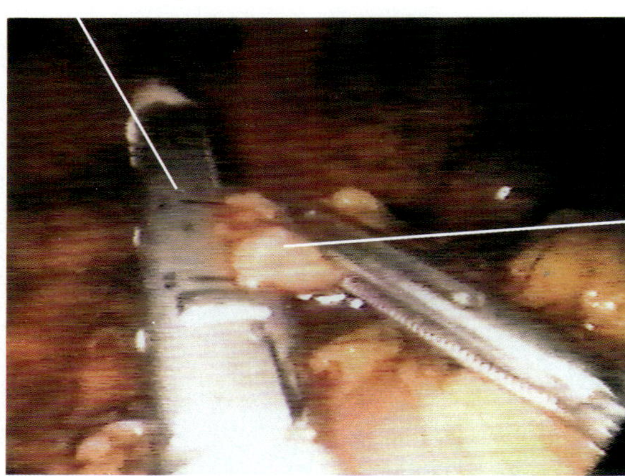

FIGURE 18-11. Endovascular stapler dividing right colic vessels.

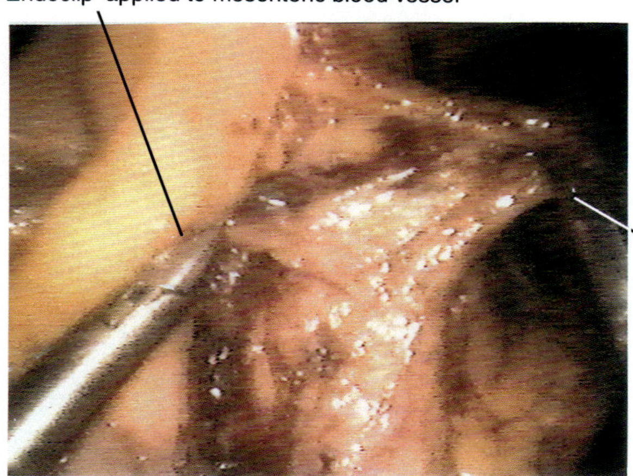

FIGURE 18-12. Retracting the ileal mesentery and the application of an Endo-Clip to the mesenteric blood vessel.

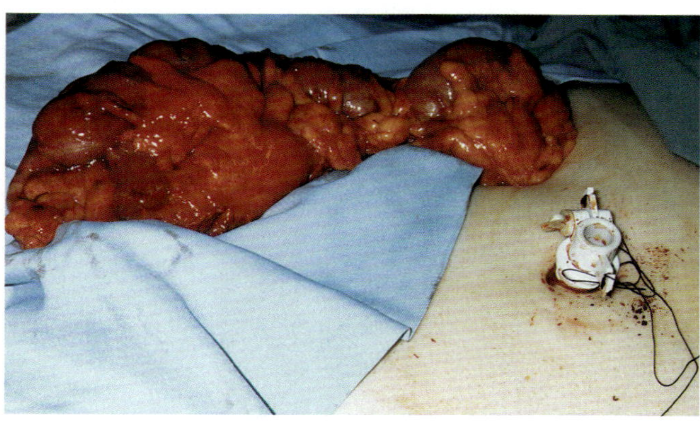

FIGURE 18-13. Exteriorized specimen.

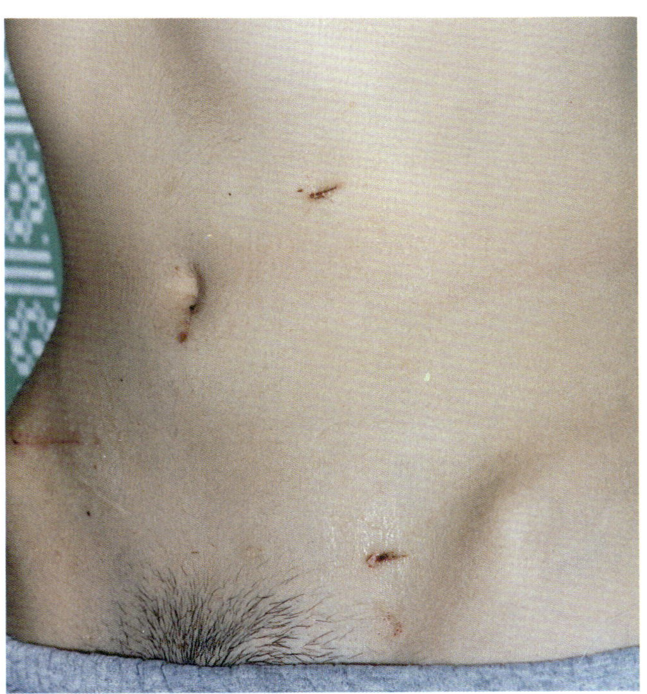

FIGURE 18-14. Abdomen of a 21-year-old patient 3 weeks after right hemicolectomy for Crohn's disease.

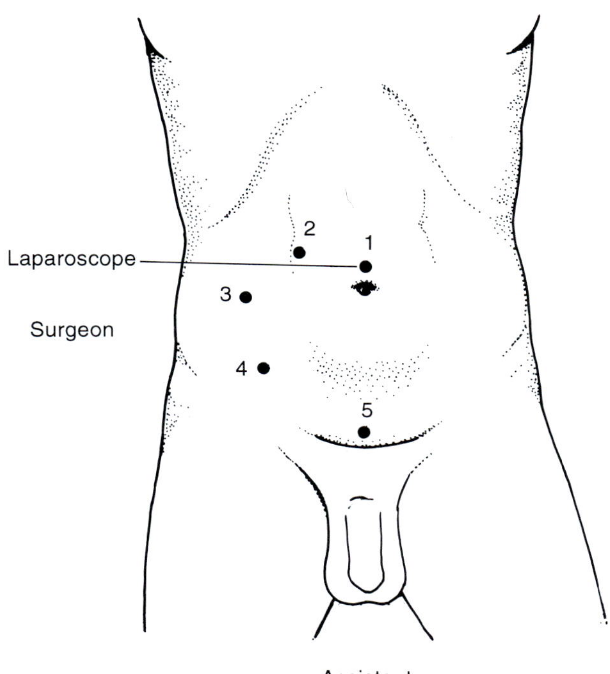

FIGURE 18-15. Position of surgeon, assistant, and five port sites.

ports 4 and 5 and retracted toward the midline and caudally. One may need to reposition the camera to a port more distant from the operating site. The greater omentum is elevated (through port 2) and dissection (through port 3) proceeds in the plane between the omentum and the colon. The dissection continues to the left to expose the apex of the splenic flexure (Fig. 18-16).

The lateral peritoneal attachments of the upper descending colon are divided by retracting the colon medially. Retraction may be switched to ports 2 and 3, with dissection using grasper and endoshears with cautery through ports 2 and 3. The line of dissection progresses proximally around the apex of the flexure to complete its mobilization (Fig. 18-17).

Mobilization of Sigmoid and Descending Colons. The sigmoid colon is triangulated and retracted medially. Retraction is best performed through ports 2 and 3, with dissection through ports 4 and 5. The developmental adhesions to the lateral abdominal wall are divided. The gonadal vessels are identified, and the dissection continues medial to them to expose and identify the left ureter (Fig. 18-18). Sharp dissection proceeds caudally along the white line to complete mobilization of the colon. This dissection is best accomplished using blunt forceps and scissors with electrocautery.

Division of Inferior Mesenteric Vessels. The mobilized sigmoid colon is held up with bowel clamps passed through ports 2 and 3, to demonstrate the peritoneal fold over the inferior mesenteric vessels (Fig. 18-19). Scissors (through port 4) are used to develop a window on either side of the vessels, which are then divided using a vascular Endo-GIA stapler (port 5; Fig. 18-20). Before firing the stapler, the position of the left ureter is checked.

Exteriorization of Specimen and Colocolic Anastomosis. The specimen is exteriorized through a small and appropriately placed muscle-splitting incision. The remaining mesenteric vessels are ligated and divided extracorporeally, and the specimen is resected. A colocolic anastomosis is performed, via the surgeon's preferred technique.

LAPAROSCOPIC-ASSISTED HIGH ANTERIOR RESECTION

Mobilization of the Upper Rectum. Trocar placement is the same as for left colon resection (see Fig. 18-15). The left colon is mobilized as described above. The upper rectum is retracted to the right and a peritoneal incision is continued on the left side into the pelvis, to the level of the mid-rectum (Fig. 18-21). The incision is made sharply with cautery scissors inserted through ports 4 and 5. The left branch of the hypogastric nerve is identified. The soft areolar tissue plane between the nerve and the rectal mesentery is developed by sharp

(text continues on page 175)

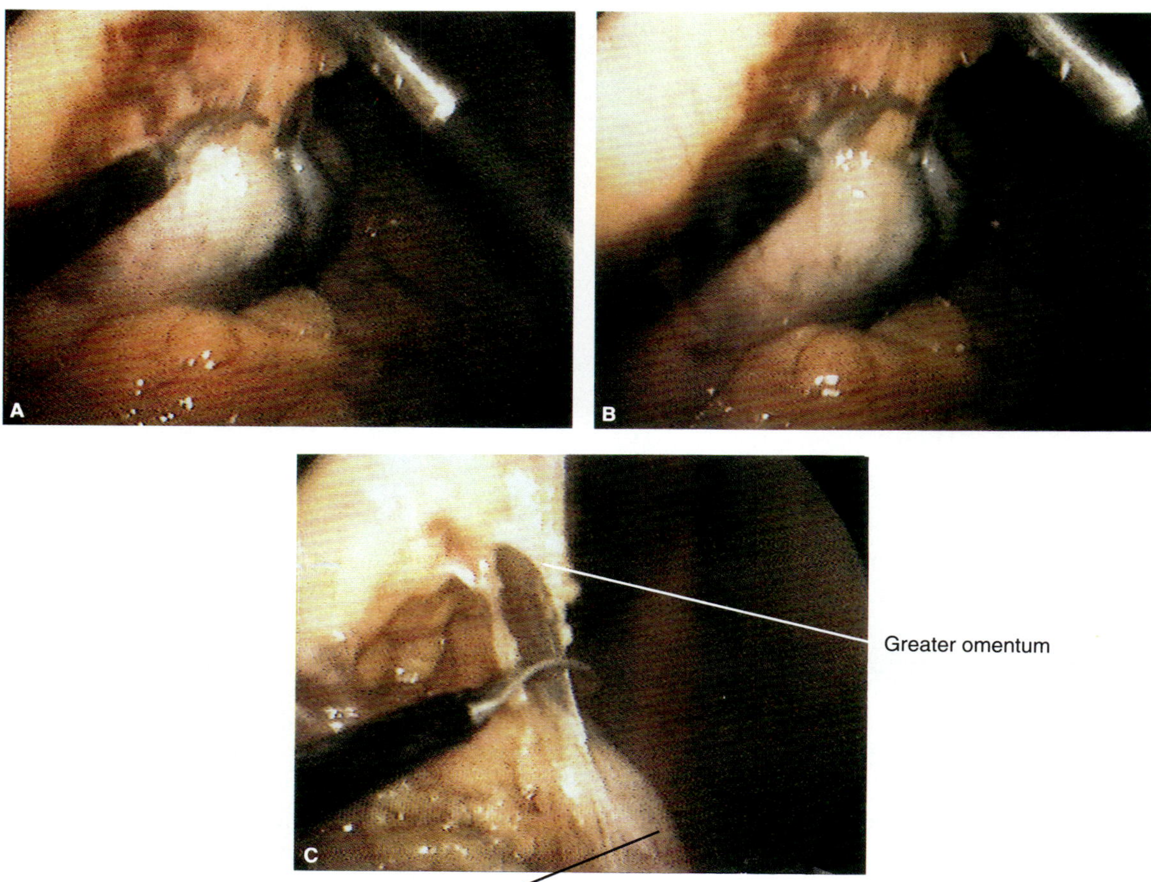

FIGURE 18-16. (A–C) Dissection of the greater omentum and the distal transverse colon in order to expose the apex of the splenic fixture.

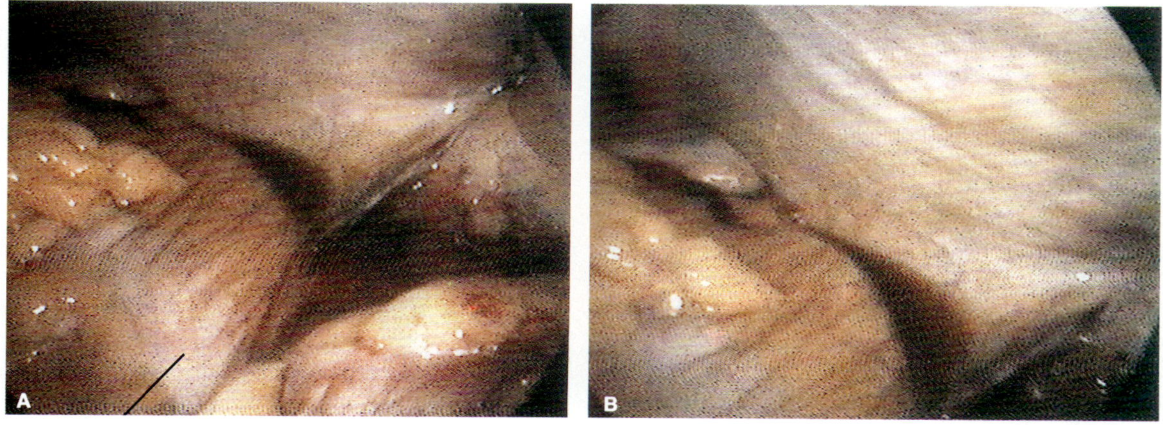

FIGURE 18-17. (A, B) Splenic flexure.

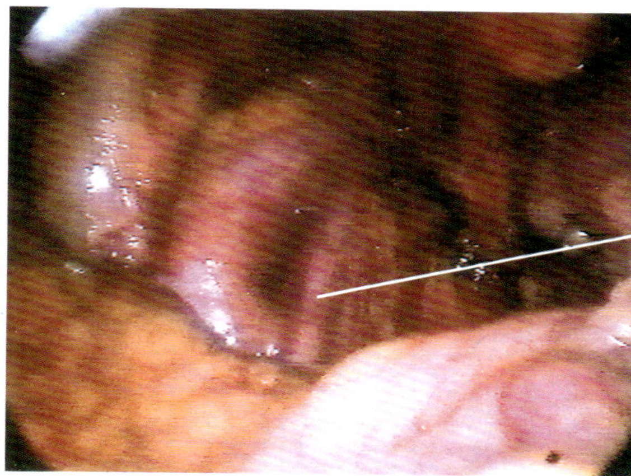

FIGURE 18-18. Left ureter crossing the common iliac artery.

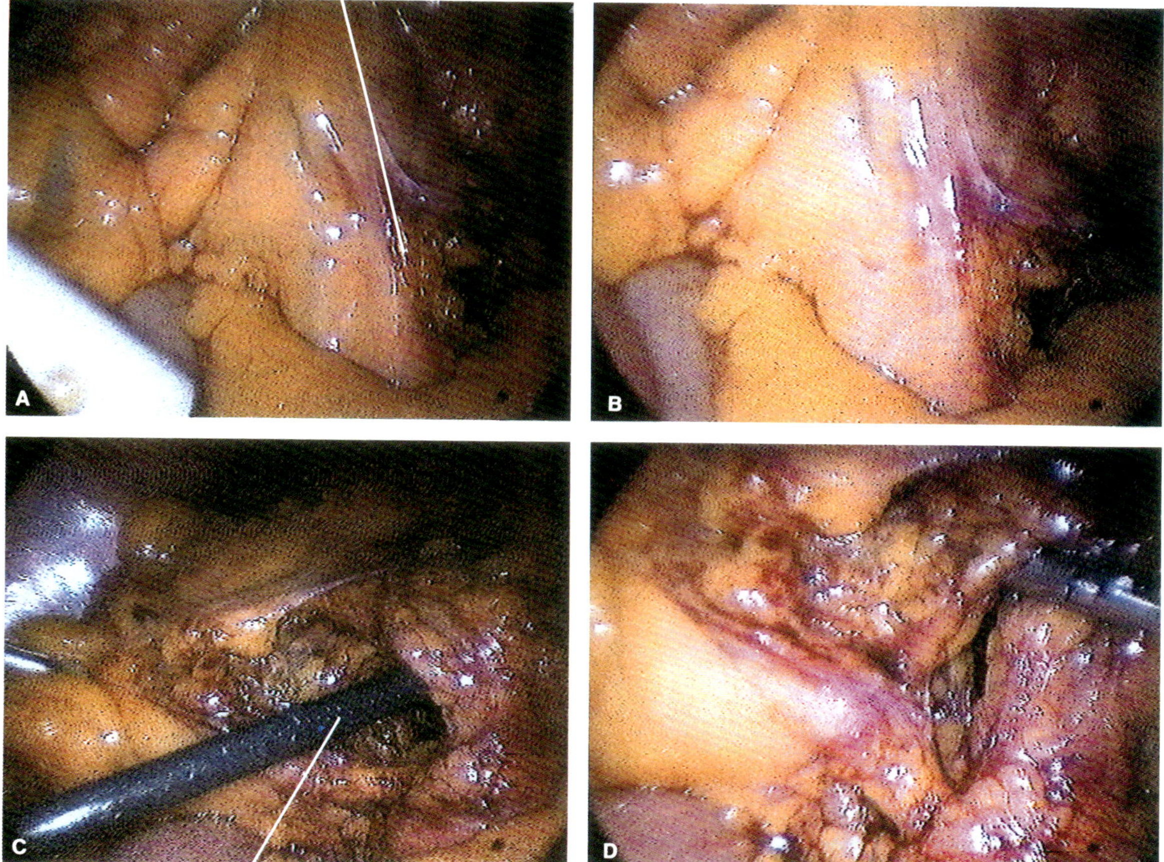

FIGURE 18-19. (A, B) Peritoneal fold over the inferior mesenteric vessels. (C, D) A grasper behind the inferior mesenteric vessels.

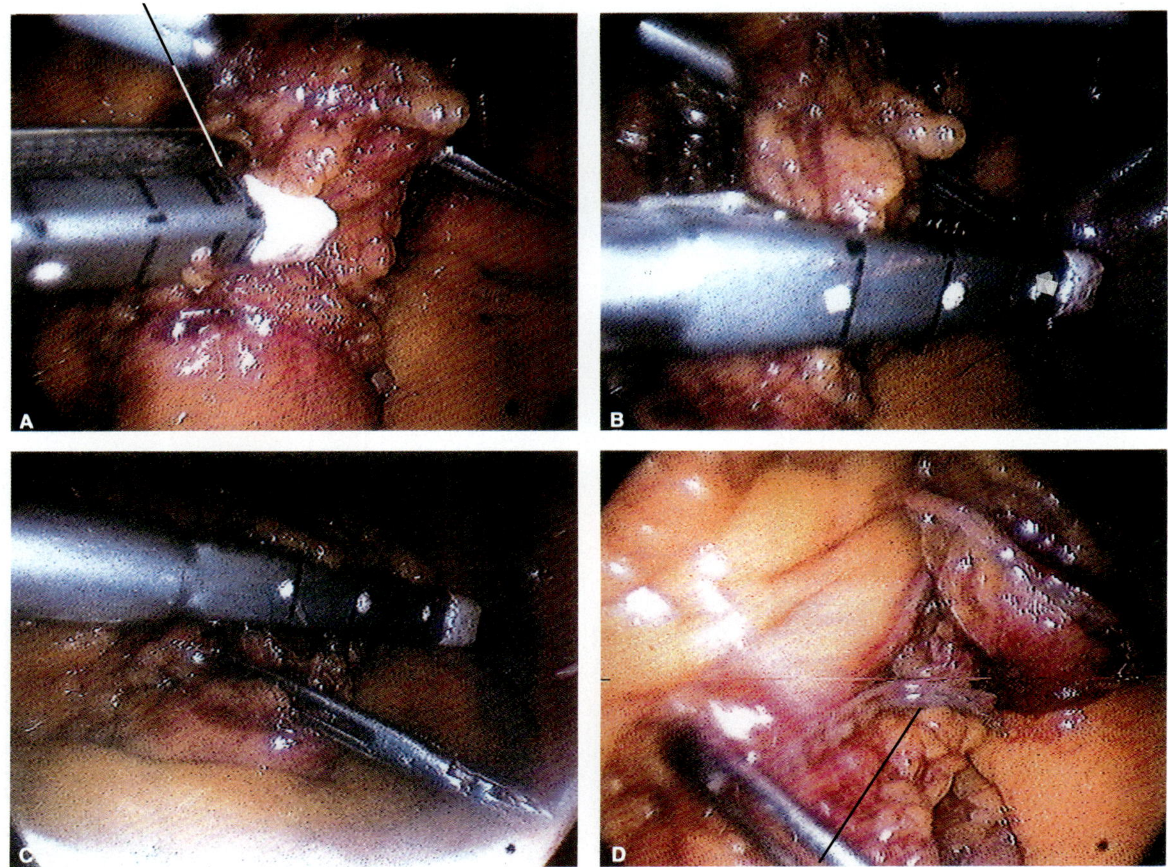

FIGURE 18-20. (A–C) Endovascular stapler. (D) Stapled and divided inferior mesenteric vessels.

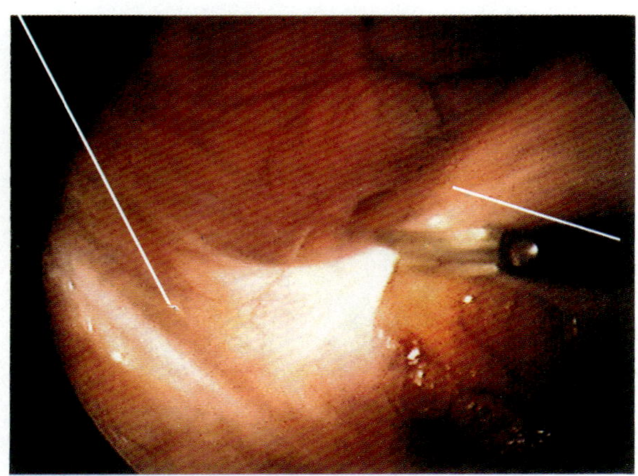

FIGURE 18-21. Pelvic side-wall with the rectum retracted to the right.

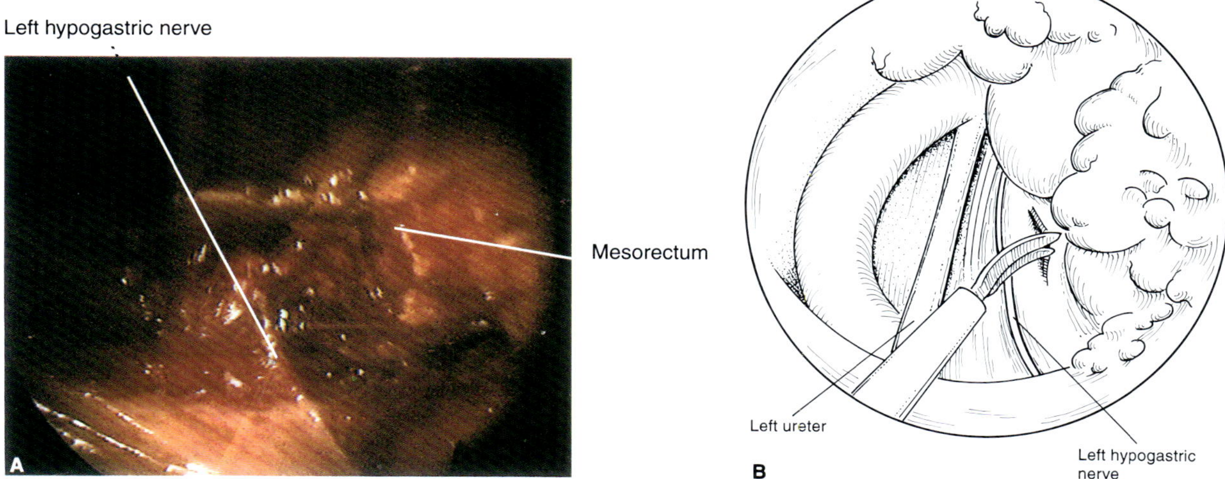

FIGURE 18-22. (**A**) Photograph of a dissection of the rectum off the sacrum. (**B**) Drawing of the dissection of the rectum off the sacrum.

dissection (again using the scissors) and with forward retraction with a bowel clamp inserted through port 3, the rectum is dissected off the sacrum (Fig. 18-22).

The rectum is then retracted to the left and a peritoneal incision is continued on the right side into the pelvis (Fig. 18-23). The right branch of the hypogastric plexus is identified and the rectal mesentery is dissected from it, as described.

Dividing Inferior Mesenteric Vessels. The inferior mesenteric vessels are identified and divided with an Endo-GIA vascular stapler inserted through port 3, as described. The left ureter is identified before dividing the vessels. Blunt dissection of the ureter may be accomplished by using a small gauze-tipped dissector passed through port 4 or 5.

Division of the Rectal Mesentery. The overlying peritoneum is incised with electrocautery, using the hook or scissors. The superior rectal vessels are demonstrated, a window is made in the mesentery, and the vessels are divided using an Endo-GIA vascular stapler inserted through port 4 or 5 (Fig. 18-24). The remaining blood vessels of the mesentery are divided after double application of Endo-Clips (U.S. Surgical, Norwalk, CT).

Division of Rectum. An Endopath Endolinear cutter 60 (Ethicon Endo-Surgical) is used to staple and divide the rectum (Fig. 18-25). Depending on individual anatomy, the trocar in position 4 or 5 is replaced with an 18-mm trocar to accomplish this procedure.

Exteriorization of the Proximal Colon. A small incision is made in the left iliac fossa. The specimen is exteriorized and resected.

Application of Pursestring Suture. A pursestring suture is applied to the proximal colon and the anvil of an intraluminal stapler is secured in place (Fig. 18-26).

Proximal Colon and Anvil Returned to Abdominal Cavity. The colon is returned to the peritoneal cavity. The abdominal wall incision is closed and pneumoperitoneum reestablished.

Colorectal Anastomosis. The shaft of the instrument is introduced into the rectum. The perforating rod is extended, and a small diathermy incision is made into the stapled line, allowing the rod to advance into the pelvis.

The anvil is fitted onto the rod, and a staple-on-staple anastomosis is performed (Fig. 18-27). After filling the

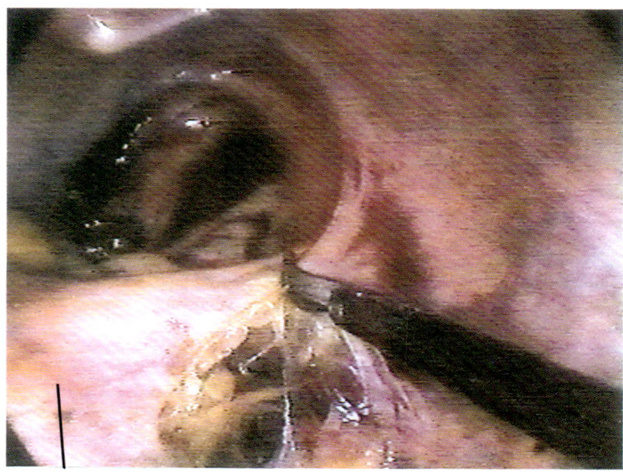

FIGURE 18-23. Rectum retracted to the left.

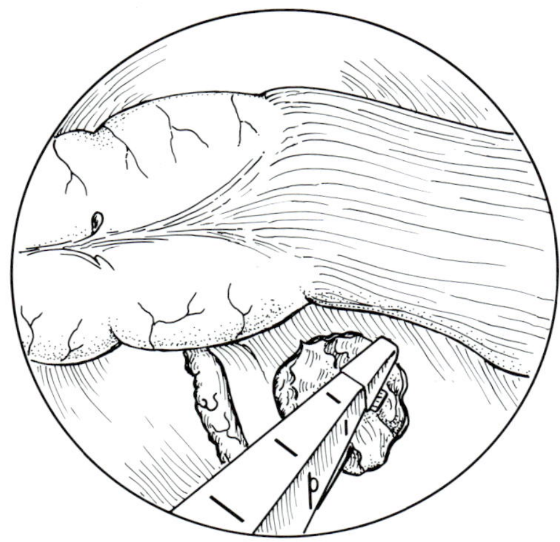

FIGURE 18-24. Division of the superior rectal vessels.

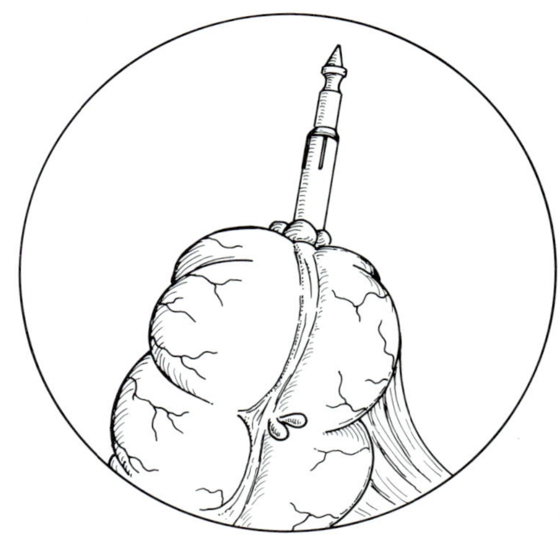

FIGURE 18-26. An intraluminal stapler anvil in place.

pelvis with saline and occluding the proximal colon, the anastomosis is tested with air.

LAPAROSCOPIC-ASSISTED ABDOMINOPERINEAL EXCISION OF THE RECTUM

Laparoscopic techniques may be suitable for patients who require an abdominoperineal resection of the rectum. We have only used this technique for relatively small tumors occurring in the lower 3 to 4 cm of the rectum.

Position of Ports. Five trocars are inserted as shown in Figure 18-28.

Mobilization of Sigmoid and Descending Colons. The sigmoid and descending colons are mobilized and the left ureter is identified.

Mobilization of the Rectum. The clue to accurate and bloodless mobilization of the rectum is the identification of the left and right branches of the hypogastric plexus. The correct plane of dissection is medial and anterior to each plexus.

Lateral Mobilization of the Rectum. The rectum is retracted to the right and the peritoneal incision is continued on the left side into the pelvis (Fig. 18-29).

The left branch of the hypogastric plexus is identified, and the rectal mesentery, enveloped in its fascia, is dissected from the nerve. This plane of dissection proceeds posteriorly to lift the mesorectum off the sacrum. This procedure is duplicated on the right side to dissect the right posterolateral aspect of the rectum. This dissection is accomplished with blunt dissectors passed alternatively through ports 2 and 4.

Posterior Mobilization of the Rectum. The rectum is retracted superiorly and by sharp dissection, the meso-

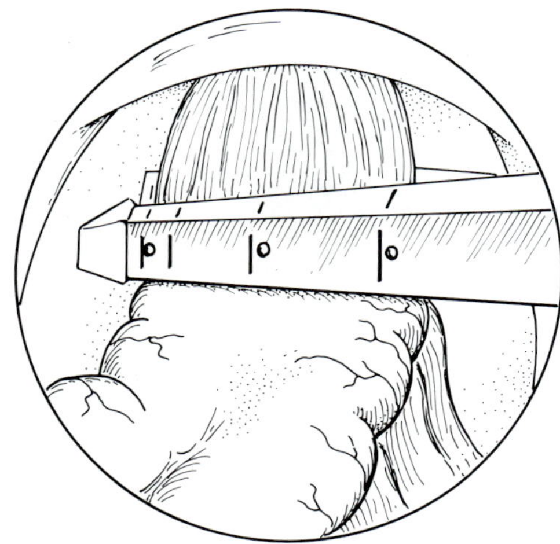

FIGURE 18-25. Division of the rectum.

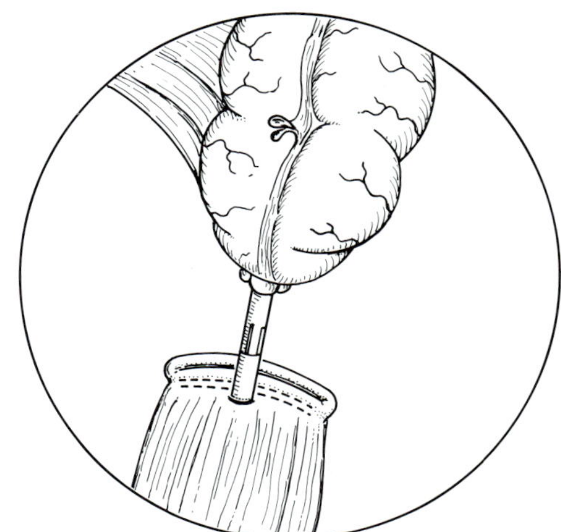

FIGURE 18-27. An anvil fitted onto a rod.

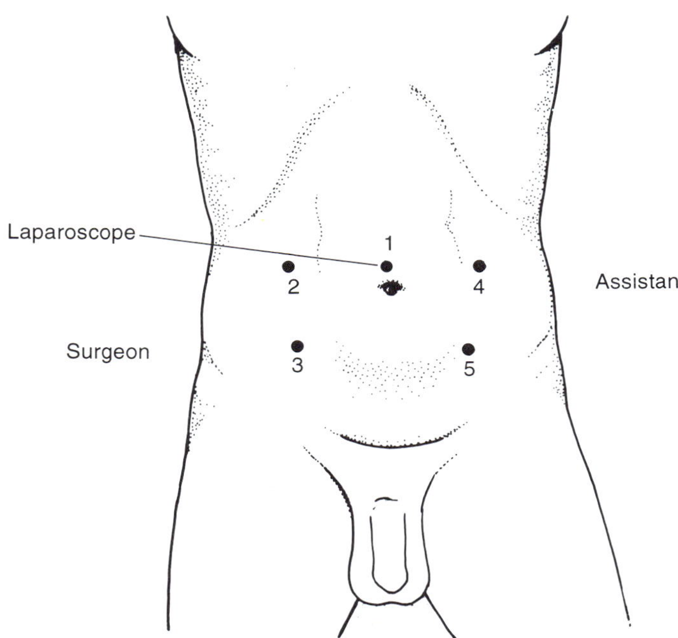

FIGURE 18-28. Position of surgeon, assistant, and port sites.

rectum is separated from the presacral fascia down to the levator muscles (Fig. 18-30).

Anterior Mobilization of the Rectum. The anterior peritoneal reflection is elevated (Fig. 18-31), and the lateral peritoneal incisions are extended anteriorly to meet in the midline (Fig. 18-32). The anterior plane is developed by sharp dissection with scissors and electrocautery through ports 2 and 4 (Fig. 18-33).

Division of Lateral Ligaments. The rectum is elevated, placing the right lateral ligament under tension. With electrocoagulation, the ligament is thinned to expose the middle rectal vessels, which are then doubly endoclipped and divided (Fig. 18-34). The procedure is repeated to divide the left lateral ligament.

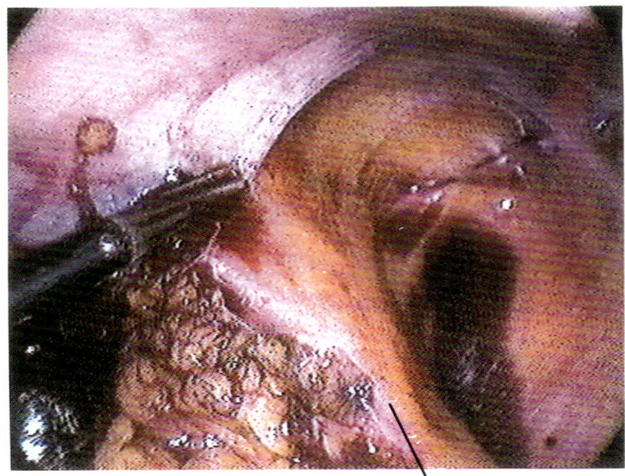

FIGURE 18-29. Rectum retracted.

Division of Inferior Mesenteric Vessels. This is described above, using an Endo-GIA vascular stapler.

Division of Mesentery and Proximal Colon. The level of resection of the proximal colon is identified. The mesentery is triangulated, defatted by electrocautery, and individual vessels divided, either with an Endo-GIA vascular stapler or a double application of Endo-Clips. The colon is divided with a single application of an Endopath Endolinear cutter 60 (Ethicon Endo-Surgical) introduced through an 18-mm port (port 4). A grasper is applied to the proximal colon to aid in subsequent identification during exteriorization.

Perineal Dissection. The perineal dissection proceeds as usual. Figure 18-35 demonstrates the operator's fingers transgressing the fascia. The perineal dissection is completed and the specimen delivered through the perineal wound, which is closed in layers around a corrugated drain. Figure 18-36 shows the completed dissection, with both hypogastric nerves well demonstrated.

The colostomy is exteriorized in the usual fashion. Partial pneumoperitoneum is reestablished and the pericolic gutter is closed with a hernia stapler.

Figure 18-37 shows the abdomen of a 52-year-old man who had a laparoscopic abdominoperineal excision 3 weeks previously.

LAPAROSCOPIC LOOP STOMA FORMATION

The patient is prepared for surgery as previously described. Preoperative siting of the stoma position is mandatory.

Pneumoperitoneum and Placement of Trocars. Pneumoperitoneum is achieved with a 10-mm Hasson trocar introduced adjacent to the umbilicus under direct vision. A second 10-mm port is placed through the selected stoma exit site. In patients having a loop ileostomy, two additional 5-mm ports are introduced in the left iliac fossa (Fig. 18-38).

The patient is placed in Trendelenburg's position, with the left side down, to enable easy identification of the cecum. The terminal ileum is located and held up by two atraumatic bowel-grasping forceps. A small window is made in the mesentery adjacent to the bowel wall. A linen tape is introduced through the 10-mm port (port 2), passed through the mesenteric defect, and secured with Endo-Clips to form a loop encircling the ileum (Fig. 18-39).

(text continues on page 181)

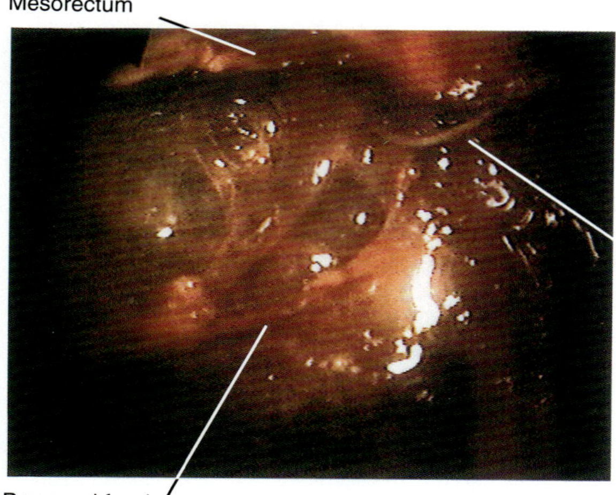

FIGURE 18-30. Separation of the mesorectum from the presacral fascia.

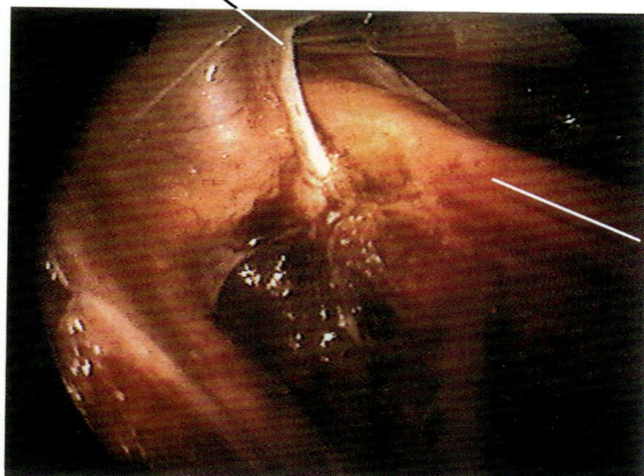

FIGURE 18-31. Elevation of the anterior peritoneal reflection.

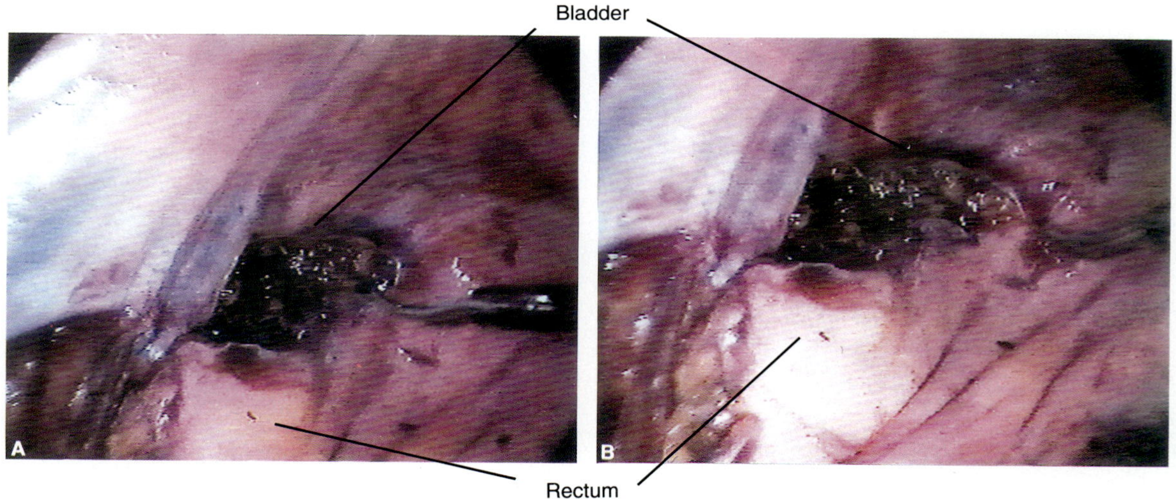

FIGURE 18-32. (A, B) Anterior extension of lateral peritoneal incisions.

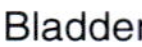

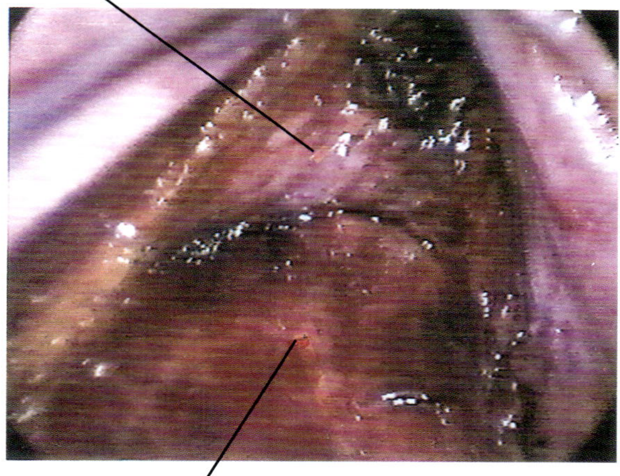

FIGURE 18-33. Bladder and retracted rectum.

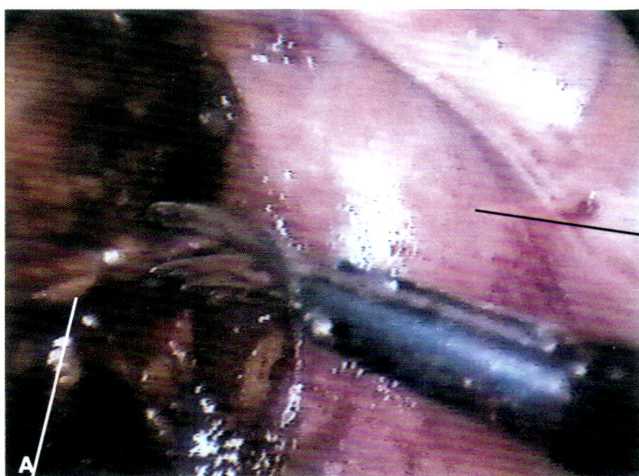

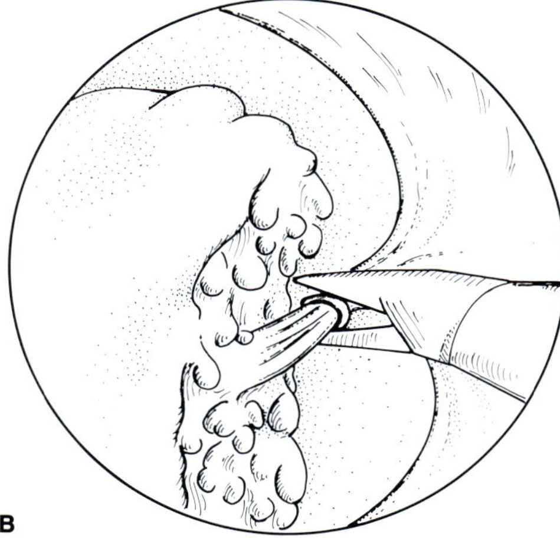

FIGURE 18-34. (**A**) Photograph of a division of the middle rectal vessels. (**B**) Drawing of the division of the middle rectal vessels.

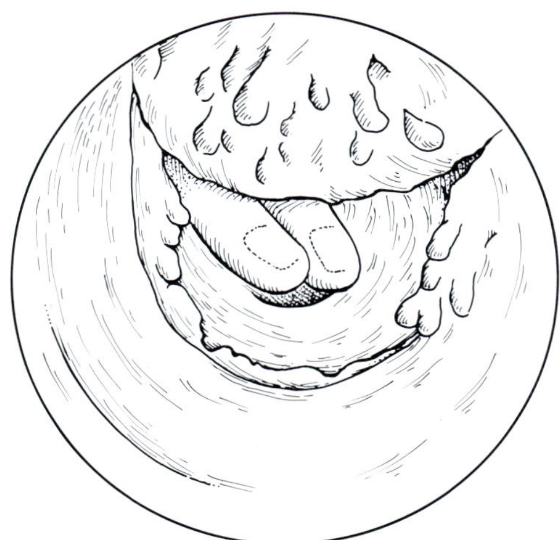

FIGURE 18-35. Operator's fingers transgressing the fascia.

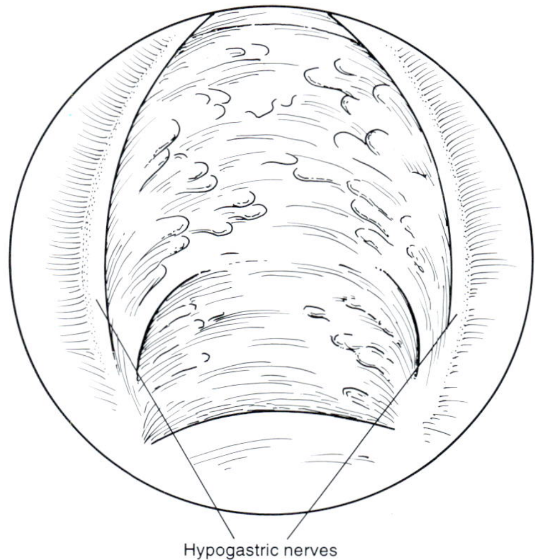

FIGURE 18-36. Right and left hypogastric nerves.

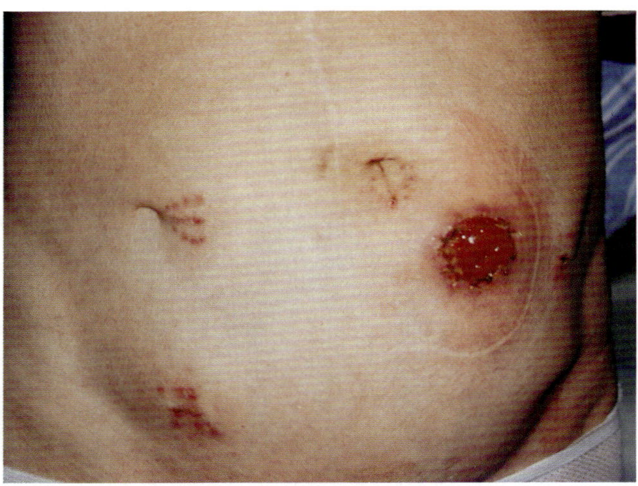

FIGURE 18-37. Abdomen of 52-year-old man 3 weeks after laparoscopic abdominoperineal excision.

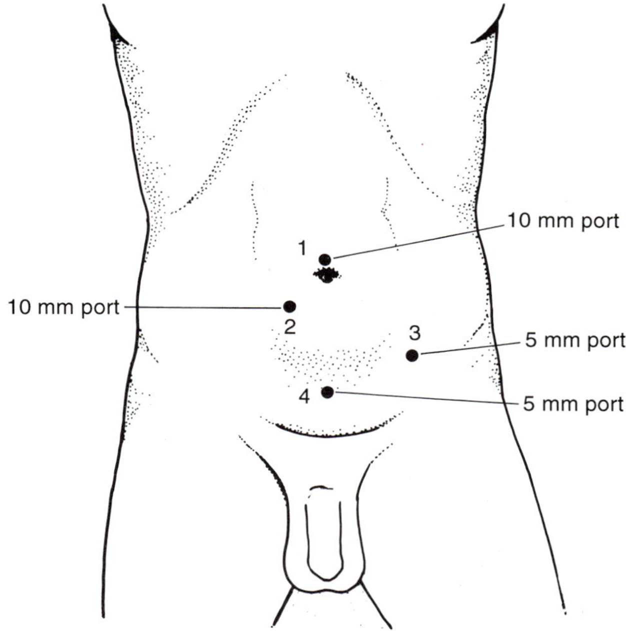

FIGURE 18-38. Port placements for loop ileostomy/colostomy.

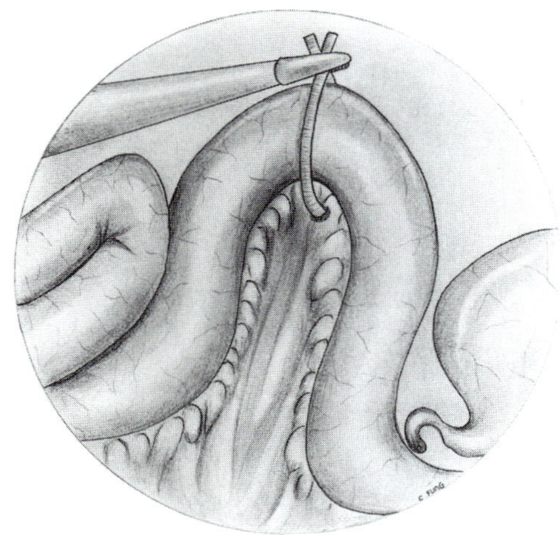

FIGURE 18-39. Loop encircling the ileum.

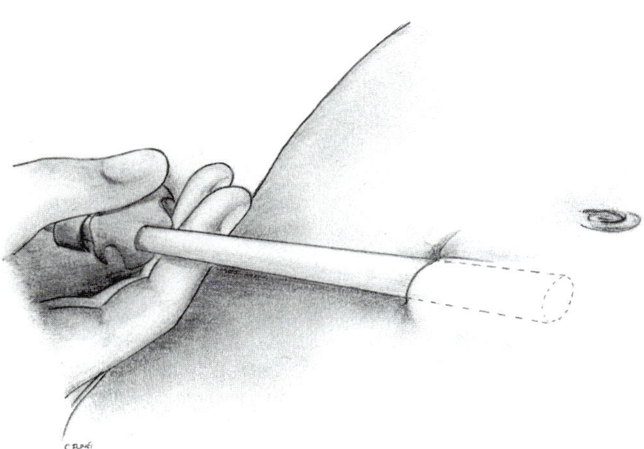

FIGURE 18-40. Port depressed against the lateral margin of the wound.

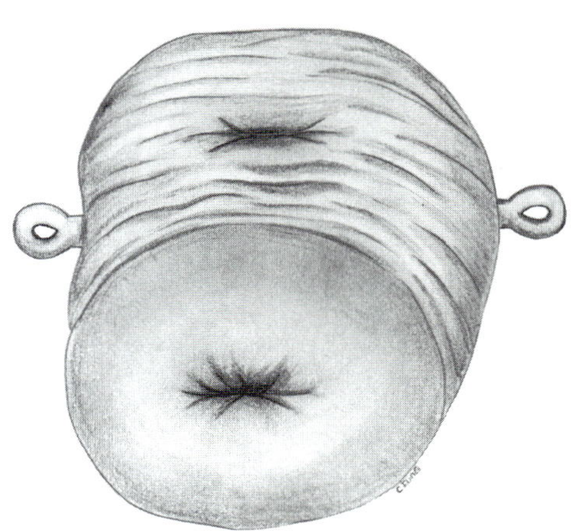

FIGURE 18-41. Proximal limb of the stoma, everted and pouting.

The trocar at the stoma site is left in place and the skin incision is lengthened transversely. The wound is deepened through the subcutaneous fat, and a cruciate incision is made in the anterior rectus sheath. The port is then depressed against the lateral margin of the wound to elevate the rectus muscle, posterior rectus sheath, and peritoneum, which are divided sequentially (Fig. 18-40).

The linen tape is grasped with endoforceps that are passed through the 10-mm port. The trocar, with forceps in place, is withdrawn from the incision and the tape brought into the wound. Gentle traction on the tape delivers the ileum onto the anterior abdominal wall. Pneumoperitoneum is reestablished and the loop is inspected intracorporeally to ensure that there is no twist and to confirm the correct orientation of the proximal limb of the stoma. The trocar entry wounds are then closed in the usual way and the ileostomy fashioned over a small rod, ensuring that the proximal limb is everted and pouting (Fig. 18-41).

Formation of the loop sigmoid is similar in principle. A 10-mm port is placed through the stoma site in the left iliac fossa. The 5-mm ports are placed in the right iliac fossa. Dissection of the lateral adhesions of the sigmoid colon to the lateral abdominal wall and mobilization of the sigmoid mesentery are required to ensure that the stoma is formed without tension.

Postoperative Care. After laparoscopic-assisted colorectal procedures, patients are managed as for the equivalent open procedure. Urinary catheters are removed postoperatively as soon as the patient has established normal urine output and is comfortable enough to void without assistance. Nasogastric tubes are removed once gastrointestinal function begins to return. Oral fluid is started soon thereafter. Our impression is that patients generally recover from these procedures quickly. This, however, needs to be confirmed by prospective controlled trials.

Chapter 19

Laparoscopic Surgery: An Atlas for General Surgeons, edited by
Gary C. Vitale, Joseph S. Sanfilippo, and Jacques Perissat.
J. B. Lippincott Company, Philadelphia, © 1995.

Highly Selective Vagotomy

Gary C. Vitale

STANDARD APPROACH

While undergoing vagotomy, the patient is supine, with legs extended and kept apart by being placed in Allen universal stirrups. This allows the operator, who is standing between the open legs, to work in a mid-plane position. The legs are relatively flat, so as not to impede the passage of instruments in and out of the abdominal ports. The pneumoperitoneum is established by inserting an insufflating needle into the left upper quadrant, 2 to 3 cm below the left costal margin in the mid-clavicular plane. At this point, the natural curve of the thoracic cage tends to bow the abdominal wall away from the visceral organs.

After insufflation to 12 mmHg CO_2 pressure, the abdominal wall is grasped and elevated. A transverse incision is made in the supra-umbilical position and a 10-mm trocar inserted. A 15° laparoscope is introduced, and all other trocar placements are performed under direct vision. When there is a long distance between the xiphoid process and the umbilicus, the trocar is inserted 5 to 7 cm above the umbilicus in the midline; sometimes a 30° laparoscope is preferable.

A 10-mm trocar is inserted in the mid-clavicular line, 2 cm below the right costal margin. This is for the introduction of a liver retractor. We use a Padron endoscopic exposing retractor, designed by Jarit Surgical Instruments (Hawthorne, NY). A 10-mm retractor is placed in the anterior axillary line, 6 to 7 cm below the right costal margin, for insertion of a Babcock retractor. Another 10-mm trocar is inserted in the left anterior axillary line, 4 cm below the costal margin, for insertion of a Babcock retractor to grasp the greater curvature of the stomach. Finally, a 5-mm trocar is inserted into the mid-clavicular line, 2 cm below the costal margin, which is used for the dissecting scissors and electrocautery hook dissector (Fig. 19-1).

A nasogastric tube is placed in the esophagus to aid in the identification of the esophagus at the hiatus. A toothed grasping forceps is used to grasp the lateral attachments of the left lobe of the liver. With downward retraction, a hook dissector is then used to divide the ligamentous attachment of the left lobe of the liver to the diaphragm. This is continued medially to the right of the esophagus. The liver retractor is then placed to push the left lobe of the liver superiorly and to the right, thus exposing the hiatus. In some cases, the left lobe of the liver may be pushed upward without dividing this attachment. The hook dissector and a grasping forceps are then used to elevate and divide the peritoneum overlying the esophagus; this is done in a transverse fashion from 2 cm to the left to 1 cm to the right of the esophagus (Fig. 19-2). The esophagus is identified at this point by palpation with a blunt-tipped forceps to locate the nasogastric tube. Alternatively, a pediatric endoscope may be placed to illuminate the gastroesophageal junction.

The blunt-tipped duckbill forceps is used to spread tissue to the right and left of the esophagus, just medially to the inner border of the right and left crura (Figs. 19-3 and 19-4). The right posterior vagus nerve is usually identified at this point and isolated from the esophagus (Fig. 19-5). The Babcock retractors are placed distally on the greater and lesser curvatures of the stomach and retracted inferiorly. This spreads the lesser curvature, thus exposing the anatomy of the anterior nerve of Latarjet. We usually complete the posterior dissection of the esophagus, allowing the passage of a blunt duckbill-type dissector posterior to the esophagus. An elastic vessel loop is then passed around the esophagus and brought

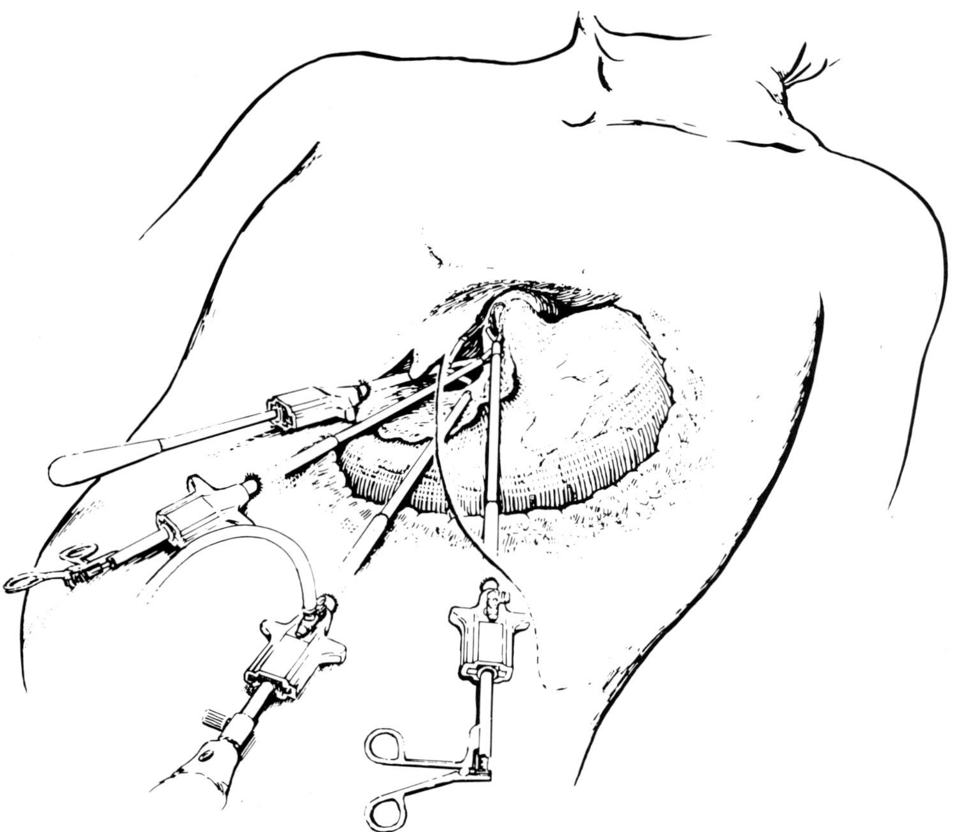

FIGURE 19-1. Overview showing port and instrument placement.

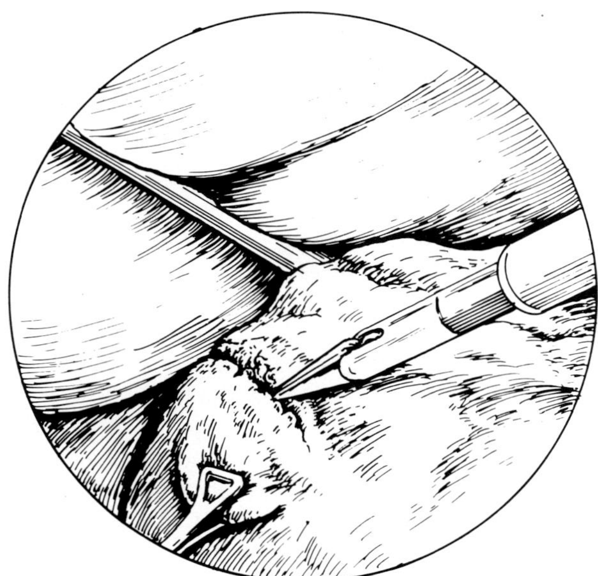

FIGURE 19.2. Peritoneum is divided over esophagus.

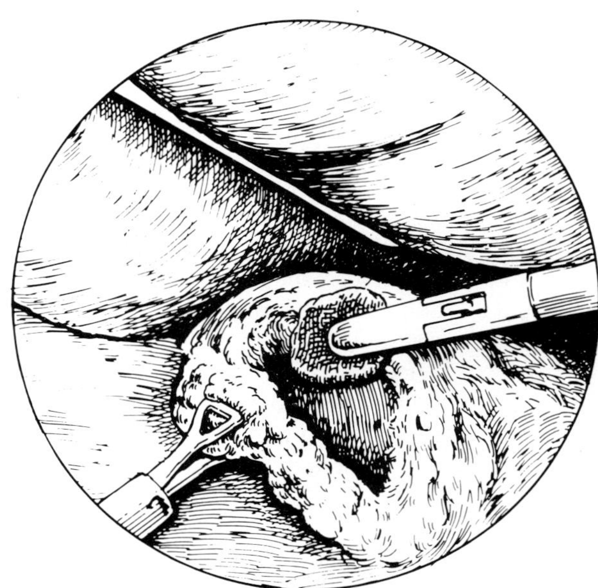

FIGURE 19-3. Right lateral wall of esophagus exposed by blunt dissection.

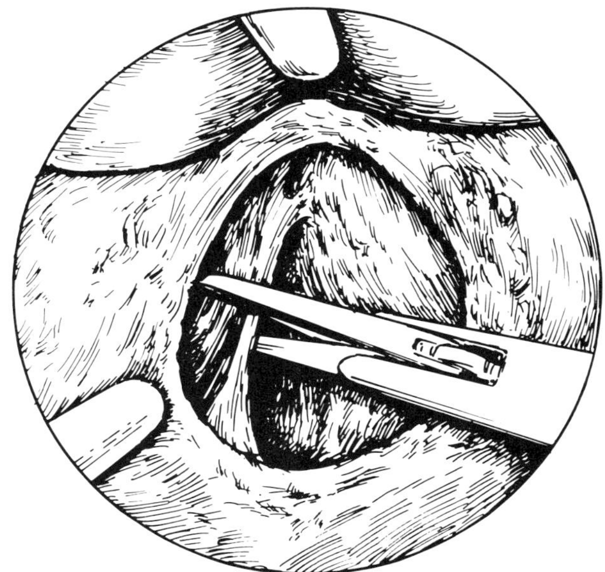

FIGURE 19-4. Connective tissue divided from hiatus to gastroesophageal junction. Scissors shown cutting phrenicoesophageal strand.

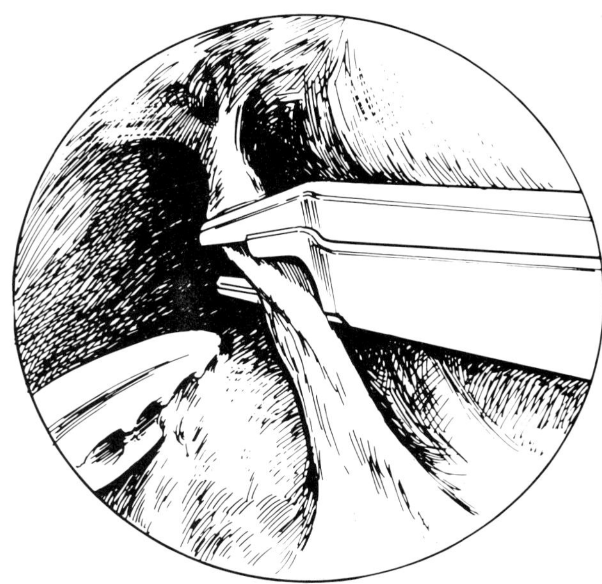

FIGURE 19-6. Posterior vagal trunk is clipped.

out through a 5-mm port, which is placed right below the xiphoid process. With retraction on the elastic vessel loop, the esophagus is raised, thus creating tension at the superior aspect of the dissection. This facilitates the performance of the highly selective vagotomy.

At this point, a decision is made whether to perform a posterior truncal vagotomy with an anterior highly selective vagotomy or a complete highly selective vagotomy. In the former case, a posterior truncal vagotomy is performed and a segment is sent for pathologic evaluation. We use clips proximally and distally on the nerve and divide between them (Figs. 19-6 and 19-7). The anterior nerve is identified and traced to its root along the lesser curvature of the stomach. The nerve of Latarjet is carefully examined at its distal insertion and the proximal branches of the nerve of Latarjet are marked for division.

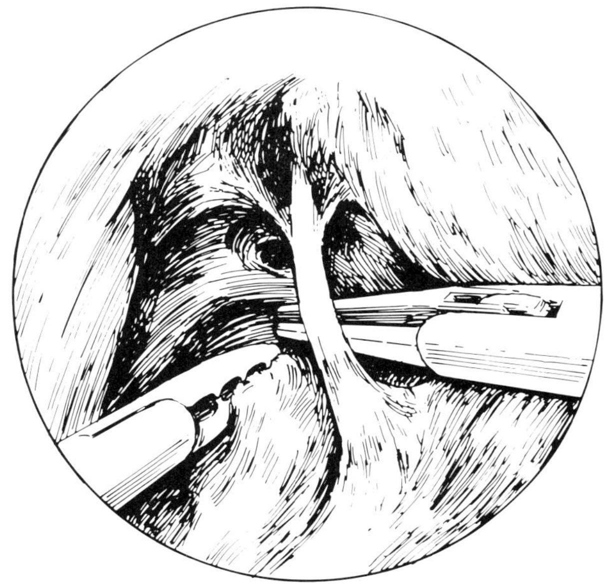

FIGURE 19-5. Dissection of right vagal trunk from posterior esophagus.

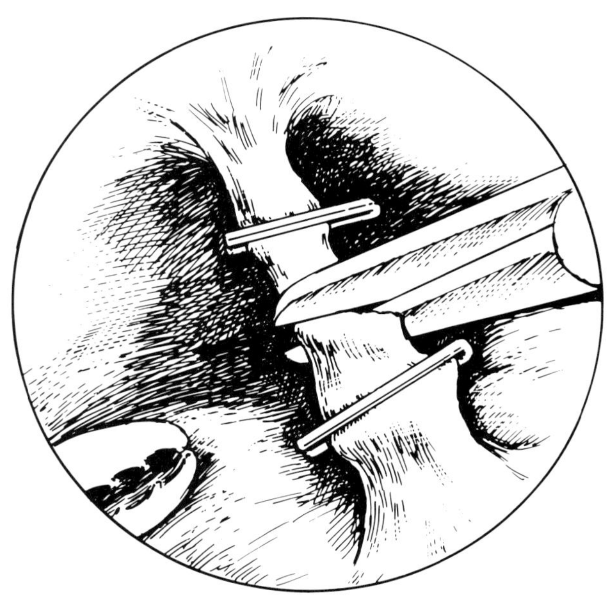

FIGURE 19-7. Posterior vagal trunk divided between clips.

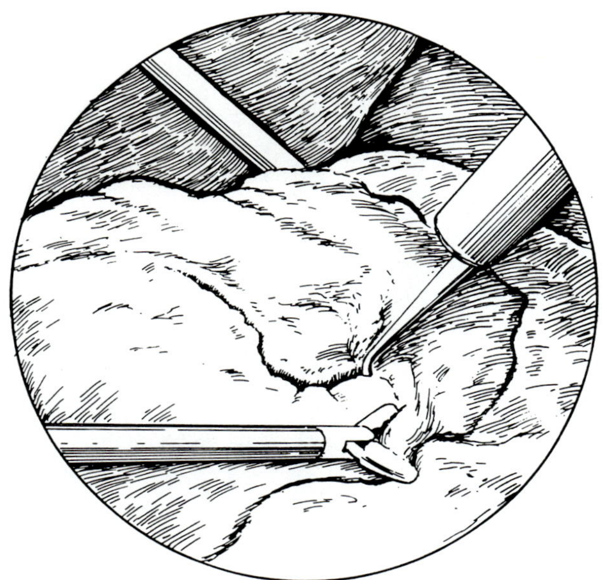

FIGURE 19-8. Superficial marking cut defining extent of seromyotomy.

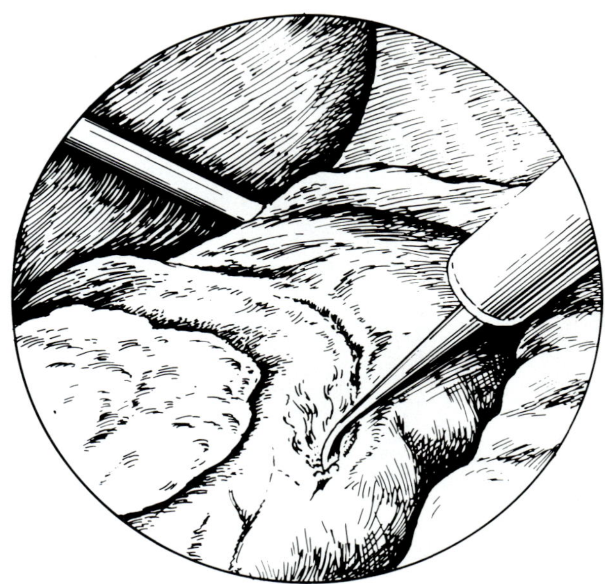

FIGURE 19-9. Seromyotomy cut is deepened using cautery scissors or hook dissector. Incision is stopped at level of mucosa.

The branch that continues straight and the two branches that curve toward the pylorus are preserved. The one or two branches that curve toward the antrum and greater curvature are divided. The Babcock retractors are positioned to stretch the lesser curvature. The inserting branches of the nerve of Latarjet are identified and doubly clipped and divided. The hook dissector is used to divide the visceral peritoneum and fatty tissues between vessels. The anterior leaf of the lesser curvature of the gastric mesentery is divided to the mid-plane of the stomach and the posterior branches are left intact because the posterior nerve has already been divided. In the case of a full highly selective vagotomy, the dissection is continued to reach the posterior surface of the stomach; division of the anterior and posterior branches of the nerve of Latarjet is accomplished—first distally and then continued proximally to the esophagus.

The dissection of the anterior nerve is continued well up on the esophagus, and all nerve branches exiting to the left are divided, particularly those at the junction of the cardia of the stomach and the esophagus. A short serosal myotomy is performed at this superior level to ensure complete division of the nerves of Grassi, which may travel subserosally to this portion of the stomach.

Finally, after completion of the vagotomy, the area is irrigated until the return runs clear, the pneumoperitoneum is evacuated, and the trocars are removed. It should be noted that great care is taken during the dissection to divide the branches of the nerves of Latarjet close to the stomach to avoid injury to the main trunk innervating the pylorus. Additionally, these small branches are divided after placement of clips, without application of cautery, again to avoid cautery burn to the main trunk through conduction along the nerve or coagulation of tissue surrounding the clips. In obese patients, maintenance of a dry operating field during division of the branches of the nerve of Latarjet is often difficult, and in this case, suture ligatures of 3-0 silk may be used to ligate some branches that are imbedded in fat tissue and are difficult to clip or coagulate. The advantage of the ligature is that it allows encircling of a larger cross section of tissue, thus including smaller vessels that may otherwise bleed.

POSTERIOR TRUNCAL VAGOTOMY AND ANTERIOR SEROMYOTOMY

The patient is placed in a supine position, with legs held open by Allen Universal stirrups. The operating surgeon stands between the patient's legs. The pneumoperitoneum is created by placing a Veress needle in the umbilicus, and the intraabdominal pressure is maintained at 12 mmHg. A total of five ports are used. First, a 10-mm trocar is placed through the umbilicus and a 15° laparoscope is introduced. Second, a 5-mm port is placed 5 cm to the right of the xiphoid process for insertion of a suction irrigator. This device also retracts the left lobe of the liver. A third trocar, 5 mm in size, is inserted in the mid-clavicular line, two fingerbreadths below the right costal margin. A fourth trocar, also 5 mm, is placed in the mid-clavicular line, 2 cm below the left costal margin. A 10-mm trocar (the fifth port) is placed 6 cm to the left of the umbilicus. This channel is used for the dissecting scissors, the hook cannula, and the clip appliers.

The lesser omentum is opened, using the hook dissector. The left gastric vein is clipped and divided. A pediatric endoscope can be placed into the esophagus to the level of the gastroesophageal junction. This aids in the identification of the esophagus at the hiatus. The hook cannula is then used to free the hiatus by first incising the overlying peritoneum and then dissecting the plane between the esophagus and the right and left crura. At this point, the right vagus nerve is identified; it is usually easier to see than at open laparotomy. The nerve is divided between metallic clips and a short segment is excised for histologic examination.

The anterior lesser curvature seromyotomy begins at the cardia and is extended to about 6 cm from the pylorus. The incision is made using the hook electrocautery, with an atraumatic grasping forceps inserted through the subcostal ports to grasp and retract the edges of the incised serosa (Figs. 19-8 and 19-9). At the proximal end, the seromyotomy is carried to the junction of the cardia of the stomach with the esophagus. Care is taken to divide the nerves of Grassi, which insert on the stomach to the left of the esophagus. The precise distal limits of the dissection are determined by the nerve of Latarjet. We preserve the branches curving right toward the pylorus and the main nerve trunk, which continues in a straight line onto the stomach. We divide the two or three branches curving back to the left. The gastric pouch is filled with 500 mL of dilute methylene blue and the mucosa is carefully examined for perforations. If a perforation is encountered, it may be sutured, using extracorporeal knot-tying techniques. Fibrin glue is then applied

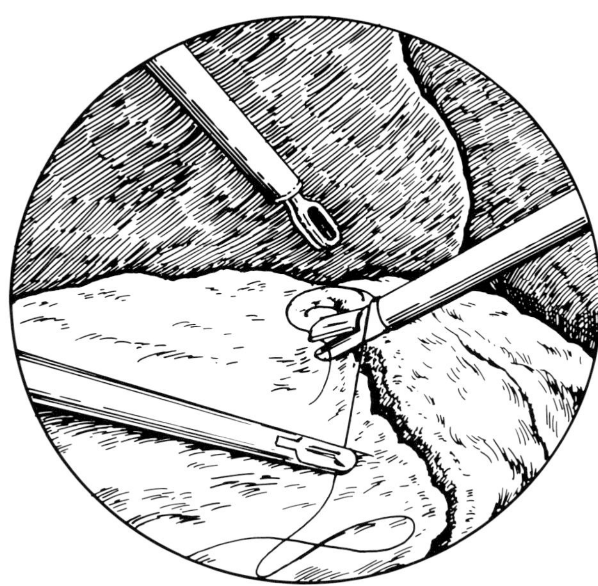

FIGURE 19-11. Knot tied after placing first suture at the apex of seromyotomy.

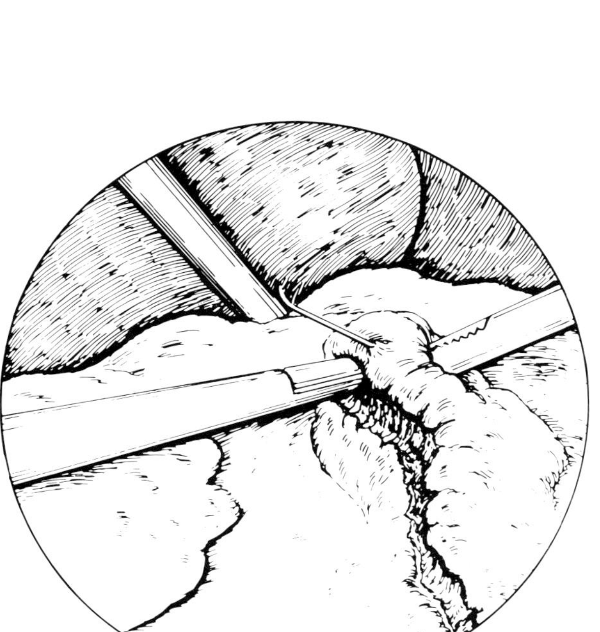

FIGURE 19-10. Counter pressure is used to separate edges of seromuscular layer and a suture is placed to approximate the cut edges.

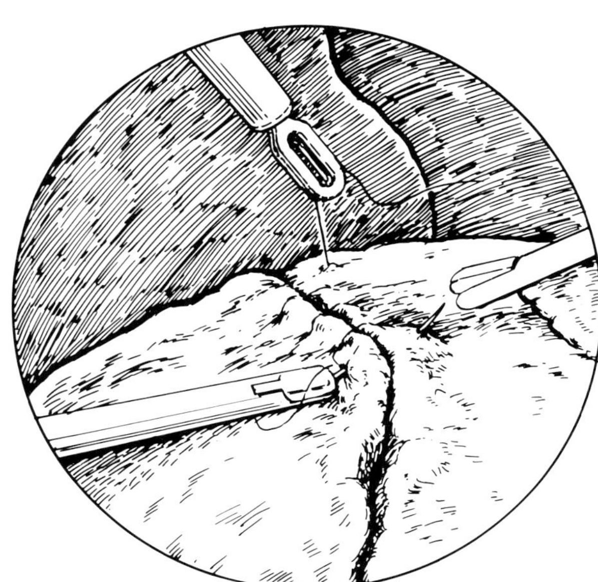

FIGURE 19-12. Tension maintained during running suture.

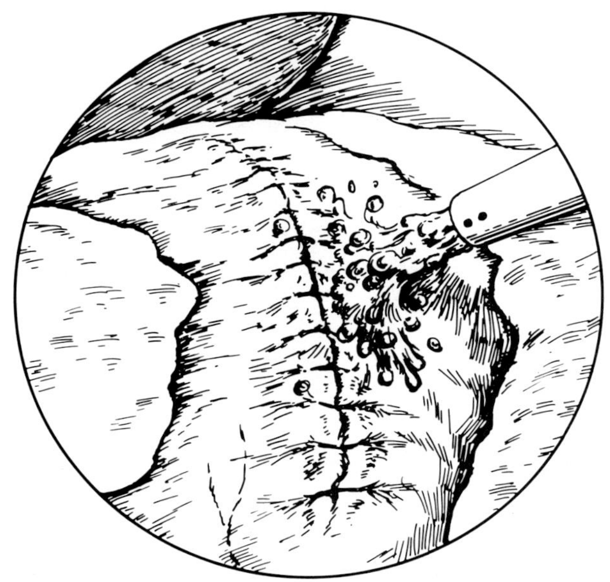

FIGURE 19-13. Irrigation and inspection of sutured seromyotomy.

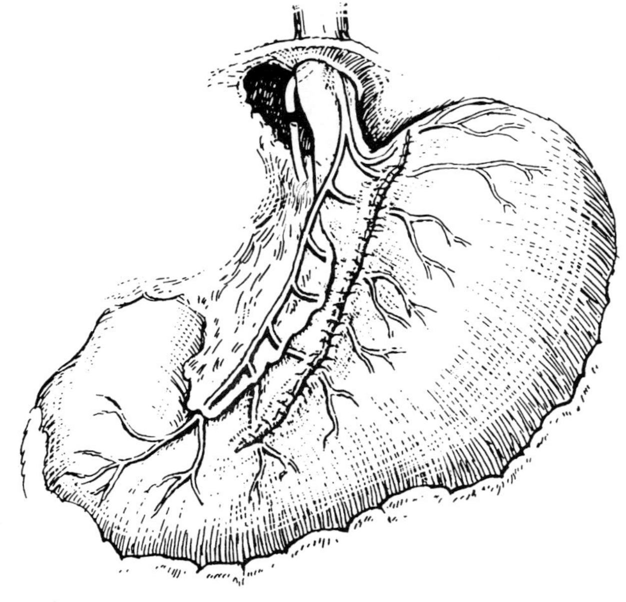

FIGURE 19-14. Posterior truncal vagotomy and anterior seromyotomy. The right posterior vagus nerve truck has been cut and the left anterior truck remains intact.

to the seromyotomy or alternatively, the edges of the serosa may be overlapped and sutured with a running 3-0 silk suture (Figs. 19-10–19-12). The area is irrigated until the return runs clear, and the trocars are then removed (Figs. 19-13 and 19-14).

Selected Readings

Branicki FJ, Nathanson LK: Minimal access gastroduodenal surgery. Aust N Z Surg 1994;64(9):589.

Katkhouda N, Heimbucher J, Mouiel J: Laparoscopic posterior vagotomy and anterior seromyotomy. Endosc Surg Allied Technol 1994;2(2):95.

Katkhouda N: A new technique of surgical treatment of chronic duodenal ulcer without laparotomy by videocoelioscopy. Am J Surg 1991;161:361.

Weerts JM, Dallemagne B, Jehaes C, Markiewicz S: Laparoscopic gastric vagotomies. Ann Chir Gynaecol 1944;83(2):118.

Zucker KA, Bailey RW: Laparoscopic truncal and selective vagotomy for intractable ulcer disease. Semin Gastrointest Dis 1994;5(3):128.

Chapter 20

Laparoscopic Surgery: An Atlas for General Surgeons, edited by
Gary C. Vitale, Joseph S. Sanfilippo, and Jacques Perissat.
J. B. Lippincott Company, Philadelphia, © 1995.

Laparoscopic Nissen Fundoplication

Gary C. Vitale

Antireflux procedures are ideally suited to a laparoscopic approach. The operations require dissection and freeing of tissue at the gastroesophageal junction, with a subsequent wrap of gastric fundus partially or completely around the esophagus, with crural repair of the esophageal hiatus. Although there are clearly some dangers associated with dissection of the esophagus, both in laparoscopic and open surgery, not opening the gastrointestinal tract—necessitating a subsequent anastomosis and need to remove tissue—makes it ideally suited to a laparoscopic approach. The Nissen fundoplication is probably the simplest of the antireflux procedures. There are good long-term follow-up data supporting its use and it is the procedure that we use most commonly to treat reflux disease.

Symptoms of gastroesophageal reflux disease can be nonspecific; the process may mimic a variety of other intra-abdominal pathologies. Thus, it is important to document the absence of hepatobiliary or pancreatic pathology and peptic ulcer disease before Nissen fundoplication. Although cholecystectomy may be accomplished simultaneously with reflux, again, clear documentation of the importance of the reflux to the patient's constellation of symptoms is important before choosing an operative approach to this disease process. Endoscopic and histologic documentation of persistent esophagitis despite adequate medical management is a standard indication for surgery. We prefer to document the extent of gastroesophageal reflux, using ambulatory 24-hour pH monitoring for all patients who are selected to undergo operative repair. In some cases, the pattern of reflux can be clearly identified, with 24-hour reflux monitoring allowing adjustment in the nonsurgical management of the disease, thus avoiding operative intervention. There are several settings in which an operative approach should be considered, even in the absence of acid reflux. Strictures can form due to bile or trypsin reflux without acid being detected. This occurs in a subset of patients with gastroesophageal reflux. This condition is indicated by a lack of response to H_2-blockers, with progressive narrowing or esophagitis of the gastroesophageal junction and neutral pH recordings. Additionally, there are patients who have severe gastro-oral reflux, such that pulmonary complications result from nocturnal aspiration. Indeed, reflux of this sort may mimic chronic obstructive pulmonary disease or asthma. Some patients may even have sleep apnea that is not recognized to be a result of significant nocturnal gastroesophageal reflux. In these patients, repair of the gastroesophageal junction to prevent reflux is indicated, even in the absence of esophagitis or narrowing of the distal esophagus.

The concept of the Nissen fundoplication repair is simple. The esophagus is dissected free from its retroperitoneal attachments in a fashion similar to that for vagotomy. Care must be taken to preserve the phrenicoesophageal ligament, extending from the diaphragm onto the esophagus. Next, the stomach is freed from its posterior attachments to the retroperitoneum and pancreas. In most instances, this allows adequate mobilization of the fundus of the stomach, so that it may be pushed posterior to the esophagus and brought around anteriorly to make the circumferential Nissen wrap. Division of the short gastric vessels to the spleen is sometimes necessary to obtain an adequate wrap. The left gastric artery should always be preserved because it serves to some extent as a barrier for slippage of the wrap onto the body of the stomach. Thus, in dissecting the lesser curvature to allow the fundus of the stomach to pass posterior to the esophagus, one should dissect only as much as is required to bring the stomach through and no more. Several points are important. First, the plicated fundus must be attached to the esophagus with several of the sutures that are used in the plication. This helps to prevent slippage of the Nissen wrap, which could have the disastrous result of causing obstruction with severe vomiting. Second, we perform the wrap over a Maloney dilator, 44 French.

Alternatively, the repair may be performed over a manometric catheter and the wrap tightened to increase pressures 10 to 15 mmHg. An excessively tight or long fundoplication may cause a relative obstruction. Third, about four or five sutures (for a total plication distance of about 3 cm) are usually adequate. We favor the creation of a relatively loose or floppy Nissen fundoplication; in our opinion, this prevents pathologic reflux but reduces the chance of dysphagia and may allow some eructation. Fourth, there is no indication for associated vagotomy with this procedure when it is used exclusively for gastroesophageal reflux disease with esophagitis. If the patient has recalcitrant peptic ulcer disease, one should consider operative treatment for this disease alone, with observation of the effect on the esophagitis. A Nissen fundoplication may be added at a later date in a sequential fashion to treat the reflux if it remains a major symptomatic problem. If the vagus nerve is inadvertently damaged during the Nissen fundoplication, a pyloroplasty should be added. Fifth, it is my opinion that reduction of the hiatal hernia is necessary with crural repair. Leaving the Nissen wrap in the chest, although potentially necessary in some cases of severe esophageal shortening, is not optimal and may promote recurrent reflux. Competence of the gastroesophageal junction in preventing reflux may depend partly on restoring an intra-abdominal segment of distal esophagus.

The Nissen fundoplication as described herein has an excellent record of short- and long-term results for gastroesophageal reflux disease. With an average follow-up of 10 years, the cure rate for refractory esophagitis is 93% to 95%. Thus, the advent of laparoscopy should make this a reasonable and successful approach for severe gastroesophageal reflux disease. The indications for an operative approach should not change, however, based on the advent of minimal-access surgery. All efforts to control the disease with nonsurgical management should be employed emphatically before consideration of an operative approach.

PATIENT POSITIONING AND TROCAR INSERTION

The patient is placed in the supine position, with his or her legs in Allen stirrups. This position allows the operator to stand between the patient's legs, which facilitates the use of both of the surgeon's hands during the operation. An Elmed adjustable arm (Elmed Inc., Attison, IL) is used to hold the laparoscope and attached camera. The lack of motion provided by a fixed camera holder is highly desirable when working on the esophageal hiatus. Although a forward viewing telescope may be used, the view is improved with a 15° (or in some cases, 30°) viewing-angle laparoscope.

Five 10-mm trocars are used for this procedure:

- Port 1: The laparoscope is inserted through a trocar placed 3 to 4 cm above the umbilicus (several centimeters higher if the patient is long from xiphoid to umbilicus).
- Port 2: One trocar is placed in the mid-clavicular line a few centimeters below the left costal margin is for the Endopath Babcock forceps (Ethicon-Endosurgery, Cincinnati, OH), which is used to retract the stomach and push it inferiorly.
- Port 3: A trocar is inserted in the left anterior axillary line, again several centimeters below the rib margin; it is used for dissection of the esophageal hiatus, using various instruments such as a pair of scissors or a hook dissector.
- Port 4: Trocar 4 is placed in the right mid-clavicular line, through which a retracting device is inserted. It is used to hold the left lobe of the liver away from the esophageal hiatus. We prefer to use a Padron endoscopic exposing retractor (Jarit Instruments, Hawthorne, NY), which comes in two sizes: 5 mm and 10 mm. For smaller patients, a 5-mm Padron endoscopic exposing retractor may be used; therefore, the trocar used can be 5 mm (Fig. 20-1).
- Port 5: The fifth and final trocar is placed in the right anterior axillary line, several centimeters below the right costal margin. This is for insertion of the instruments used to dissect the gastroesophageal junction and ultimately for passage of an Endopath Babcock forceps behind the esophagus, which is used to grasp the left portion of the gastric fundus and pull it posteriorly, to and around the esophagus for the wrap. Depending on patient anatomy, the liver retractor may be placed through either port 4 or port 5, whichever gives the best result (Fig. 20-2).

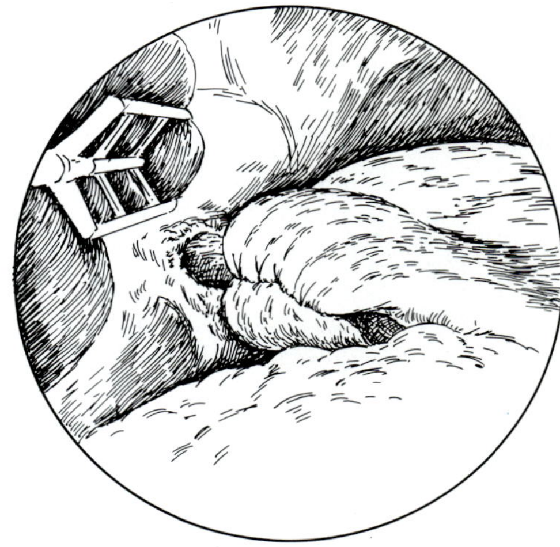

FIGURE 20-1. Completed fundoplication. Liver retracted using Padron endoscopic exposing retractor.

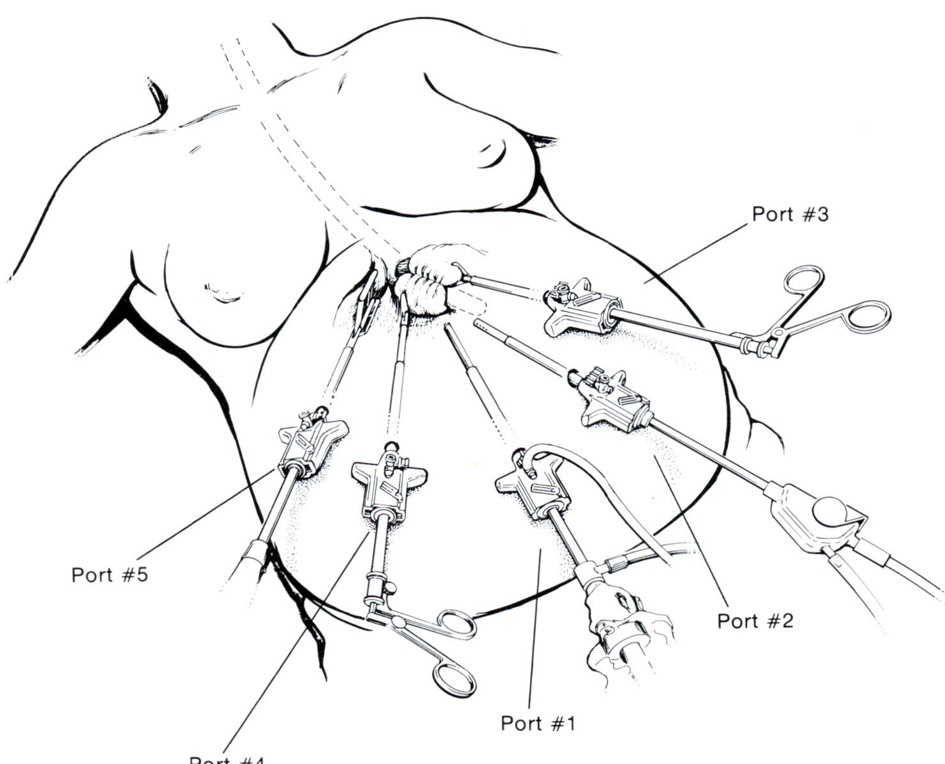

FIGURE 20-2. Overview of port placement and instrument positioning.

EXPOSURE OF ESOPHAGEAL HIATUS

After positioning the laparoscope, the left lobe of the liver is inspected. The left lobe may sometimes be retracted superiorly without detaching it from the diaphragm (Fig. 20-3). Occasionally, particularly when the attachment to the diaphragm consists of a thin peritoneal reflection, detachment is desirable. A grasping forceps is inserted through one of the right subcostal ports (port 5), and the attachment of the left lobe to the diaphragm is grasped and pulled inferiorly. A hook dissector with cautery or scissors with cautery is inserted through the most lateral left upper quadrant port (port 3) and used to detach the liver from the diaphragm (Fig. 20-4). Once this is accomplished, a Padron endoscopic exposing retractor is inserted through the medial right upper quadrant port (port 4) and the liver is lifted superiorly and laterally. This may be performed by an assistant who stands on the patient's right. An Endopath Babcock clamp or other atraumatic grasping instrument is passed

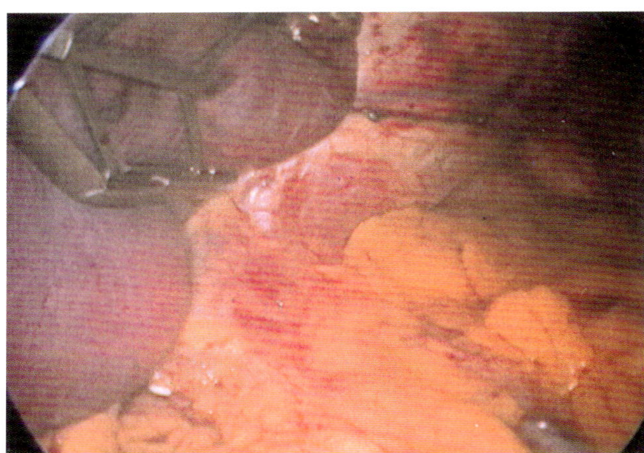

FIGURE 20-3. Left lobe of liver, retracted to expose esophageal hiatus at diaphragm.

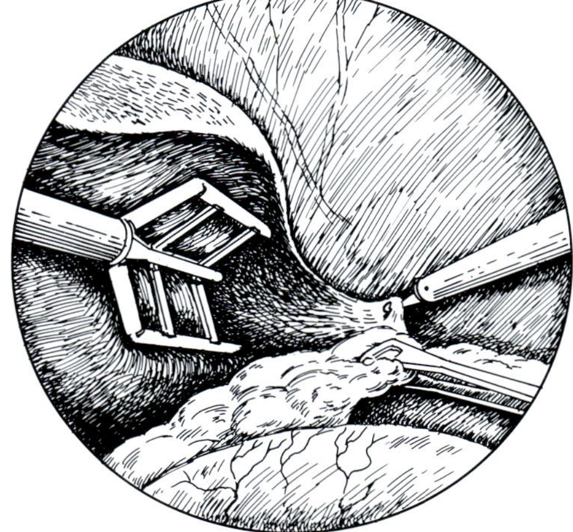

FIGURE 20-4. Hook dissection, used to divide attachment of the left lobe of the liver.

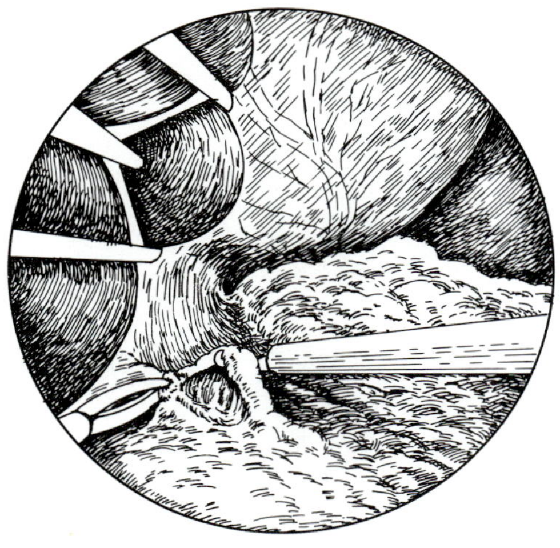

FIGURE 20-5. Initial dissection of the esophagus: peritoneum is divided at esophagus junction and anterior vagus nerve is identified.

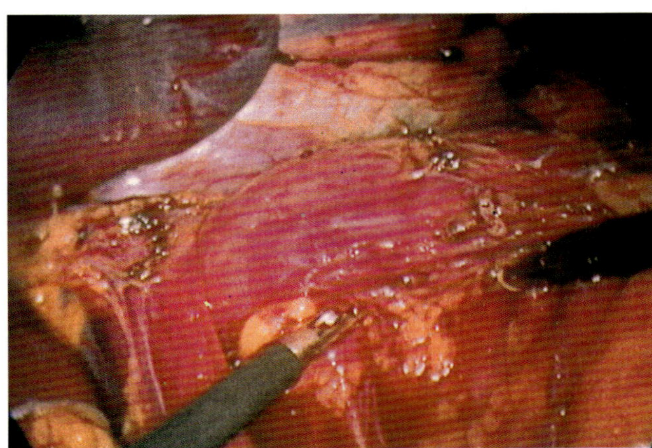

FIGURE 20-7. A plane is created between the esophagus and aorta.

through the medial port (port 2) in the left upper quadrant, and the greater curvature of the stomach is grasped and pushed inferiorly. The area of the esophageal hiatus should be exposed. Two dissecting instruments are placed through the lateral right and left port sites (ports 3 and 5). A hook dissector or scissors with cautery is generally placed in the lateral left port (port 3) for use with the operating surgeon's right hand. In the lateralmost right port (port 5), a grasper or dissecting forceps is passed for use with the surgeon's left hand. The phrenicoesophageal ligament is identified, and the peritoneum is carefully incised just inferior to it. This peritoneum, along with the phrenicoesophageal ligament, is pushed and dissected superiorly, which exposes the anterior surface of the esophagus and usually the anterior vagus nerve (Fig. 20-5). Dissection is continued for several centimeters to the right and left of the esophagus; dissection then begins on the lesser curvature of the stomach at the gastroesophageal junction (Fig. 20-6). A plane is created between the esophagus and the aorta and using a dissecting forceps, a space is created (Fig. 20-7). One must take care not to injure the posterior vagus nerve, which is identified and dissected to stay with the esophagus (Fig. 20-8). It is easy to separate the posterior vagus nerve from the esophagus at this point because its course may take it a centimeter or more away from the esophagus as it traverses downward onto the stomach. The dissection posterior to the esophagus should be posterior to the vagus nerve, so that the fundic wrap can encompass the posterior vagus nerve rather than pushing it laterally and potentially damaging it. Dissection of the esophagus at greater curvature of stomach is now begun (Fig. 20-9).

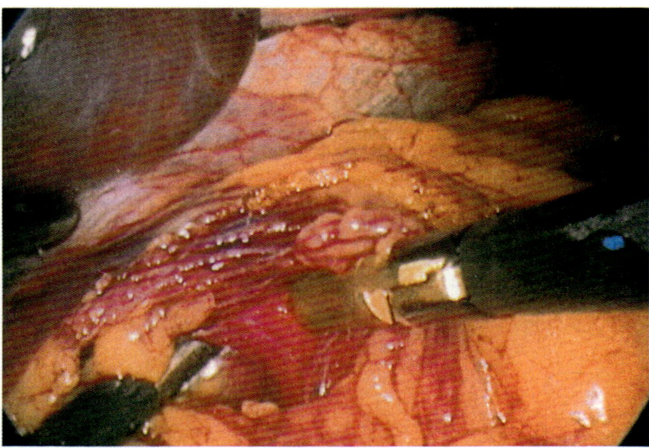

FIGURE 20-6. Esophagus is exposed by opening peritoneum with dissection beginning at the gastroesophageal junction on the lesser curvature of the stomach.

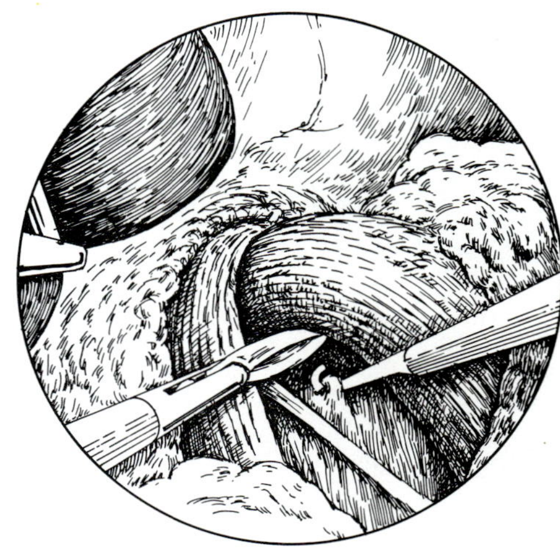

FIGURE 20-8. Esophagus is lifted anteriorly and dissected free from posterior connective tissue. The vagus nerve is identified and dissected to stay with the esophagus.

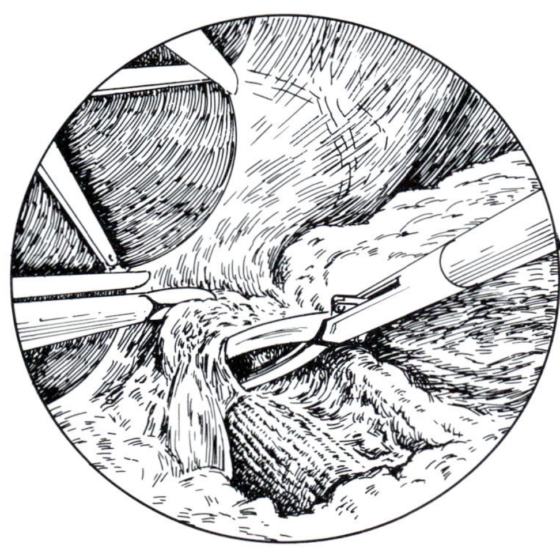

FIGURE 20-9. Dissection of esophagus, using scissors and dissector to gently tease away surrounding tissue. Short gastrics are divided with clips, as necessary.

DISSECTION OF GASTROESOPHAGEAL JUNCTION

After an instrument has been passed completely behind the esophagus, it may be useful to pass a vessel loop behind the esophagus and bring it out through the medial left port (port 2). A heavy elastic vessel loop is passed behind the esophagus and is brought out initially through the port. The trocar sleeve is then removed and a clamp placed on the elastic vessel loop at the exit point from the abdominal cavity to create the minimal tension necessary to pull the esophagus forward. Care is taken not to pull this too tightly. The sleeve can then be replaced and the stomach retracting device, an Endopath Babcock forcep, can be passed again through the sleeve and the stomach regrasped. In some cases, because of the angles of the costal margin, a 5-mm trocar must be placed in the midline or to the left of midline for passage of the vessel loop. In many cases, the dissection can be completed without the necessity of pulling the esophagus anteriorly.

RETROGASTRIC DISSECTION AND EVALUATION OF SHORT GASTRIC VESSELS

At this point in the dissection, a space must be created between the posterior wall of the stomach and the pancreas (Fig. 20-10). The retrogastric tissue is usually flimsy and is easily divided. The difficulty is to obtain anterior traction on the posterior wall of the stomach to allow visualization of these points of attachment, so that they may be lysed. Because the gastric retractor grasps only the anterior surface of the stomach, it is difficult to obtain this necessary countertraction by pulling anteriorly on the stomach but the elastic band around the esophagus

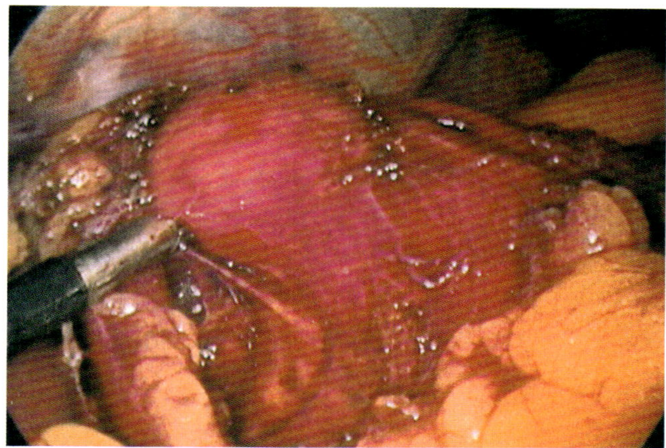

FIGURE 20-10. A plane is created between the posterior wall of the stomach and the anterior surface of the pancreas.

helps to accomplish this goal. A grasping instrument may be passed from one of the ports on the patient's left (usually port 3) to grasp either the stomach or perigastric tissue on the lesser curvature, just below the gastroesophageal junction, which is retracted laterally to the left and anteriorly. The instrument being passed through a port on the patient's right (port 5) can be used to dissect this retrogastric space, either bluntly or by directly cutting with coagulation current. After this is accomplished, the posterior fundus is grasped near the greater curvature, usually with an Endopath Babcock forcep passed through port 5, and it is pulled posterior to the esophagus (Fig. 20-11). This allows evaluation of the size of the space to make sure that it is adequate for passage of the fundus; one can also evaluate the mobility of the fundus vis-à-vis the necessity for the division of the short gastric vessels. In some patients, the fundus of the stomach is so firmly associated with the splenic hilum that division of the short gastric vessels is advisable. This is accomplished by careful dissection along the greater curvature of the stomach, beginning at the gastroesopha-

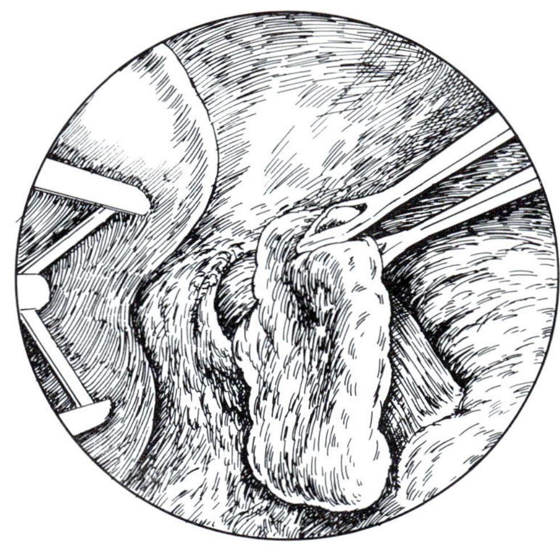

FIGURE 20-11. Fundus is pulled through, behind the esophagus.

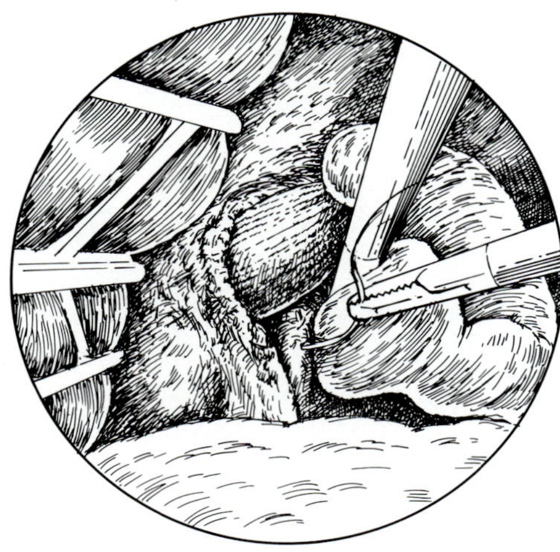

FIGURE 20-12. The crura are exposed by pushing the fundus and gastroesophageal junction inferiorly and anteriorly.

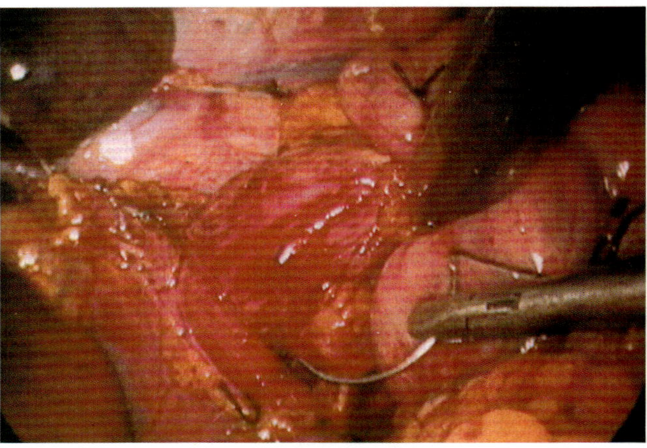

FIGURE 20-14. Suturing of crura.

geal hiatus. Thin tissue may be coagulated and divided, whereas vessels should be doubly clipped on both sides and divided sharply. The propensity of the short gastric vessels to bleed is such that simple coagulation and division of them is not advisable, even if the vessels appear well-coagulated at the time of operation. After division of the short gastric vessels, the posterior gastric fundus should again be grasped and brought posterior to the esophagus to assess mobility. If the retrogastric space and mobility of the fundus are both considered to be adequate, the fundus is let loose and attention is turned to the esophageal hiatus.

CRURAL CLOSURE

Assessment is made of the gastroesophageal junction in relation to the hiatus. In some patients, foreshortening of the esophagus has occurred due to severe inflammation, and the gastroesophageal junction has a tendency to ride up into the hiatus. The gastroesophageal junction must be grasped and pushed inferiorly and anteriorly while the crural edges are approximated (Figs. 20-12 and 20-13). The crural edges are sutured together with 2-0 silk. One needle holder is passed through the left lateral port (port 3); a second needle holder is passed through the lateral right (port 5) for grasping of the needle. The needle is passed through the port (port 3), using a special sleeve. It is grasped by the other needle holder, which is held in the surgeon's left hand, and the needle is then positioned in the needle holder held by the surgeon's right hand (Fig. 20-14). A good bit of muscle and surrounding fibrous tissue is pierced when passing the needle through first the left crus and then the right (Fig. 20-15). Internal knotting is performed and a second suture is then passed and placed in a similar fashion about 1½ cm from the first. Usually, two sutures in the crura are adequate to close this space.

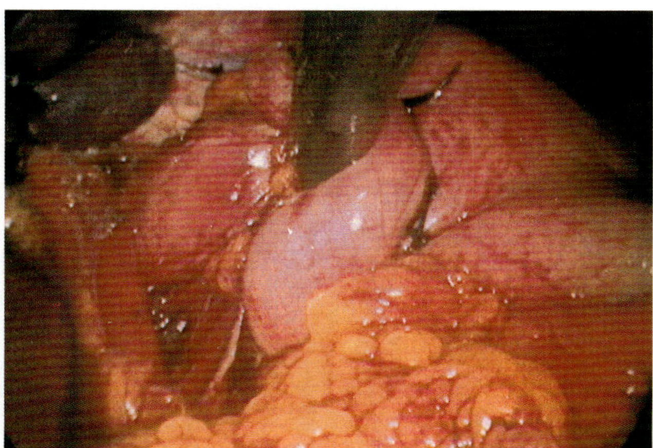

FIGURE 20-13. Exposure of crura.

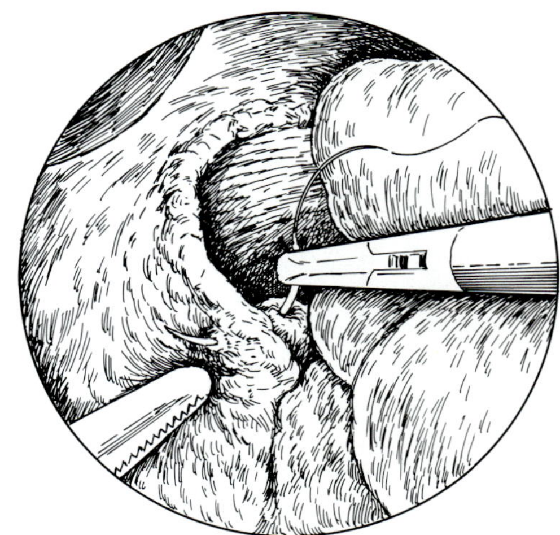

FIGURE 20-15. Crural closure.

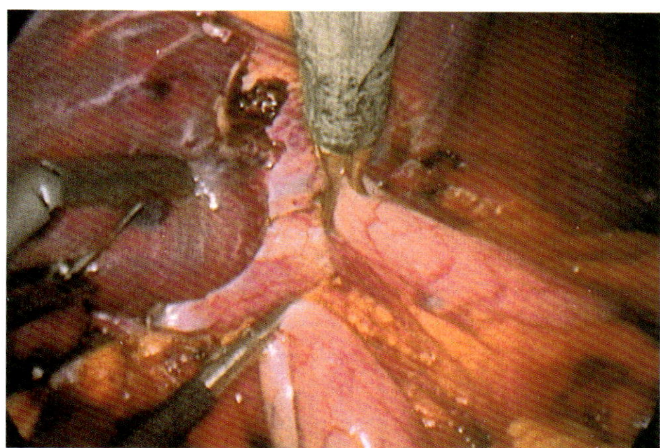

FIGURE 20-16. Endo-Babcocks are used to grasp the fundus of the stomach, wrapping it around the esophagus to meet the greater curvature anteriorly.

PLICATION OF FUNDUS

Fundoplication is then performed. First, a 44-French Maloney dilator is passed through the mouth into the esophagus and stomach. An Endopath Babcock forcep is passed through the lateral right port (port 5) posterior to the esophagus and the fundus is grasped adjacent to the greater curvature. The fundus is then pulled behind the esophagus and brought to an anterior position adjacent to the gastroesophageal junction (Fig. 20-16). A second Endopath Babcock forcep is then used to grasp the fundus anteriorly adjacent to the greater curvature, and this is pushed medially to meet with the portion of the fundus that has been passed posteriorly (Fig. 20-17). A third Endopath Babcock forcep is then passed, usually through the medial left upper quadrant port (port 4), and is used to grasp these two portions of the fundus anteriorly to allow the release of the other two Endopath Babcock forceps, which are holding the stomach wrap in position (Fig. 20-18). This frees the two lateral ports (ports 3 and 5) for insertion of needle holders. A 2-0 silk suture is passed, and the first fundoplication stitches are placed (Fig. 20-19). Depending on the position of the Endopath Babcock forceps, a second suture may be placed and tied also. At this point, the last Endopath Babcock forcep is removed and the final sutures are placed. When placing the most superior stitch, the suture is passed through the fundic tissue on the left, through some of the fibrous or serosal tissue at the gastroesophageal junction, and finally through the fundic tissue on the right (Figs. 20-20 and 20-21). This serves to anchor the plication. Sutures are left long to grasp and hold traction for the next suture (Figs. 20-22 and 20-23). Additionally, this may be done with the lowermost one or two sutures, thus tacking the fundus securely in this position. During the entire process of wrapping the fundus around the esophagus, a 44-French Maloney dilator has been in place to prevent the Nissen fundoplication from becoming too tight. The Maloney dilator can be removed at this point, while the

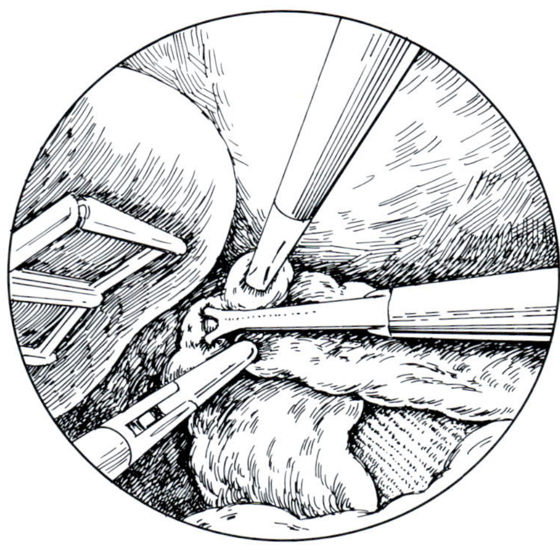

FIGURE 20-18. Fundus is approximated and endo-Babcock is used to grasp both edges of the stomach, freeing a port for a needle holder.

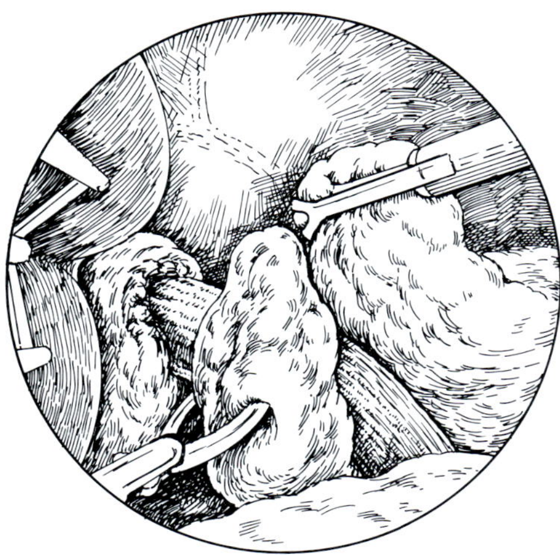

FIGURE 20-17. Fundus segments are approximated without tension; 44-French Maloney dilator is in place.

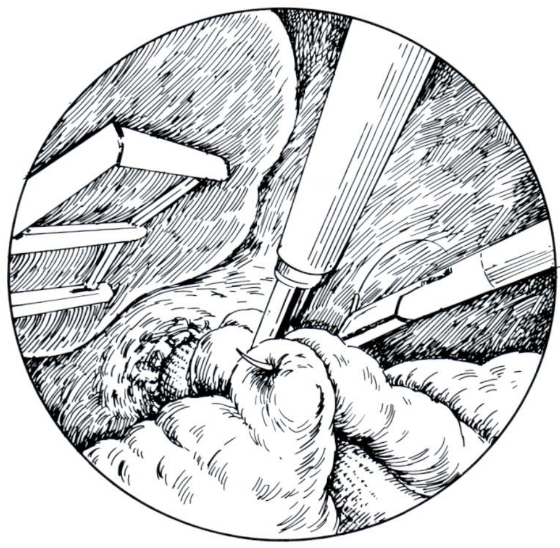

FIGURE 20-19. First suture is placed, securing the wrap.

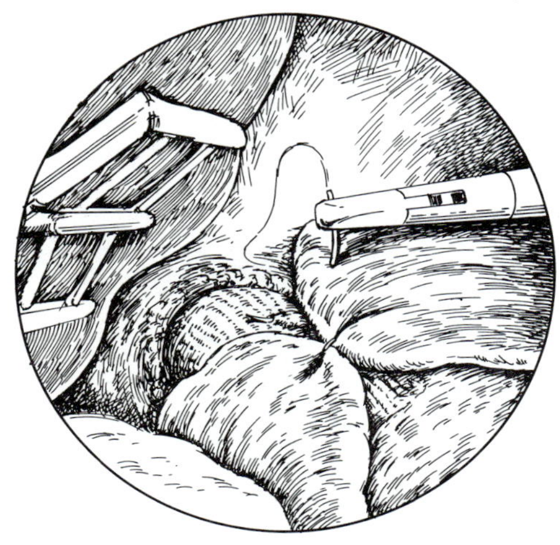

FIGURE 20-20. Superior suture is taken through periesophageal tissue to secure wrap.

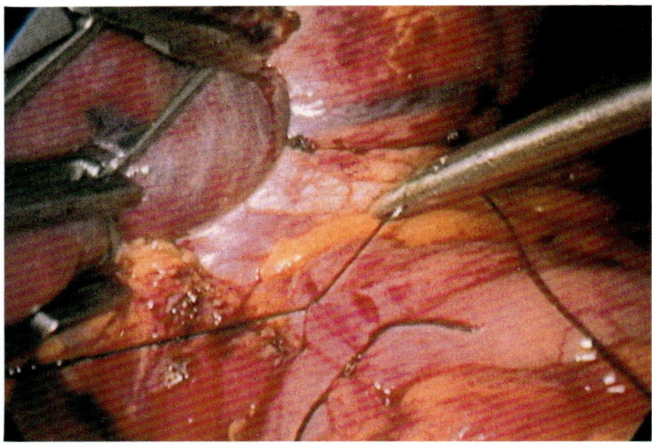

FIGURE 20-21. The fundoplication is performed by suturing fundus anteriorly, with superior sutures anchored through serosa at gastroesophageal junction.

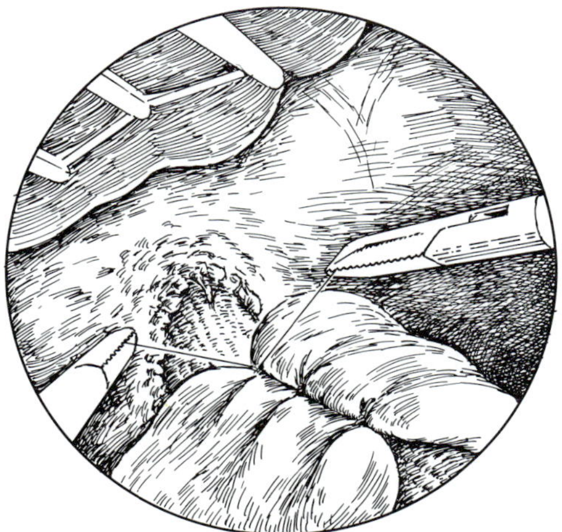

FIGURE 20-22. Tightening the knot in fundoplication wrap.

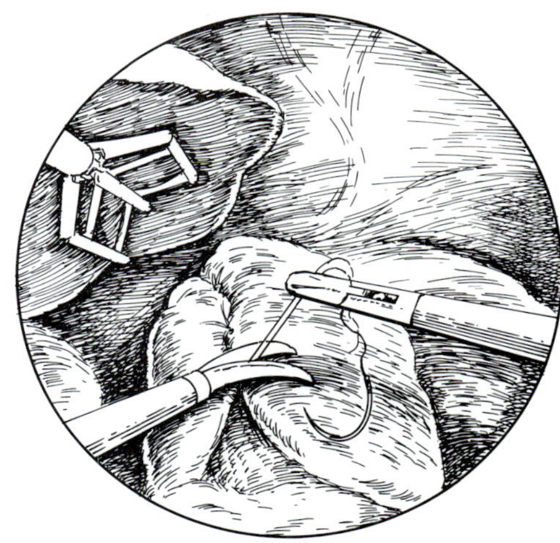

FIGURE 20-23. Prior suture is always left for traction until wrap is completed.

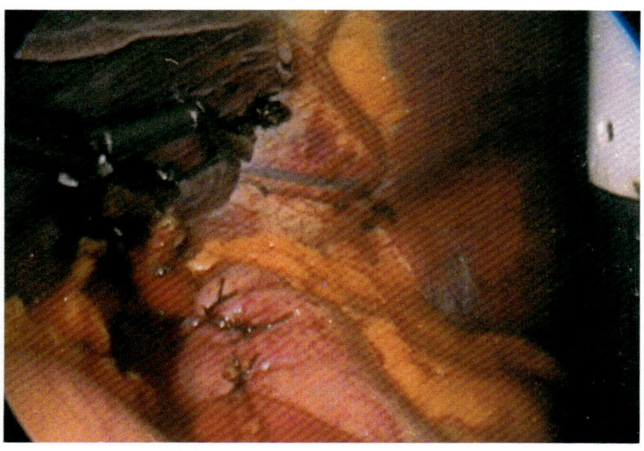

FIGURE 20-24. Completed Nissen fundoplication.

nasogastric tube is left in place. Gentle traction can then be placed on the fundoplication circumferentially to ensure that it is loose enough. One should be able to slide a blunt instrument along the plicated fundus and create a space of about 0.5 cm. If the fundoplication does not admit the tip of an instrument, it may indeed be too tight and consideration should be given to redoing it. The decision in this instance is the same as for open surgery. Most surgeons having experience in open Nissen fundoplication should not have difficulty in assessing the adequacy of the wrap when performed laparoscopically.

The fundoplication is complete, the area is irrigated with normal saline until clear, and the liver and spleen are inspected for any evidence of injury or bleeding (Fig. 20-24). If there is any question about injury to the esophagus, methylene blue may be inserted through the nasogastric tube to just above the gastroesophageal junction while gently placing pressure at the gastroesophageal junction inside the abdomen. This creates a small pool of blue dye in the esophagus at this level to help identify potential leaks. The pneumoperitoneum is deflated and the trocars removed.

Selected Readings

Geagea T: Laparoscopic Nissen-Rossetti fundoplication. Surg Endosc 1994;8(9):1080.

Hinder RA, Filipi CJ, Wetscher G, Neary P, DeMeester TR, Perdikis G: Laparoscopic Nissen fundoplication is an effective treatment for gastroesophageal reflux disease. Ann Surg 1994;220(4):472.

Kraemer SJ, Aye R, Kozarek RA, Hill LD: Laparoscopic Hill repair. Gastrointest Endosc 1994;40(2 Pt 1):155.

Pitcher DE, Curet MJ, Martin DT, et al: Successful management of severe gastroesophageal reflux disease with laparoscopic Nissen fundoplication. Am J Surg 1994;168(6):547.

Watson DI, Reed MW, Johnson AG, Stoddard CJ: Laparoscopic fundoplication for gastro-oesophageal reflux. Ann R Coll Surg Engl 1994;76(4):264.

Chapter 21

Laparoscopic Surgery: An Atlas for General Surgeons, edited by Gary C. Vitale, Joseph S. Sanfilippo, and Jacques Perissat. J. B. Lippincott Company, Philadelphia, © 1995.

Laparoscopic Splenectomy

A. Cuschieri

The first reports of laparoscopic splenectomy in the human appeared in 1992.[1–4] Since then, there have been many presentations at various conferences and additional publications on laparoscopic splenectomy but no substantive report on the indications, limitations, and outcome of splenectomy performed by the laparoscopic approach.[5,6] Indeed, a definitive review of the role of laparoscopic splenectomy in the management of splenic disorders is not possible because of the limited experience worldwide for this procedure. In this chapter, the selection of patients and the details of the operative technique of laparoscopic splenectomy as practiced in Dundee over the past 3 years are outlined.

Nowadays, splenectomy is indicated for trauma, in the management of patients with certain hematologic disorders, in some patients with acquired immunodeficiency syndrome, and in the staging of a subset of patients with Hodgkin's disease. In the trauma situation, the tendency during the last decade has been toward splenic preservation, with repair or segmental resection, as dictated by the nature of the injury, splenectomy being reserved for severe grade IV lesions.[7] The argument for splenic preservation is based on the risk of severe postsplenectomy sepsis due to encapsulated organisms, predominantly *Streptococcus pneumoniae*.[8,9] A collective review of the literature, however, shows that this risk is mainly confined to infants and children and is significantly influenced by the nature of the underlying disease for which the splenectomy is performed.[10] In the elective situation, vaccination with polyvalent pneumococcal vaccine is practiced, although the evidence for effective protection by this measure is lacking.[11,12] Vaccination is likely to stimulate the memory T-independent lymphocytes only when it is begun before the spleen is removed. The use of prophylactic penicillin therapy is advisable in infants and children.

INDICATIONS AND CONTRAINDICATIONS FOR LAPAROSCOPIC SPLENECTOMY

Although minor injuries of the splenic poles have been repaired laparoscopically by the use of omentum and fibrin glue, laparoscopic splenectomy has been undertaken in our institution only in the elective situation. The assessment of splenic size, which is important in case selection for laparoscopic splenectomy, is conducted by physical examination and splenic ultrasonography (Fig. 21-1). Laparoscopic splenectomy is difficult when the spleen is large, in the presence of significant perisplenitis, and with foreshortening of the short gastric vessels. Undoubtedly, dissection and extraction become increasingly difficult when the splenic weight exceeds 500 g. Care is needed to avoid capsular disruption and bleeding in patients with malignancy (usually lymphomas).

For two reasons, the ideal patients for elective laparoscopic splenectomy are those suffering from idiopathic thrombocytopenic purpura (ITP). In the first instance, the splenic enlargement in these patients is only moderate and secondly, the risk of postsplenectomy sepsis is minimal.[10] Laparoscopic splenectomy has also been performed in our institution for acquired hemolytic anemia that is unresponsive to steroid therapy, lymphomas (excision of primary splenic B-cell lymphoma), and in the staging of extra-abdominal Hodgkin's disease.

PREOPERATIVE WORKUP AND PREPARATION

The preoperative workup includes full hematologic testing (including platelet count and bleeding time) and splenic ultrasound examination. For large spleens, arteri-

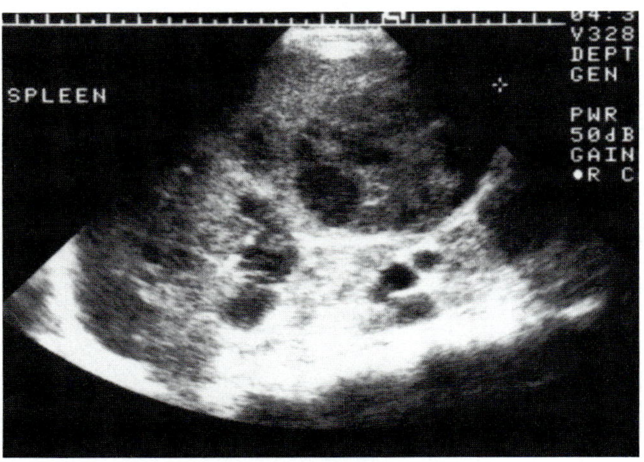

FIGURE 21-1. Splenic ultrasound examination in a patient with primary lymphoma. The substantial splenomegaly precludes safe laparoscopic splenectomy because of major difficulties with the dissection of the splenic pedicle and extraction of the malignant organ.

ography with embolic occlusion is helpful; when considered to be necessary, it is best conducted 12 to 24 hours before the planned procedure.

In patients who have been exposed to steroid therapy, parenteral hydrocortisone is used during the perioperative period. There is no indication for preoperative platelet transfusions when the platelet count is 50,000 or more. Chemoprophylaxis with subcutaneous heparin is recommended in all patients undergoing laparoscopic splenectomy because of the rebound thrombocytosis encountered in the postoperative period in most patients. The first subcutaneous dose (5000 to 8000 U) is administered with induction of anesthesia. Antithrombosis graduated elastic stockings are also used in all patients.

ANESTHESIA

Laparoscopic splenectomy is performed under general anesthesia with endotracheal intubation. The exact details and premedication vary with the practice of the anesthetist. Antibiotic prophylaxis is administered routinely, using a single injection of a cephalosporin given after induction of anesthesia. A size 14-French Salem (Sherwood Medical Co., St. Louis, MO) sump nasogastric tube is inserted and kept on continuous low suction to ensure total and continued deflation of the stomach throughout the procedure.

PATIENT POSITIONING AND SKIN PREPARATION

The two positions that may be used are the supine hyperextended position and the modified lateral kidney position (Fig. 21-2).

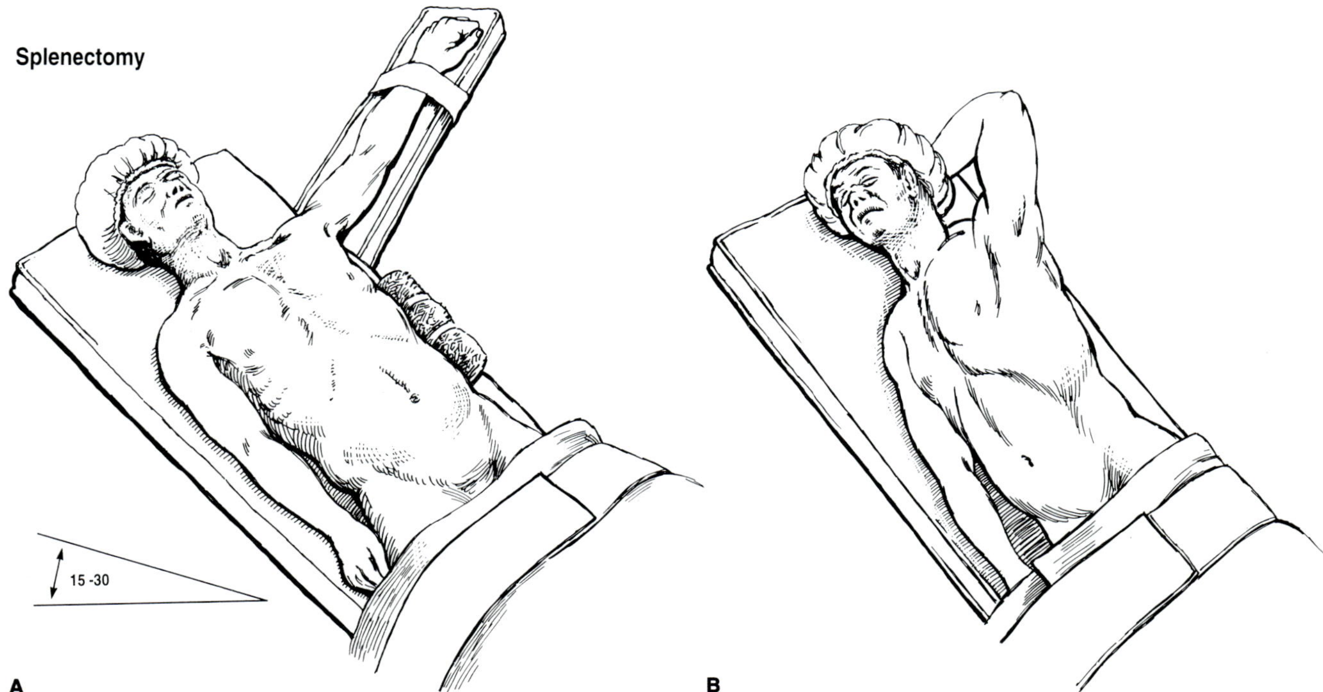

FIGURE 21-2. Positions for laparoscopic splenomegaly. (**A**) Supine hyperextended position. (**B**) Modified kidney position.

Supine Hyperextended Position

This was the original position that we adopted and is ideal when removing minimally to moderately enlarged spleens.[1] Its main advantage is the greater ease of port placement and external surgical manipulation. The left lower rib cage and loin are arched forward by a 7.5 cm deep sand bag placed posteriorly under the 12th rib. The operating table is set at a moderate (15° to 30°) head-up tilt. In addition, a slight lateral tilt of the operating table to the right, which elevates the left subdiaphragmatic recess, also improves exposure of the spleen.

Modified Kidney Position

This is similar to the split lateral decubitus position used for nephrectomy, except that the tilt is short of full lateral. It provides excellent exposure of the spleen because the stomach and omentum fall away from the spleen, which remains suspended by its parietal and diaphragmatic attachments. For this reason, it is referred to as "the hanging spleen technique" by French surgeons. Its disadvantage is that the external manipulations of the surgeons are more restricted than when the supine hyperextended position is used. For this reason, accurate port placement is crucial.

The area of skin disinfection extends from the nipple line to the pubis and laterally, well into the flanks. Draping is such as to leave exposed the abdomen from the costal margins to the suprapubic region and extending laterally to the left flank.

POSITION OF PERSONNEL AND EQUIPMENT

The surgeon operates from the right side of the operating table. Unless an adjustable vacuum lock laparoscope holder (First Assistant, Leonard, Philadelphia, PA) is used, the camera person and the surgeon both stand on the right side of the patient, with the scrub nurse and first assistant on the opposite side. The sterile instrument—Mayo Stand—is placed by the scrub nurse. A two-monitor visual display is necessary. The electrosurgical unit, suction irrigation, insufflator, and camera unit are placed on a stack behind the surgeon.

INSTRUMENTATION AND CONSUMABLES

In addition to the basic instrumentation, the following special equipment facilitates laparoscopic splenectomy:

- 10-mm 30° forward oblique telescope
- Coaxial curved instruments and flexible trocar cannulas (Fig. 21-3); these distally curved bayonet instruments are introduced through reusable flexible cannulas and allow change of direction of the functional tip by rotation of the longitudinal axis of the instrument; they greatly facilitate dissection around the splenic poles and behind the spleen[1,13]
- Liver retractor
- Consumables: these include Dacron ligatures (120 to 150 cm) mounted on a push rod (U.S. Surgical, Norwalk, CT) and Endo-GIA stapler with vascular cartridges (U.S. Surgical, Norwalk, CT)

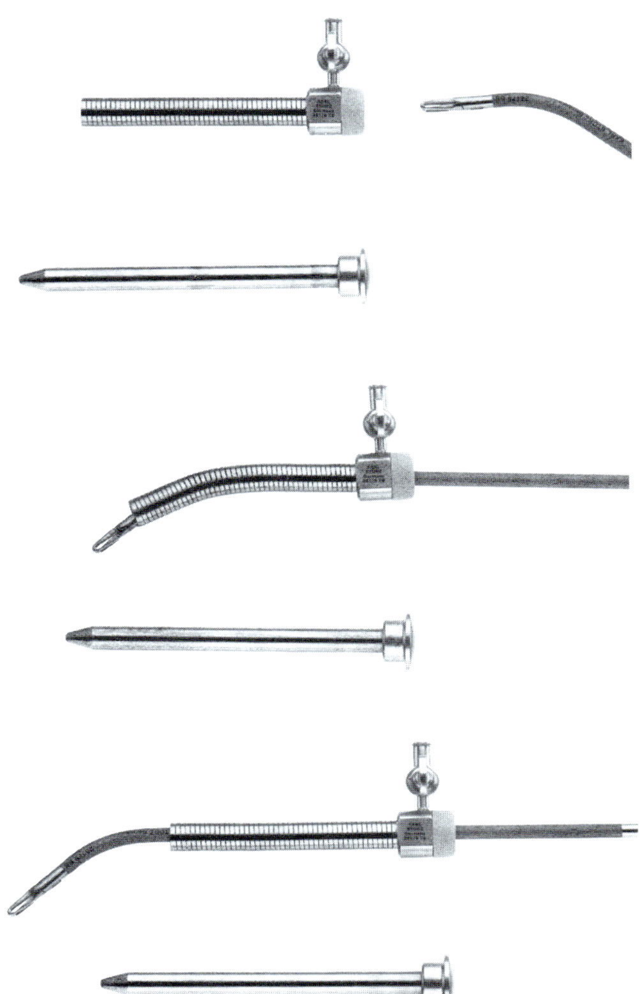

FIGURE 21-3. Coaxial curved and bayonet instruments introduced through a flexible, reusable metal cannula (Storz, Tuttlingen, Germany).

The dissection of the splenic hilar vessels from the tail of the pancreas and separation of the posterior surface of the spleen from the retroperitoneum, perirenal fat, and adrenal gland is considerably expedited by the use of ultrasonic dissection, using the Selector probe (Surgical Technology Group, Andover, UK)[14]

OPERATIVE STEPS OF LAPAROSCOPIC SPLENECTOMY

Access Ports

The positions of the five access ports for the two approaches are shown in Figure 21-4. In both positions, the telescope port (11 mm) is placed 2 cm above and to the left of the umbilicus.

Exposure of the Spleen

In some patients, the greater omentum is rolled up, obscuring the spleen; in this case, it is grasped with an atraumatic forceps and pulled down into the infracolic compartment. A coaxial curved Babcock-type grasper is placed on the proximal body of the stomach near the greater curvature and is used to retract this organ downward and to the right, to expose the anterior aspect and lower pole of the spleen. At this stage, the lower pole is attached to the splenic flexure of the colon by a vascular peritoneal fold (suspensory ligament; Fig. 21-5).

Division of Splenocolic Attachments and Devascularization of the Lower Pole

This constitutes the first step of the operation. Before scissors division of the splenocolic attachment, the leash of fine blood vessels in this peritoneal fold are electrocoagulated, preferably in the soft-coagulation autostop mode by the microprocessor-controlled ICC H-F electrosurgical unit (Erbe, Tubingen, Germany). This is an important point, considering the immediate proximity of the left colonic flexure. The incision in the peritoneum is then carried out with the coaxial curved scissors, around the lower pole of the spleen to the back of the organ, until the lower limit of the lienorenal ligament and underlying fascia are reached. The proximal ends of the vessels to the lower pole (often double) are best individually ligated proximally in continuity, using Dacron mounted on a push rod and an external slip knot (Tayside or the Melzer). The distal (splenic) ends are clipped and the vessels then divided with scissors (Fig. 21-6).

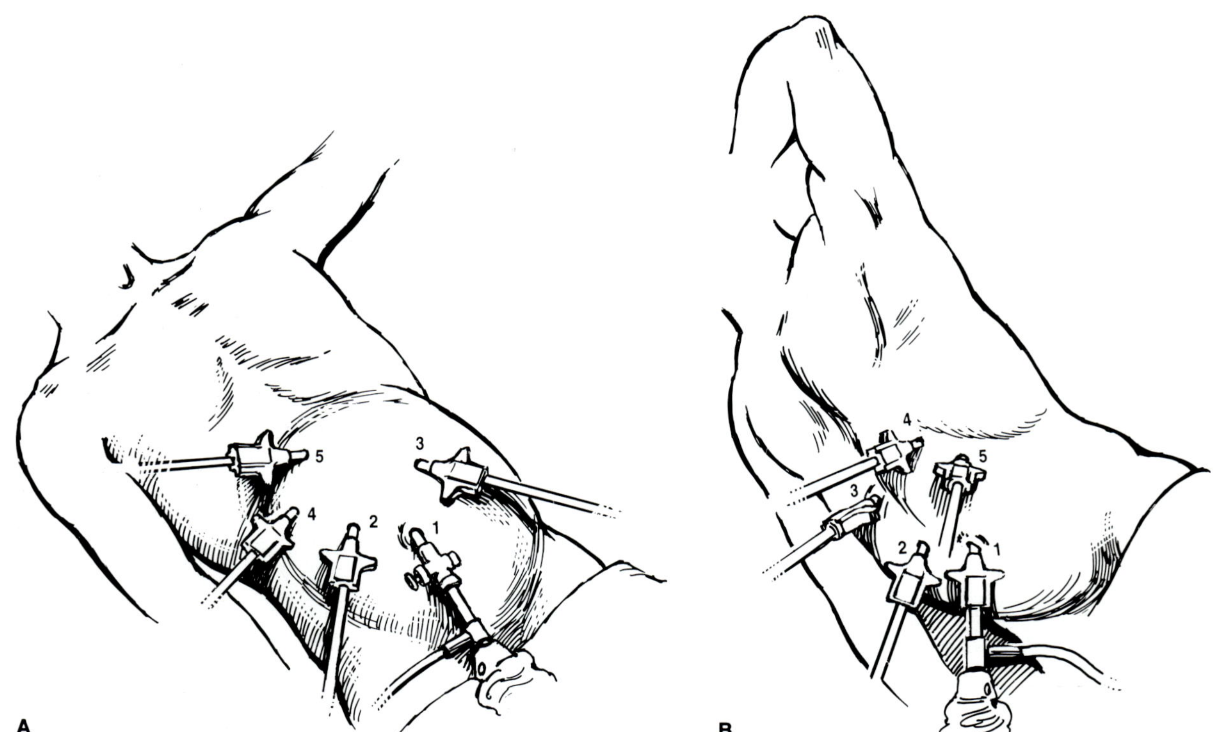

FIGURE 21-4. Access ports for laparoscopic splenectomy. (**A**) Supine hyperextended position: 1, optic port; 2 and 3, operating ports; 4, assistant's port(s); 5, cannula may be required for retraction of the left lobe of the liver. (**B**) Modified kidney position: 1, optic port; 2 and 3, operating ports; 4, assistant's port; 5, for suction-irrigation and tying/clipping.

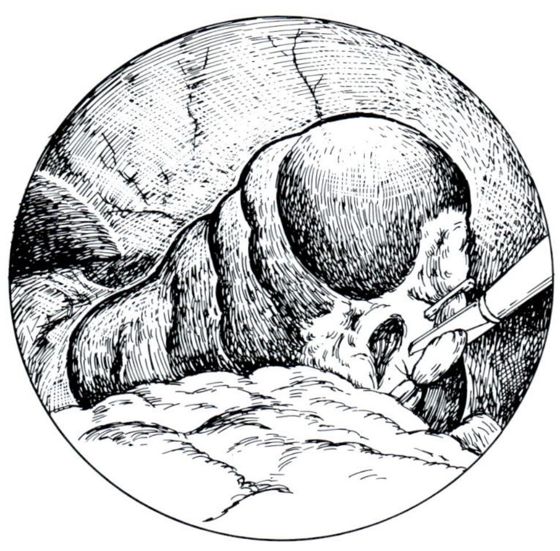

FIGURE 21-5. Dividing ligated vessels on a lower pole splenocolic junction.

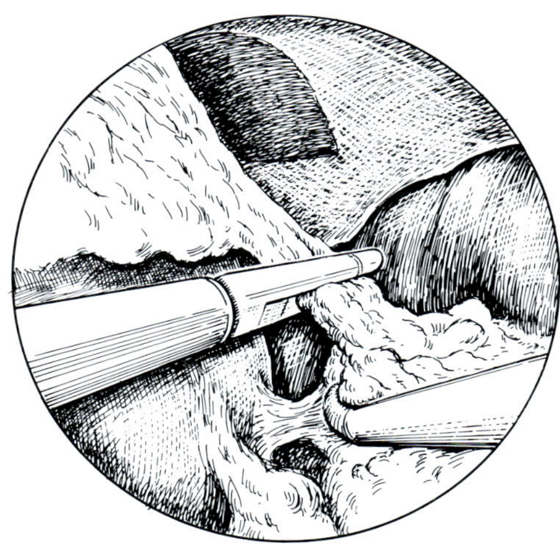

FIGURE 21-7. Stapling pedicle of gastrosplenic omentum.

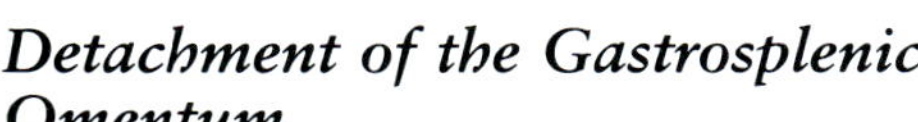

Detachment of the Gastrosplenic Omentum

The proximal greater curvature of the stomach is raised to identify an avascular window near the greater curvature below the short gastric vessels. After division of the peritoneum of this window with scissors, the coaxial curved grasper is introduced behind the stomach. The undersurface of the gastrosplenic ligament can thus be visualized. A suitable proximal avascular window is selected and opened with the coaxial curved scissors. Often, avascular adhesions between the posterior surface of the stomach and the pancreas are encountered. These are divided with the scissors until sufficient clearance is achieved. The Endo-GIA stapler with vascular cartridge (U.S. Surgical, Norwalk, CT) is then applied to the pedicle, which is then stapled and cut as the device is activated (Fig. 21-7). Proximally, there are deeper short gastric and phrenic vessels (usually two). These should not be included in the stapler but are best ligated medially and clipped laterally before being divided (Fig. 21-8).

Ligation in Continuity of the Splenic Artery Above the Tail of the Pancreas

This technique, introduced subsequent to our first three cases, has considerable advantages. It is performed routinely in all patients, except for those in whom preoperative embolization was performed. Early ligature of the splenic artery in continuity enhances the safety of the procedure because the risk of major bleeding is reduced. It also leads to a significant reduction in the size of the spleen. Because of its sinuous nature, the artery is easily mobilized at the upper border of the pancreas. A coaxial curved duckbill grasper is used to pass a Dacron ligature around the artery, which is then tied in continuity with either an intracorporeal or extracorporeal knot.

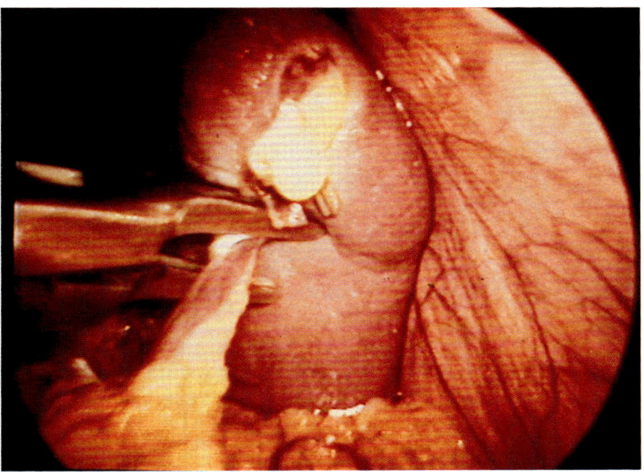

FIGURE 21-6. Distal clipping of the lower pole vessels.

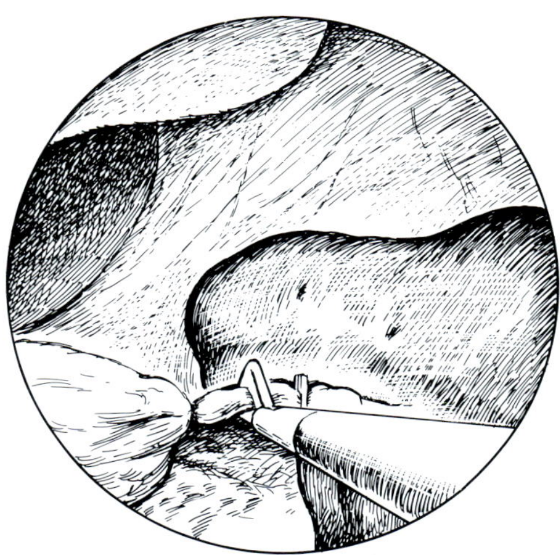

FIGURE 21-8. Dissection and division of short gastric vessels.

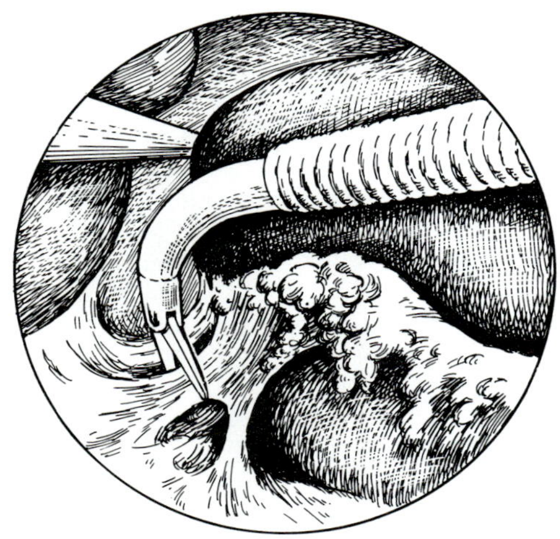

FIGURE 21-9. Mobilization of the upper pole of the spleen, using curved memory scissors.

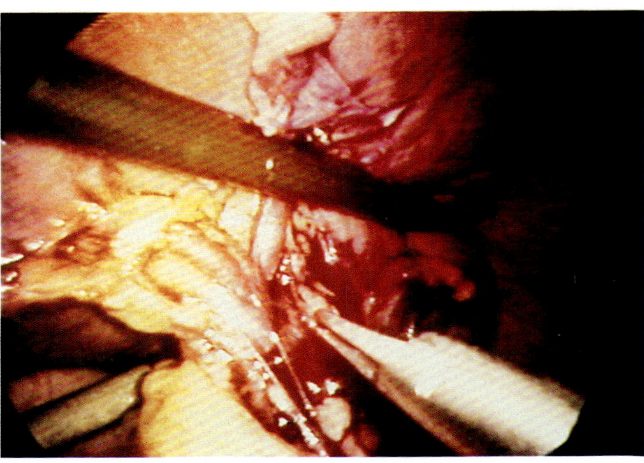

FIGURE 21-11. Dissection of the pancreatic tail from the splenic hilum.

Division of the Proximal Gastrosplenic–Phrenic Peritoneal Reflection and Mobilization of the Upper Pole of the Spleen

The peritoneal reflection between the spleen and the esophagogastric junction and between the upper pole of the spleen and the diaphragm is then divided and the dissection is extended around the upper pole (Fig. 21-9). The division of the peritoneal fold exposes the fascial layer that binds the spleen to the retroperitoneum. This too requires division with scissors. At this stage, the right adrenal gland is often identified.

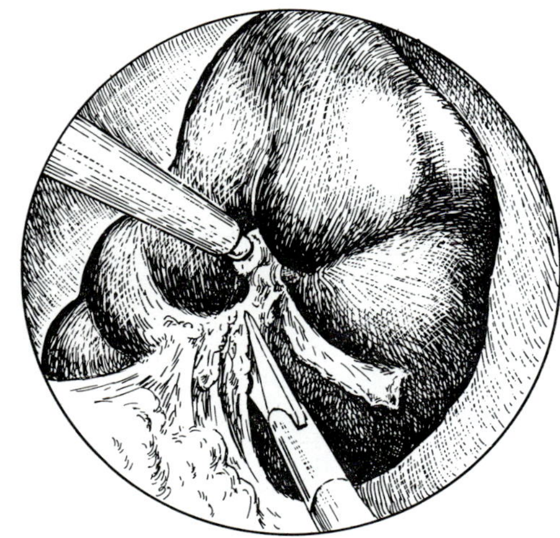

FIGURE 21-10. Division of vessels at splenic hilum after ligation in continuity. Babcock holds spleen up to assist in dividing lienorenal ligaments.

Dissection of the Pancreatic Tail and Ligature of Vessels to the Middle and Upper Splenic Segments

The detachment of the short gastric vessels (followed by retraction of the mobilized upper part of the greater curvature of the stomach upward and to the right) exposes the tail of the pancreas and the splenic hilum (Fig. 21-10). Careful dissection of the tail of the pancreas from the hilum of the spleen is necessary to avoid pancreatic injury and to identify the remaining segmental vessels to the middle and upper splenic segments (Fig. 21-11). The dissection of the splenic tail is best carried out by blunt or ultrasonic dissection (Fig. 21-12). If the latter is used, the machine should be set to deliver a low-vibration energy. A combination of both blunt and ultrasonic dissection is ideal. Once the vessels to the middle and upper segments have been separated from the tail of the pancreas, they are ligated proximally in continuity, using Dacron mounted on a push rod and an external slip knot (Tayside or Meltzer). Ligature of these vessels results in uniform dark discoloration of the entire spleen, indicating total devascularization. In patients with benign disease, the distal (splenic) ends of the vessels to the middle and upper poles are left unsecured to allow controlled splenic bleeding.

Bleeding of the Spleen After Vascular Isolation

Bleeding of the spleen is performed only in patients with benign disease; it results in a substantial reduction in the size of the spleen. A suction–irrigation device is placed in the left hypochondrium in the lateral splenic gutter. The vascular pedicles to the middle and upper segments

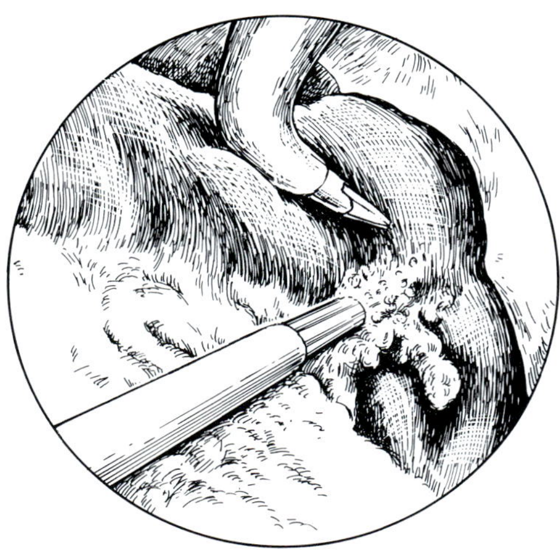

FIGURE 21-12. Hydrodissection to assist in separating the spleen from the tail of the pancreas.

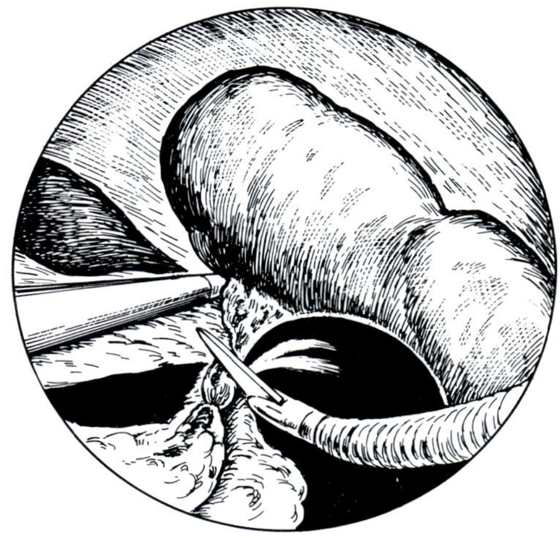

FIGURE 21-13. Controlled bleeding of the spleen to reduce size in nonmalignant cases.

are then divided by scissors, 1.0 cm distal to the proximal ligature (Fig. 21-13). As the sequestered blood in the splenic parenchyma escapes, it is sucked from the splenic fossa, which is also irrigated with warm heparinized Hartmann's solution to prevent clot formation. The process is continued until splenic bleeding has ceased and the area is dry. A greater than 50% reduction of splenic size is obtained by this simple measure (Fig. 21-14). This splenic bleeding, permissible only when the splenectomy is being performed for benign disease, is contraindicated in the presence of malignant disease.

Detachment of the Lienorenal Peritoneum and Fascia

The lienorenal ligament and underlying splenic fascia are then divided by cautery-type scissors, with coagulation of any small bleeders. During this stage, the spleen is displaced to the right by a Babcock-type grasper placed on the detached splenic hilum. Separation of the posterior surface of the spleen from the perinephric fat completes the procedure. Before extraction, a careful inspection is performed to ensure complete hemostasis and to exclude any splenunculi.

Extraction of Specimen

Half the length of a sleeve delivery system (made from rip-stop nylon) is placed inside the peritoneal cavity through the extraction port. A grasper is introduced through the sleeve and used to grab the detached spleen, which is then drawn into the sleeve. The internal open end of the sleeve is then exteriorized through an opposite port and clamped. The spleen is thereby suspended in a "third space" and the abdomen is then deflated. The extraction wound is enlarged to 3 to 4 cm, and small retractors are placed inside the sleeve. The spleen is "squeezed" toward the extraction site by twisting the opposite clamped end of the sleeve. The bulging splenic mass compressed near the exit orifice is sliced with scissors inside the sleeve; the process is repeated until the entire splenic parenchyma is extracted in segments. The opposite end of the sleeve is tied after removal of the clamp, and the sleeve is then withdrawn (Fig. 21-15). This simple technique avoids contamination of both the peritoneal cavity and the parenchyma and obviates the risk of splenosis. We have developed a superelastic shape memory alloy moving-blade tissue slicer, which is placed inside the sleeve. This allows visually controlled splenic

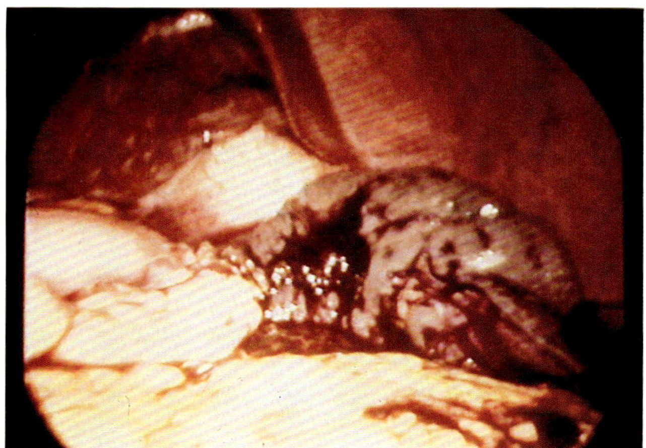

FIGURE 21-14. Exsanguinated spleen in a patient with idiopathic thrombocytopenic purpura. A greater than 50% reduction of splenic size is obtained by splenic bleeding.

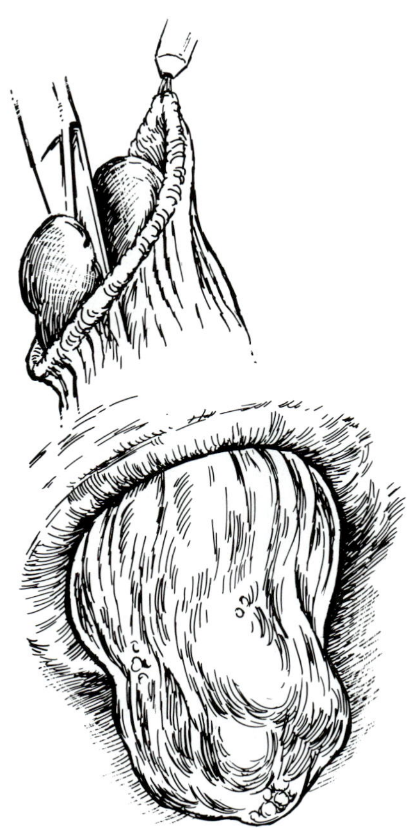

FIGURE 21-15. Removal of spleen using sleeve-delivery system.

slicing inside the third space after this space is distended with CO_2.

POSTOPERATIVE MANAGEMENT AND CLINICAL OUTCOME

The patients have done well and there have been no postoperative morbidity or mortality except for one instance of intraoperative bleeding from traction avulsion of a small venule supplying the pancreatic tail. The resulting intraoperative blood loss amounted to 500 mL, and blood transfusion was not considered necessary. The patient's postoperative hemoglobin level was 10.0 gm/dL.

Another patient developed postoperative bleeding from a segmental artery, which required reintervention. After modification of our technique to include early ligature in continuity of the splenic artery, we have not encountered any bleeding complications in 12 successive patients.

Some shoulder pain is experienced by most patients during the first 24 hours postoperatively but all are ambulatory the day after the operation. Significant ileus is absent, and clear liquids usually can be started within 24 hours. Platelet counts in excess of 300,000 are reached by the third day in all patients with ITP. The patients are usually discharged home on the fourth postoperative day on enteric-coated aspirin.

References

1. Cuschieri A: Technical aspects of laparoscopic splenectomy: hilar segmental devascularization and instrumentation. J R Coll Surg Edinb 1992;37:414.
2. Carroll BJ, Phillips EH, Semel CJ, Fallas M, Morgenstern L: Laparoscopic splenectomy. Surg Endosc 1992;6:183.
3. Delaitre B, Maignien B, Icard P: Laparoscopic splenectomy. Br J Surg 1992;79:1334.
4. Thibault CI, Mamazza J, Letourneau R, Poulin E: Laparoscopic splenectomy: operative technique and preliminary report. Surg Laparosc Endosc 1992;2:248.
5. Zornig C, Emmermann A, Peiper M, Zschaber R, Brolsch CE: Laparoskopische splenektomie. Chirurg 1993;64:314.
6. Akle CA, Wickham JE, Gravett P, Dick R: Laparoscopic splenectomy. Letter. Br J Surg 1993;80:126.
7. Oakes DD, Charters AC: Changing concepts in the management of splenic trauma. Surg Gynecol Obstet 1981; 153:181.
8. King H, Shumacker HB Jr: Splenic studies; susceptibility to infection after splenectomy performed in infancy. Ann Surg 1952;136:239.
9. O'Neal BJ, McDonald JC: The risk of sepsis in the asplenic adult. Ann Surg 1981;194:775.
10. Holdsworth RJ, Irving AD, Cuschieri A: Postsplenectomy sepsis and its mortality rate: actual versus perceived risks. Br J Surg 1991;78:1031.
11. Schlaeffer F, Rosenheck S, Baumgarten-Kleiner A, Grieff Z, Alkan M: Pneumococcal infections among immunised and splenectomised patients in Israel. J Infect 1985;10:38.
12. Giebink GS, Schiffman G, Krivit W, Quie PG: Vaccine-type pneumococcal pneumonia. Occurrence after vaccination in an asplenic patient. JAMA 1979;241:2736.
13. Cuschieri A, Shimi S, Banting S, Vander Velpen G: Coaxial curved instrument for minimal access surgery. Endoscopic Surgery and Allied Technologies 1993;1:303.
14. Cuschieri A, Shimi S, Banting S, Vander Velpen G: Endoscopic ultrasonic dissection for thoracoscopic and laparoscopic surgery. Surg Endosc 1993;7:197.

Chapter 22

Laparoscopic Surgery: An Atlas for General Surgeons, edited by
Gary C. Vitale, Joseph S. Sanfilippo, and Jacques Perissat.
J. B. Lippincott Company, Philadelphia, © 1995.

Laparoscopic Inguinal Hernia Repair

Robert J. Fitzgibbons, Jr.
José Camps
Gary C. Vitale

It is unusual for a new procedure to enjoy the rapid acceptance that was seen with the introduction of laparoscopic cholecystectomy. It became the procedure of choice for uncomplicated gallbladder disease, almost at the outset. This resulted in an attempt to adapt other abdominal procedures for laparoscopic guidance. Few of the newer laparoscopic operations have seen such a rapid rate of acceptance because the advantages over their conventional counterpart are not so obvious. Examples include laparoscopic appendectomy, colectomy, splenectomy, and the subject of this chapter, laparoscopic inguinal herniorrhaphy.

Laparoscopic inguinal herniorrhaphy is being considered because the conventional operation, although safe and effective, is not perfect. It is a relatively painful procedure, the patient is unable to work for a considerable amount of time, and the overall recurrence rate is estimated to be 10%, despite groups that specialize in herniorrhaphy reporting a lower rate of recurrence.[1] Thus, it is not surprising that many investigators are pursuing alternatives to the conventional approach.

It is unlikely that laparoscopic inguinal herniorrhaphy will replace the classic hernia repair for all patients. The primary goal for the development of the technique has been to reduce the recurrence rate and to decrease perioperative morbidity, primarily pain. It is conceivable that laparoscopic inguinal herniorrhaphy may not offer these advantages for the adolescent with a small indirect inguinal hernia or the older patient who is at risk for general anesthesia and does not have a pressing need to return to work quickly. Conversely, a patient with a recurrent hernia, bilateral hernias, or a manual laborer who desires early return to work may better be served by the laparoscopic procedure. A recommendation for laparoscopic inguinal herniorrhaphy rather than the conventional procedure must be made with consideration given to the possible complications associated with laparoscopy and a clear understanding that the benefits outweigh the risks for an individual patient. Prospective randomized trials that compare laparoscopic herniorrhaphy with the conventional procedure will be important after the laparoscopic operation becomes refined enough to be considered standardized.

CONTEMPORARY TECHNIQUES

Most laparoscopic inguinal herniorrhaphies can be classified as one of three types: the *t*rans*a*bdominal *p*re*p*eritoneal laparoscopic inguinal herniorrhaphy (TAPP) repair, the intraperitoneal onlay mesh repair (IPOM), and the totally extraperitoneal repair. Common to all three is the placement of a large prosthesis that widely overlaps the hernia defect, reinforcing all potential sites of recurrent groin herniation (i.e., direct, indirect, and femoral spaces).[2–4] Although other laparoscopic repairs have been described, such as simple ring closure for uncomplicated indirect hernias and even a formal sutured preperitoneal repair, these are in the minority and are rarely used.[5] The intraperitoneal onlay mesh repair involves the placement of a prosthetic patch within the abdominal cavity, potentially in contact with intraabdominal viscera. Thus, the possibility of prosthetic erosion exists. For this reason, we consider the operation experimental and therefore do not discuss it in detail. The purpose of this chapter is to describe the techniques known as the TAPP repair and the totally extraperitoneal laparoscopic herniorrhaphy.

Transabdominal Preperitoneal Laparoscopic Herniorrhaphy

Based on the conventional preperitoneal repairs popularized by Stoppa and Warlaumont in France and Nyhus and Condon in the United States, the TAPP herniorrhaphy is the most popular type of laparoscopic repair.[6,7] In the conventional form, the preperitoneal space is entered through a skin incision. The preperitoneal space can also effectively be entered laparoscopically by making a peritoneal incision. A prosthetic repair can then be accomplished in a manner essentially identical to the conventional approach. The potential advantages of the laparoscopic approach is that the large skin incision is avoided, decreasing postoperative morbidity. The major disadvantages are the risks of laparoscopy, which include major organ or vascular injury and possible adhesive small bowel obstruction because of adhesions at sites where the peritoneum has been breached.

TECHNIQUE

The operating setup most commonly employed for the TAPP laparoscopic herniorrhaphy procedure has the surgeon standing on the opposite side of the table from the hernia, which allows the optimal angle for dissection and staple placement. After induction of general anesthesia, a Foley catheter is placed to ensure continuous decompression of the bladder. Although diagnostic laparoscopy is possible under local anesthesia, the considerable dissection involved in this procedure precludes its use.

After creation of a CO_2 pneumoperitoneum, the laparoscope (port 1) is placed in the umbilicus, which allows generalized exploration of the abdomen. The patient is placed in Trendelenburg's position, allowing the bowel to fall away from the pelvis and permitting good access to this area. The inguinal regions are then inspected to confirm the pathology and to check the contralateral side (Figs. 22-1 and 22-2).

Two more ports are placed lateral to the rectus sheath at the level of the umbilicus under direct vision: one (port 2) 12 to 15 cm to the right and the other (port 3) 12 to 15 cm to the left of the umbilicus (Fig. 22-3). All three are large cannulas (i.e., 10 to 12 mm), permitting free movement of the laparoscope and the stapler to any position, depending on the patient's anatomy.

A toothed grasper is inserted through port 2 and a scissors through port 3. The peritoneum is opened by making an incision at the medial umbilical ligament, at least 2 cm above the hernia defect (Fig. 22-4). The incision is extended laterally to the anterior superior iliac spine, allowing the peritoneum to be dissected free from the overlying abdominal wall (Fig. 22-5). The preperitoneal space is exposed by traction with the grasper in port 2 while using sharp and blunt dissection with the scissors in port 3. Intermittently, coagulation current is used through the scissors to obliterate small vessels. The inferior epigastric vessels, symphysis pubis, transversalis fascia, and cord structures are exposed (Figs. 22-6 and 22-7).

The peritoneal flap is mobilized downward until the hernia defect and the space around it are denuded circumferentially—a distance of 4 to 5 cm. Cooper's ligament inferomedially and the iliopubic tract laterally are visualized (Fig. 22-8). For direct hernias, the sac and preperitoneal fat are reduced from the hernia orifice by using gentle traction. The thinned out transversalis fascia (the so-called pseudosac) lining the defect is left behind—if necessary, separating it by sharp dissection. An indirect inguinal hernia sac extending through the internal ring is inverted into the peritoneal cavity and mobilized from the cord structures (Fig. 22-9). The hook dissector with cautery is helpful in accomplishing this dissection. If, however, an indirect hernia sac is large,

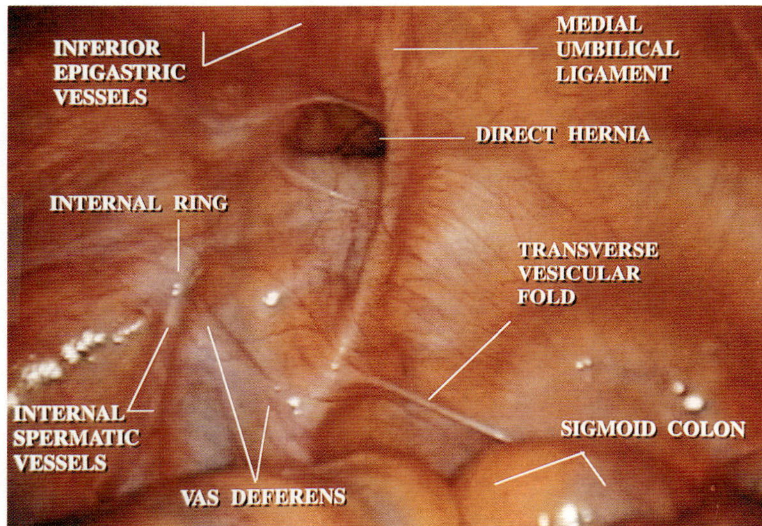

FIGURE 22-1. Laparoscopic view of a left direct hernia.

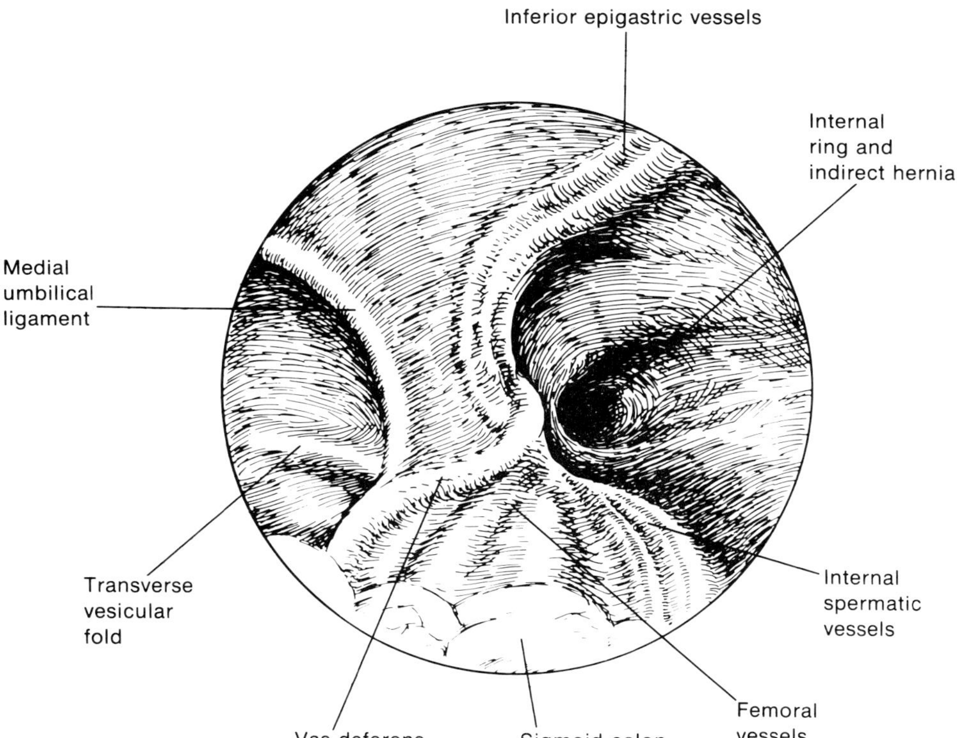

FIGURE 22-2. Laparoscopic view of a right direct hernia.

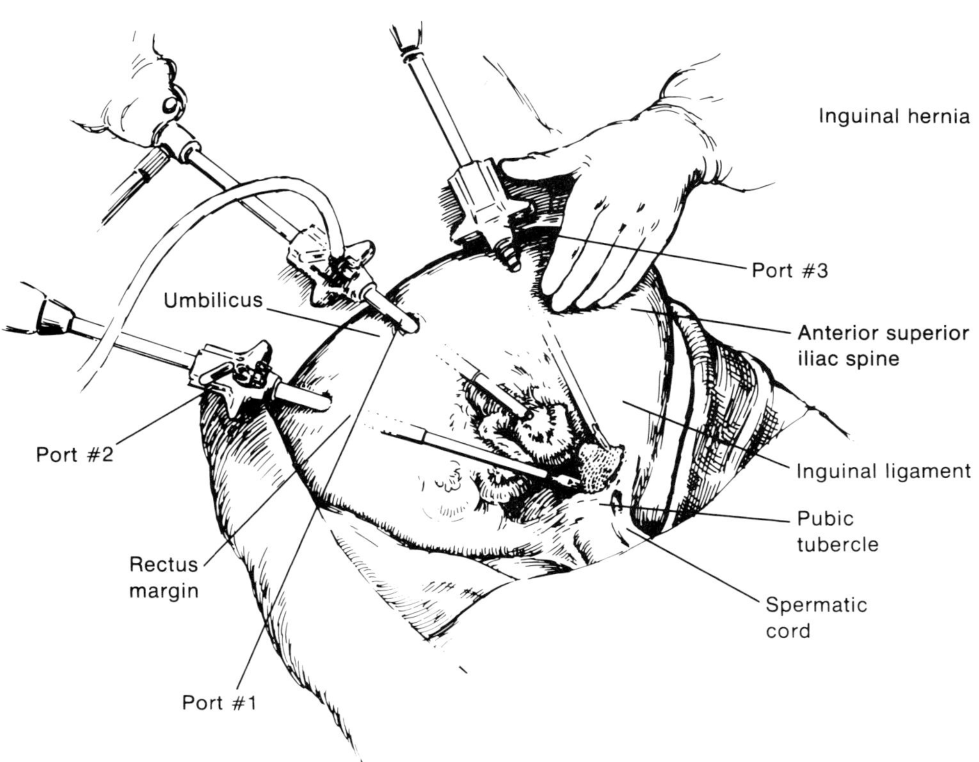

FIGURE 22-3. Overview of port placement for repair of a left inguinal hernia.

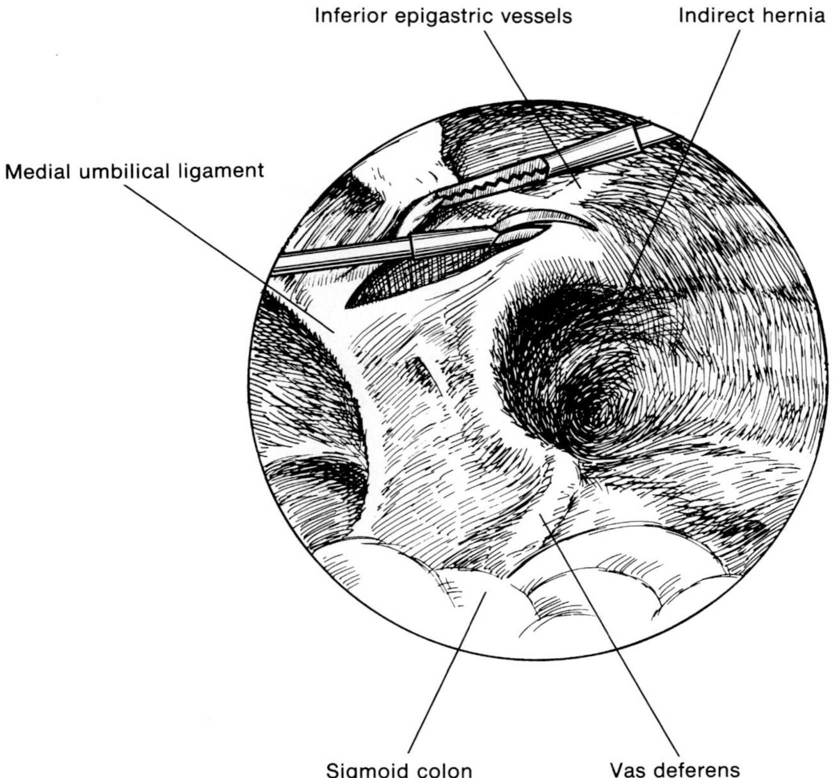

FIGURE 22-4. Peritoneum is opened starting near the medial umbilical ligament. A right indirect inguinal hernia is pictured.

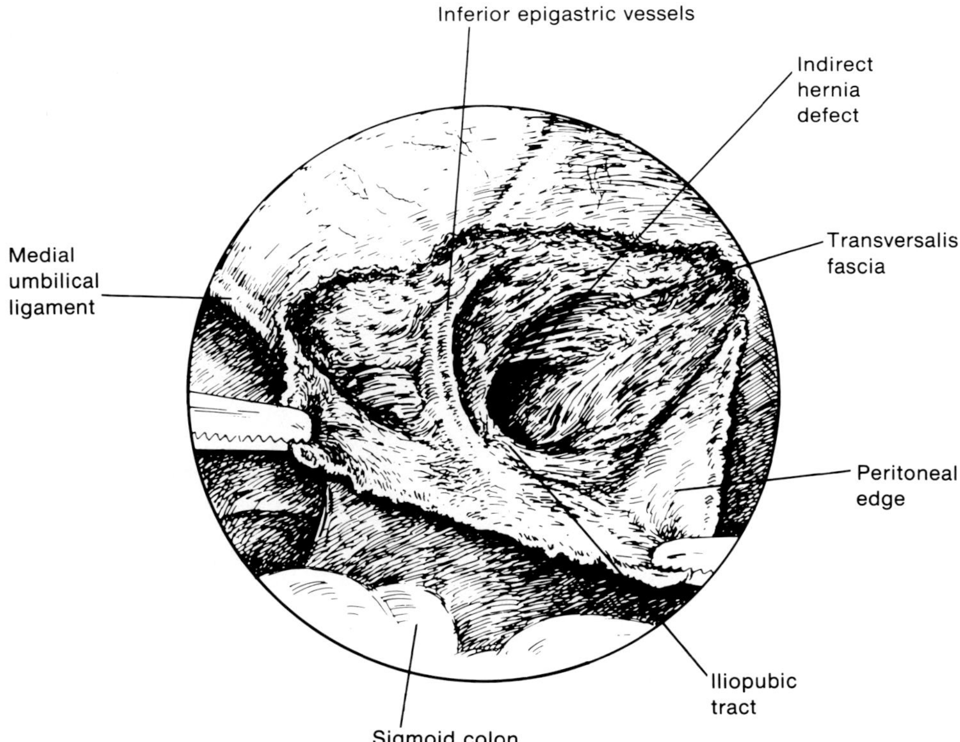

FIGURE 22-5. Peritoneum is dissected back to expose retroperitoneal anatomy. A right indirect inguinal hernia is pictured.

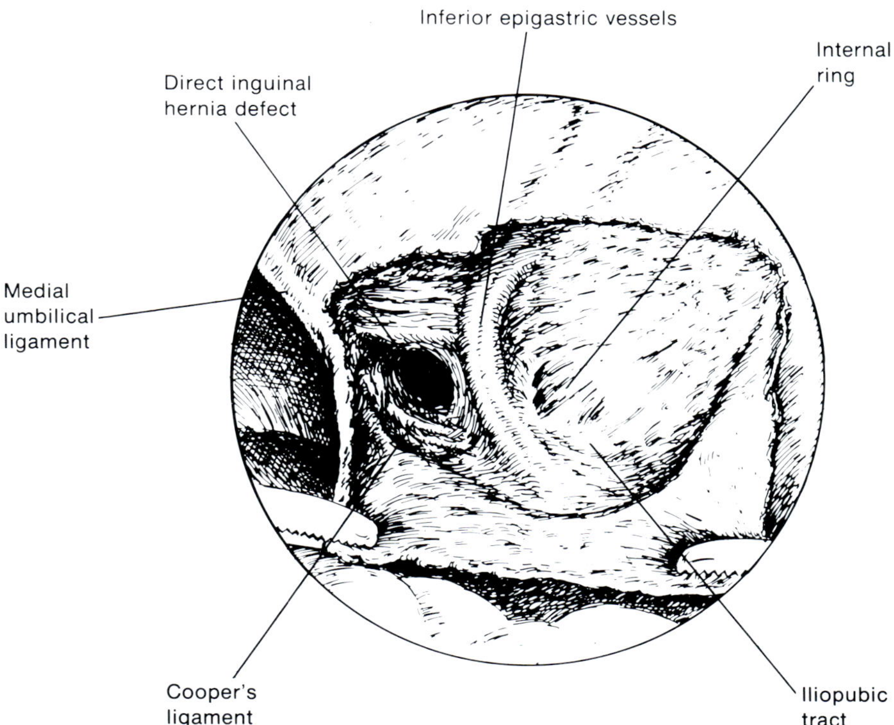

FIGURE 22-6. Peritoneum is dissected back to expose retroperitoneal anatomy. A right direct inguinal hernia is pictured.

extending into the scrotum, its complete mobilization may result in an increased incidence of spermatic cord or testicular complications, and the hernia is best treated by dividing the sac at the internal ring, leaving the distal part in situ, with dissection of the proximal sac away from the cord structures. Care must be taken to identify the vas deferans; it is located inferomedially to the internal ring and crosses the origin of the inferior epigastric vessels from the external iliac artery and vein, just before it enters the internal ring.

After completely dissecting the preperitoneal space and identification of the critical anatomic structures, the repair is commenced. Repair of a small indirect hernia (i.e., Nyhus type 1) may be performed by directly suturing the iliopubic tract to the transversalis fascia, beginning at the lateral aspect of the internal ring. A suture is passed through port 2 with a needle holder while the edge of the iliopubic tract is grasped using port 3. The needle is passed from posterior to anterior through the iliopubic tract and the transversalis fascia. Knots are

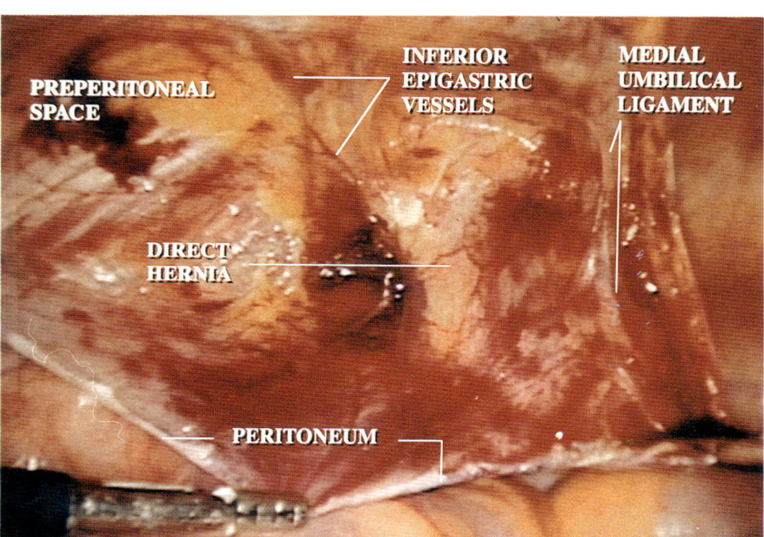

FIGURE 22-7. Peritoneum is dissected to demonstrate anatomy of a left direct hernia.

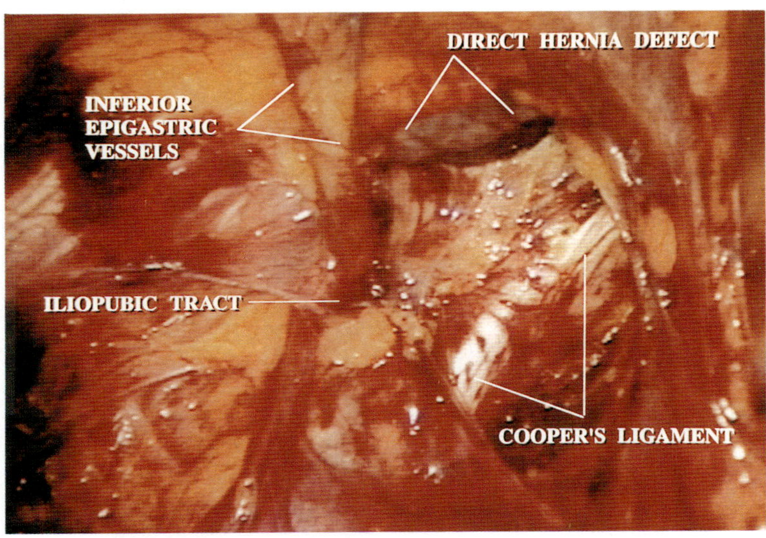

FIGURE 22-8. The peritoneal flap is dissected downward further to expose Cooper's ligament inferomedially and the iliopubic tract laterally. A left direct hernia is pictured here.

tied intracorporeally, and the peritoneum is then closed over the repair, using either sutures or staples (Fig. 22-10). In this particular case, a radical dissection of the preperitoneal space may not be necessary.

For larger indirect hernias or for direct hernias, a mesh prosthesis is preferable to direct suture, to allow tension-free repair. A polypropylene prosthesis is most popular (Marlex, Prolene, Surgipro), although some surgeons prefer polyester (Dacron, Mersilene) or expanded polytetrafluoroethylene (ePTFE; Gore-Tex). The size of the prosthesis that is used is important because many of the earlier recurrences with laparoscopic herniorrhaphy are thought to be due to inadequate coverage of all of the potential sites of recurrent groin herniation.[8,9] As an absolute minimum, it is important that the size of the prosthesis be no less than 10 × 5 cm. It must be sufficiently large to cover the defect and provide an extensive overlap. This allows the intra-abdominal pressure to act on an area of the prosthesis that overlies strong healthy tissue, thus tending to keep it in position rather than encouraging it to herniate through the defect.

The prosthesis is inserted into the abdominal cavity through either of the two lateral laparoscopic cannulas. We find it best not to roll the prosthesis before inserting it. A corner is grasped with a 5-mm instrument, the prosthesis is quickly placed through one of the 10-mm or 11-mm lateral cannulas, and the instrument is promptly withdrawn so that excessive CO_2 loss does not occur. It is then positioned (Fig. 22-11). The prosthesis can either be slit to accommodate the cord structures or simply be placed over them, depending on the surgeon's preference. Most surgeons prefer the latter because this avoids a dissection, which increases the incidence of cord or testicular complications. Proponents of the former argue

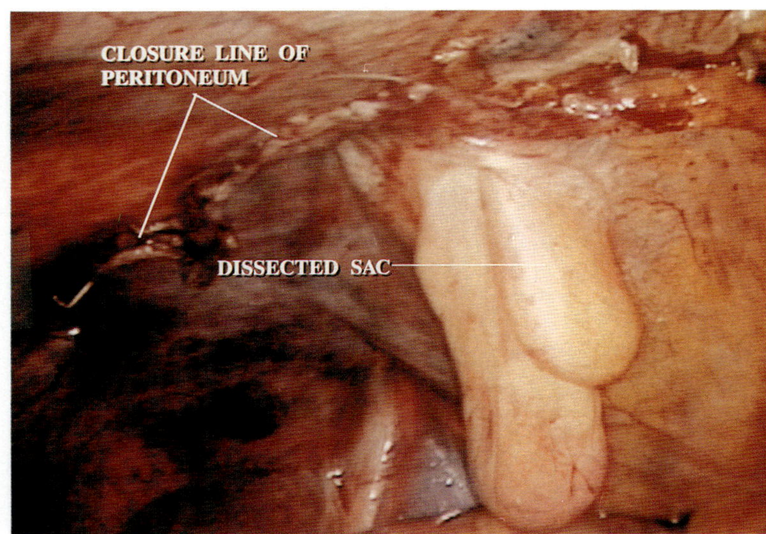

FIGURE 22-9. Dissected hernia sac and cord lipoma after it has been mobilized from the cord structures and inverted into the peritoneal cavity. A left indirect hernia is shown here after the repair has been completed and the peritoneum closed.

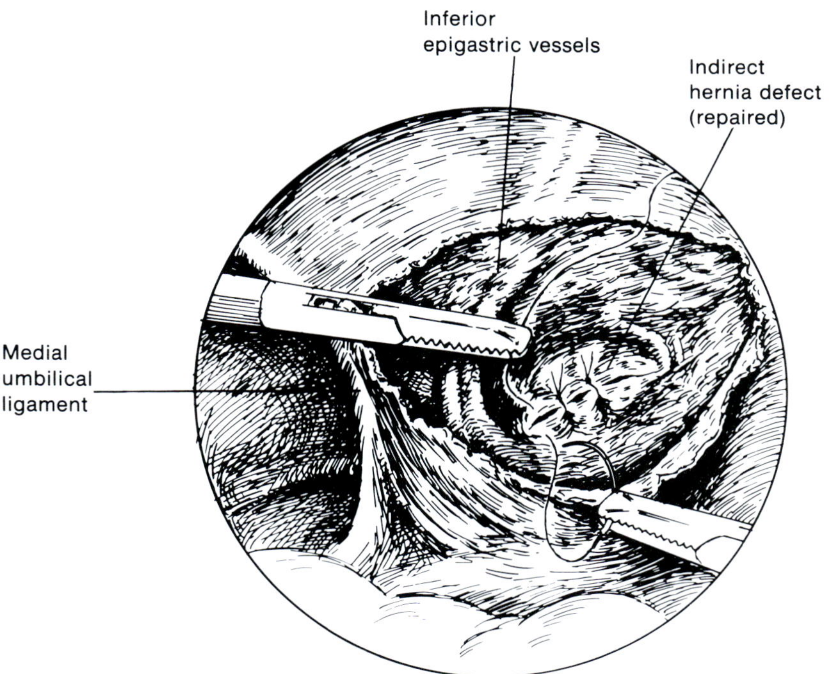

FIGURE 22-10. Simple suture repair of a small indirect inguinal hernia. A right indirect inguinal hernia is shown here.

that this maneuver adds stability to the prosthesis and in effect creates a new internal ring. Optionally, the epigastric vessels also may be dissected free from the anterior abdominal wall, with the prosthesis passed behind the vessels after making a split in the mesh. This allows the mesh to lie flush against the posterior abdominal wall fascia in those cases wherein the epigastric vessels are prominent or bowed outward from the anterior abdominal wall. In most cases, the prosthesis may be fixed as a solid sheet over the vessels.

Once the mesh is positioned, it is stapled in place using a hernia stapler. Rarely, individual interrupted tacking sutures are used, but suturing in this area is difficult. The following landmarks are used:

- Medially, the symphysis pubis
- Superiorly, the abdominal wall, at least 2 cm above the defect
- Laterally, a point about 1 cm medial to the anterior superior iliac spine
- Inferolaterally, the iliopubic tract
- Inferomedially, Cooper's ligament

Care must be taken not to staple below the iliopubic tract when lateral to the internal spermatic vessels to avoid injury to the lateral cutaneous nerve of the thigh or the femoral branch of the genitofemoral nerve.[10,11] A

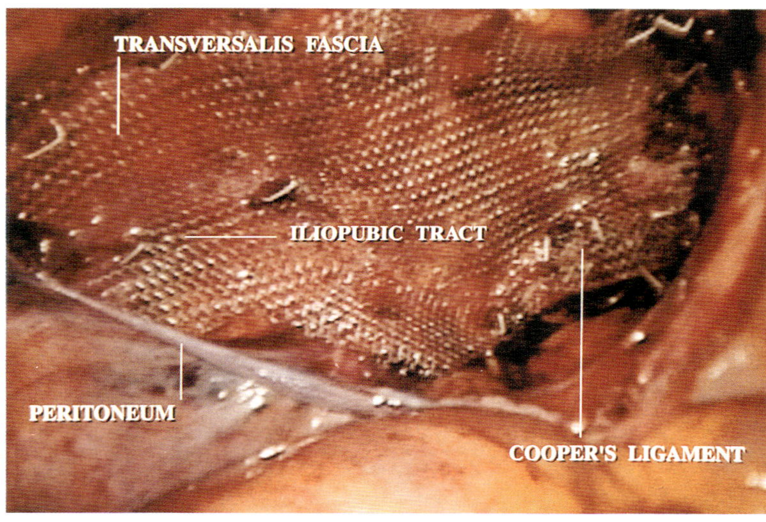

FIGURE 22-11. Mesh positioned with a few tacking staples.

helpful maneuver in this situation is to use a bimanual technique. Staples are not placed without being able to palpate the head of the stapler; this ensures that the surgeon is above the iliopubic tract. Staples should be oriented vertically when stapling inferiorly because the laterocutaneous nerve of the thigh and the femoral branch of the genitofemoral nerve course in this direction (Fig. 22-12). This allows parallel staple placement. Superiorly and laterally, staples should be oriented horizontally, corresponding to the direction of the ilioinguinal and iliohypogastric nerves, which lie in a plane superficial to the preperitoneal space but nevertheless can be damaged with a too vigorous bimanual technique (Fig. 22-13). During the course of staple placement, excess mesh is trimmed in situ, so that the prosthesis is tailored to the preperitoneal space perfectly.

After the prosthesis is fixed in place, the peritoneum is closed over it to eliminate the possibility of direct contact with intraabdominal viscera, using either staples or interrupted sutures. It is important not to leave gaps between the staples because bowel has been reported to slip into them, causing obstruction (Fig. 22-14).[11] Partial reduction of the pneumoperitoneum to lower abdominal pressure may be necessary to make the peritoneal edges coapt. Instruments are removed and the port sites closed. An attempt should be made to close the fascia of the trocar sites because there have been increasingly frequent reports of trocar-site hernias where larger cannulas have been placed, especially in the lower abdomen.[11]

Bilateral hernias can be repaired using one long transverse peritoneal incision. A single prosthesis (at least 20 × 6 cm) can be used to cover both defects, fashioned similar to that described for the preperitoneal bilateral conventional repair. Two separate pieces of prosthetic material are preferred by some authorities because it is easier to manipulate the smaller prostheses. This may avoid the theoretic complication that might be encountered if the urachus is patent and an incision is made across it and not recognized.

This approach to herniorrhaphy has—at least on short-term follow-up—an acceptably low recurrence rate and good patient acceptance.[11] Considerable dissection is required, but with experience, the operating time is similar to that for a conventional herniorrhaphy. The peritoneal dissection leads to some pain, but the tension-free nature of the repair means that it is not prolonged, and most patients return to normal activities within a week.

Totally Extraperitoneal Herniorrhaphy

The totally extraperitoneal herniorrhaphy is not truly laparoscopic because the abdominal cavity is not entered. Nevertheless, because laparoscopic instrumentation and techniques are used, it is appropriate to discuss this with the other procedures. It is gaining in popularity because by avoiding entering the abdominal cavity, the complication of bowel obstruction secondary to adhesions at sites where the peritoneum has been breached is avoided. A word of caution is in order for surgeons planning to perform a totally extraperitoneal laparoscopic herniorrhaphy. A thorough understanding of the preperitoneal space, as observed during the TAPP procedure, is essential because the field of vision and working

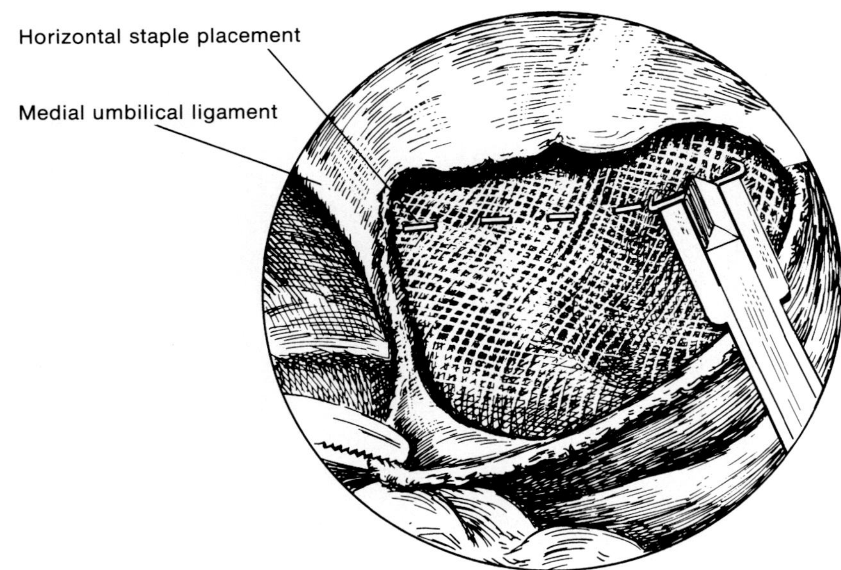

FIGURE 22-12. Mesh being stapled in place with inferior row of staples placed vertically.

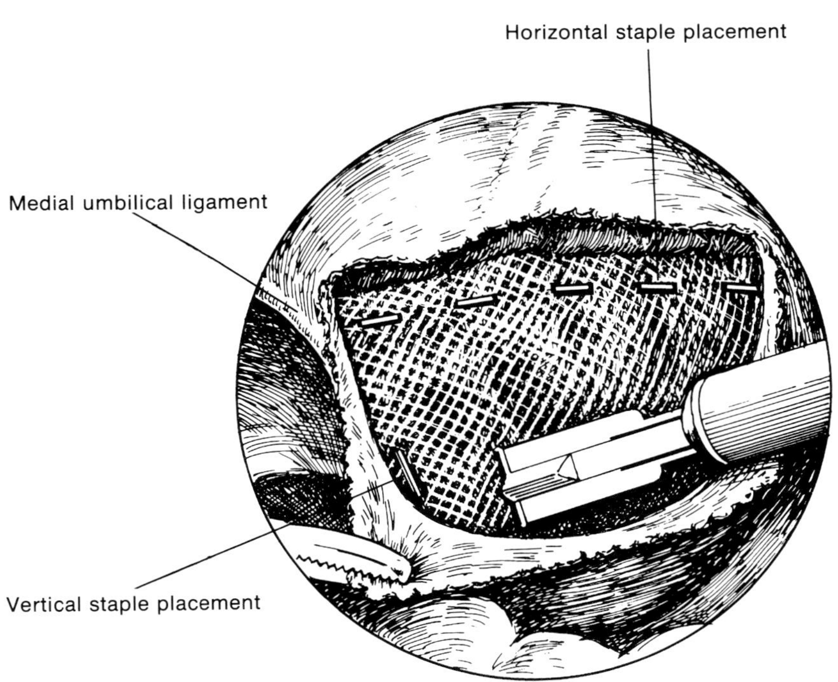

FIGURE 22-13. Mesh being stapled in place with superior row of staples placed horizontally.

space is smaller than that seen with the other laparoscopic techniques.

TECHNIQUE

An incision is made in the umbilicus and a dissection through the fascia begun as if performing an open laparoscopy. The peritoneum is not entered. A laparoscopic cannula is placed between the transversalis fascia and the peritoneum, and an operating laparoscope introduced. The operating laparoscope allows both the optics and an instrument to be passed through the same 10-mm cannula. The dissection of the preperitoneal space can be commenced using blunt and sharp dissection, creating a CO_2 "pneumo-extraperitoneum." Once the space is enlarged sufficiently, accessory cannulas can be placed. A large cannula is placed between the umbilicus and the

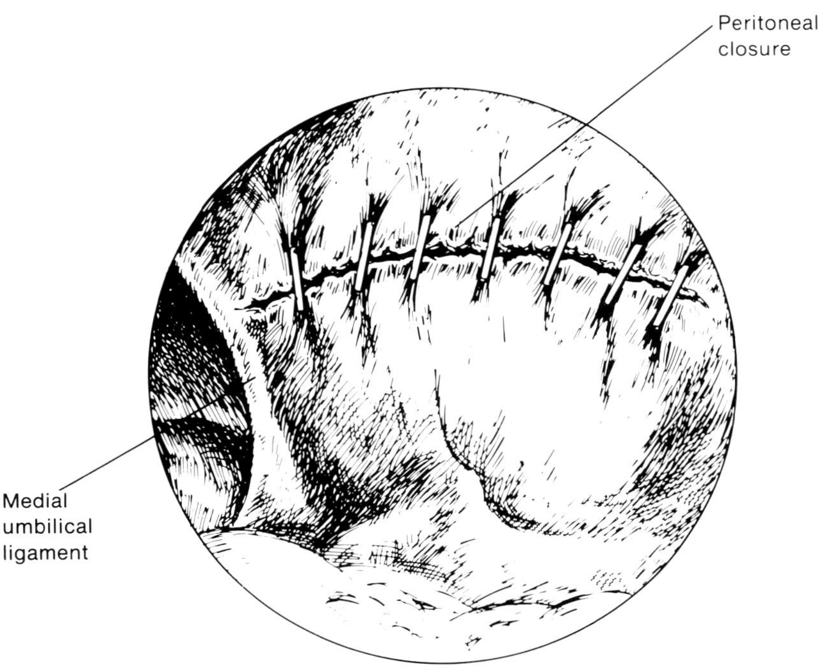

FIGURE 22-14. Peritoneal closure over mesh. No gaps are left to minimize opportunity for bowel to be caught in this area.

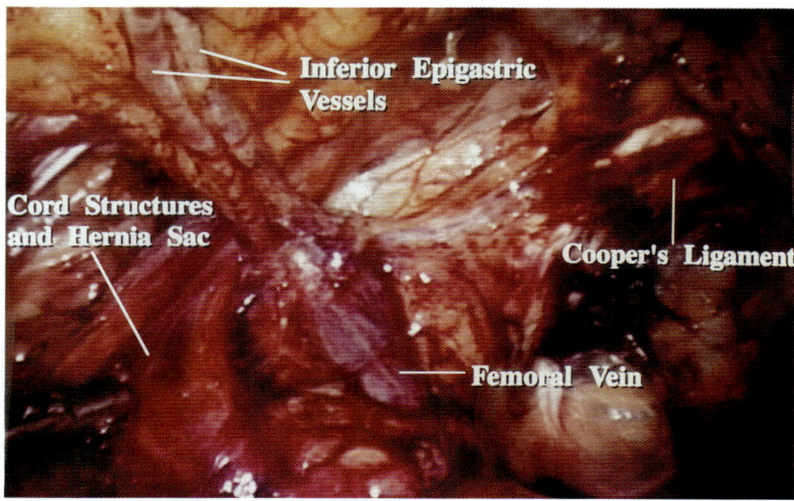

FIGURE 22-15. Preperitoneal anatomy as viewed during the totally extraperitoneal herniorrhaphy.

symphysis pubis and a 5-mm cannula is inserted, either just above the symphysis pubis or lateral to the rectus sheath at about the level of the umbilicus, depending on the surgeon's preference. The operating laparoscope is replaced with a conventional 10-mm instrument, and dissection of the preperitoneal space continues. Once the preperitoneal space in the area of the inguinal region is entered, the dissection continues in an identical fashion to that described previously for the TAPP operation, with the same critical landmarks being identified (Fig. 22-15).

The totally extraperitoneal laparoscopic inguinal herniorrhaphy has been facilitated by the introduction of air- or water-filled balloon dissectors that can accomplish preperitoneal dissection. The technique for insertion of the balloon is as follows. Again, an incision is made at the umbilicus as if performing an open laparoscopy. The dissection then proceeds to one side or the other of the midline, exposing the anterior rectus sheath, which is opened. The rectus muscle is retracted laterally and the balloon placed over the posterior rectus sheath and advanced to the midline between either symphysis pubis. The reason that the rectus sheath placement is preferred is that placement of the balloon in the midline commonly results in peritoneal perforation. This rarely occurs if the balloon is passed over the posterior rectus sheath.

After the balloon has been inflated and the dissection completed, the balloon is deflated and withdrawn. It is replaced with a laparoscopic cannula and a pneumoextraperitoneum is produced. Laparoscopic cannulas can then be placed under direct vision in the accessory positions described above, because characteristically, a nearly complete dissection of the preperitoneal space occurs. When placing the accessory cannulas, it is important that an incision be made in both the skin and the fascia, so that the cannulas can be placed with minimal pressure. Excessive pressure commonly results in traversing the preperitoneal space and entering the abdominal cavity because the space is relatively small.

For patients with uncomplicated hernias, the totally extraperitoneal procedure offers a distinct advantage over the TAPP procedure. Difficulties can be encountered with several different types of patients, however. First are those patients who have had previous lower abdominal surgery (e.g., appendectomy). The scar tissue associated with the abdominal wall closure with these procedures invariably results in peritoneal perforation. Peritoneal perforation increases the difficulty with the totally extraperitoneal operation because it results in a competing pneumoperitoneum, which compromises the size of the extraperitoneal space. Second is the patient with a large indirect inguinal hernia. It may not be practical to dissect the entire sac from the cord structures for fear of cord or testicular complications. If the sac is divided in situ, it must be closed proximally expeditiously and effectively or the patient will develop a pneumoperitoneum, resulting in the same problem described above.

SUMMARY

The key factors that have resulted in the development of the TAPP and the totally extraperitoneal laparoscopic inguinal hernia repairs are the acceptance of prosthetic materials to produce a tension-free herniorrhaphy, the apparent efficacy of the preperitoneal repair, and the development and widespread use of therapeutic laparoscopy in general surgery.

Laparoscopy affords excellent exposure of the preperitoneal space, which can be useful in repairing many inguinal hernias, especially those that are recurrent or otherwise complicated. It seems that laparoscopy will certainly have a place in the armamentarium of general surgeons treating inguinal hernias, although it is unlikely that every inguinal hernia will be best repaired laparoscopically. Preliminary results, however, suggest that further investigation is indicated.

References

1. Rubinstein RS, Beck S, Lohr KN, Kamberg CJ, Brook RH, Goldberg GA: Conceptualization and measurement of physiologic health for adults. Surgical conditions. Rand Health Insurance experiment series 1985;15:14.
2. Corbitt JD Jr: Transabdominal preperitoneal herniorrhaphy. Surg Laparosc Endosc 1993;3:328.
3. Fitzgibbons RJ Jr, Salerno GM, Filipi CJ, Hart R: Laparoscopic intraperitoneal onlay mesh technique for repair of an indirect inguinal hernia (intraperitoneal onlay mesh procedure). Ann Surg 1994;219(2):144.
4. McKernan JB, Laws HL: Laparoscopic repair of inguinal hernias using a totally extraperitoneal prosthetic approach. Surg Endosc 1993;7:26.
5. Gazayerli MM: Anatomical laparoscopic hernia repair of direct and indirect inguinal hernias using the transversalis fascia and iliopubic tract. Surg Laparosc Endosc 1992;1:49.
6. Stoppa RE, Warlaumont CR: The preperitoneal approach and prosthetic repair of groin hernia. In: Nyhus LM, Condon RE, eds. Hernia. 3rd ed. Philadelphia: JB Lippincott, 1989:199.
7. Nyhus LM: The preperitoneal approach and iliopubic tract repair of inguinal hernia. In: Nyhus LM, Condon RE, eds. Hernia. 3rd ed. Philadelphia: JB Lippincott, 1989:154.
8. Schultz L, Graber J, Pietrafitta J, Hickok D: Laser laparoscopic herniorrhaphy: a clinical trial preliminary results. J Laparoendosc Surg 1990;1:41.
9. MacFadyen BV Jr, Arregui ME, Corbitt JD Jr, et al: Complications of laparoscopic herniorrhaphy [see comments]. Surg Endosc 1993;7:155.
10. Kraus MA: Nerve injury during laparoscopic inguinal hernia repair. Surg Laparosc Endosc 1993;3:342.
11. Fitzgibbons RJ Jr, Camps J, Nguyen N, et al: Laparoscopic inguinal herniorrhaphy: results of a multi-center trial. Ann Surg 1995.

Chapter 23

Laparoscopic Surgery: An Atlas for General Surgeons, edited by Gary C. Vitale, Joseph S. Sanfilippo, and Jacques Perissat. J. B. Lippincott Company, Philadelphia, © 1995.

Thoracoscopic Esophageal Myotomy

William G. Cheadle

Surgical treatment for both achalasia and diffuse esophageal spasm involves myotomy of either the lower portion of the esophagus or the entire esophagus, respectively. This disease spectrum is thought to be due to Wallerian degeneration of the vagus nerve, which arises in the dorsal motor nucleus of the tenth cranial nerve. This subsequently leads to loss of ganglion cells, with degeneration atrophy of the smooth muscle and a hypersensitivity brought on by this degeneration. Heller first described esophageal myotomy in 1914. He used both an anterior and a posterior muscle-splitting incision to allow the mucosa to protrude through these incisions. Zaaiger modified this procedure in 1919 to include just the anterior incision, which has become the standard surgical treatment for achalasia.

With the advent of efficient optics and proper instrumentation, this procedure is being performed under thoracoscopic guidance. Diagnosis is generally entertained by barium swallow. It is confirmed by esophageal manometric study, which demonstrates failure of the lower esophageal sphincter to relax on swallowing in addition to tertiary nonpropagative waves throughout the body of the esophagus. Although dilation has become the initial treatment of choice for achalasia, the recurrence rate can reach 30%. When surgical treatment follows repeated dilations, it is performed with more difficulty than when done primarily. Esophageal myotomy under thoracoscopic guidance avoids the morbidity of thoracotomy and usually results in permanent cure because recurrence rates are extremely low. Consequently, thoracoscopic esophageal myotomy should be considered as primary therapy or after one or two attempts at pneumatic esophageal dilation for achalasia.

TECHNIQUE

The patient is placed in the right lateral decubitus position, so that the left side is exposed (Fig. 23-1). After induction of anesthesia, a double lumen endotracheal tube is inserted, which facilitates ventilation of the right lung while allowing the left lung to collapse. After this is in place, a standard upper endoscope is advanced into the esophagus for about 35 cm, to the area of dissection. The light is left on to facilitate identification of the distal esophagus through the thoracoscope.

Not only is it unnecessary to maintain a pneumothorax by insufflation, it is actually dangerous because there is a risk of tension pneumothorax. Consequently, arterial-line monitoring should be done throughout the procedure to assist in rapid identification of the development of this potential complication. A 10-mm trocar (trocar 1) is placed in the mid-axillary line through the left seventh interspace to facilitate passage of the thoracoscope, which is attached to the camera. This is done by first making an incision through the skin with a knife, followed by blunt dissection through the chest wall with a Kelly clamp, and then blunt penetration of the pleura. The patient is then ventilated only by the right lung, allowing the left lung to collapse. Two 5-mm trocars (trocars 2 and 3) are placed in the anterior and posterior axillary lines at the sixth interspace. These trocars will contain grasping forceps that will be used to retract either side of the esophageal muscle as needed, before and during the myotomy. The final 5-mm trocar (trocar 4) is then placed in the mid-axillary line through the fourth interspace; this will contain the primary dissecting instrument. Each of the four trocar sites is then cauter-

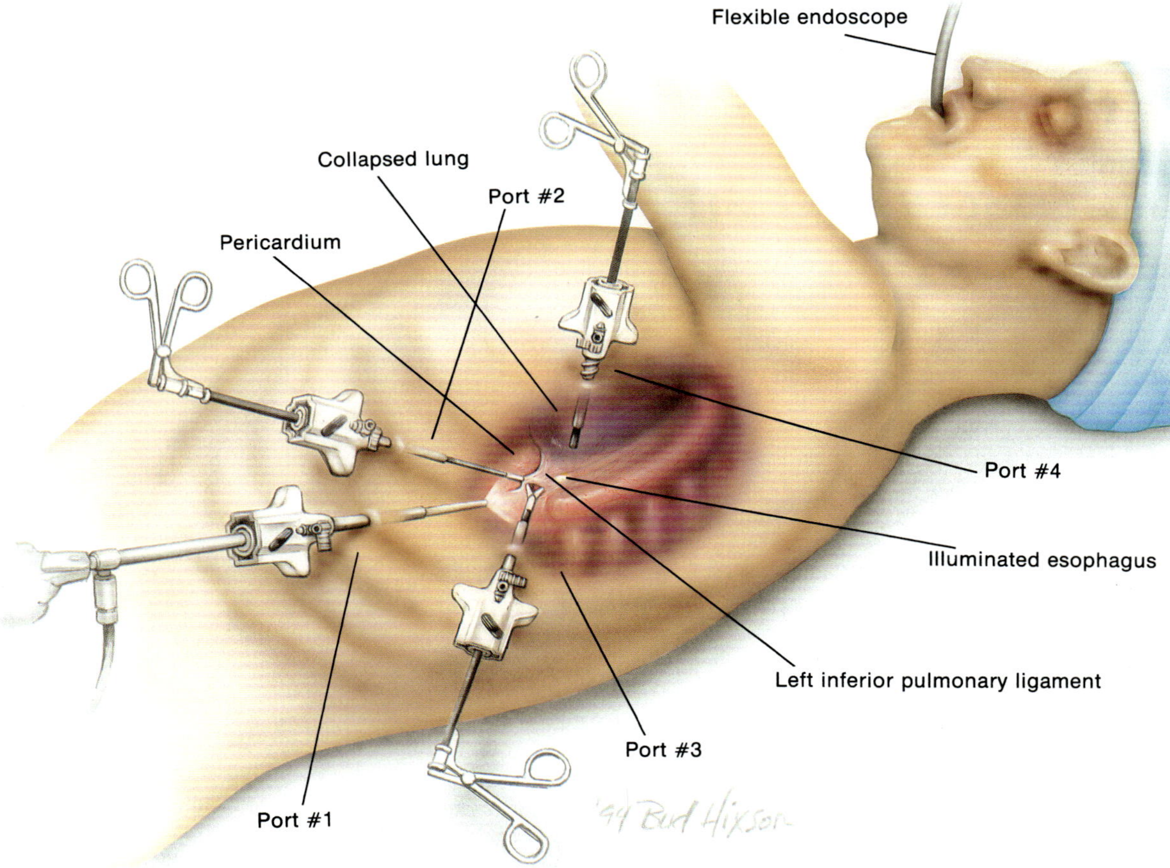

FIGURE 23-1. A patient in the right lateral decubitus position, with the appropriate placement of the trocars. The esophagus is illuminated with the use of a flexible endoscope placed after the patient has been intubated and positioned as shown.

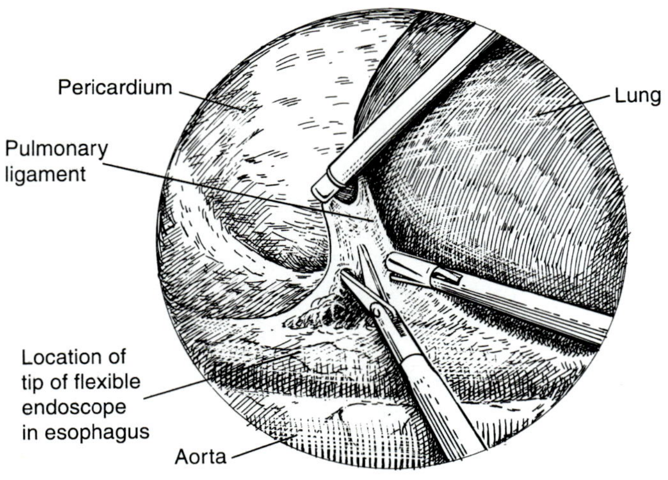

FIGURE 23-2. Exposure of the esophagus by incising the inferior pulmonary ligament.

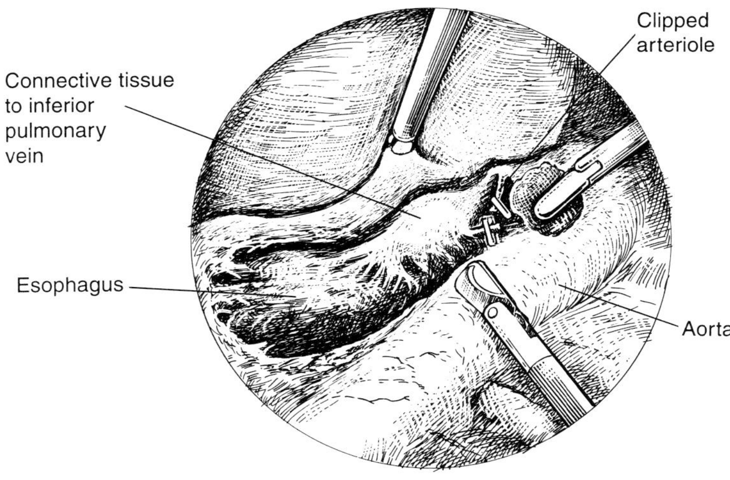

FIGURE 23-3. The esophagus is mobilized to the inferior pulmonary vein proximally when a lower esophageal myotomy is performed for achalasia.

ized through all layers to prevent blood dripping onto the camera.

The inferior pulmonary ligament is transected from its attachment to the diaphragm and mediastinum cephalad to the inferior pulmonary vein (Fig. 23-2). This allows exposure of the most proximal portion of the distal esophagus to facilitate a complete myotomy (Fig. 23-3). This portion of the procedure often is performed with a dissecting instrument in either of the inferior 5-mm trocar sites. To provide appropriate countertraction, the lung is grasped with the grasping forceps during this part of the procedure. The esophagus is then mobilized to the gastroesophageal junction (Fig. 23-4).

The esophagus is identified by visualizing the endoscopic light, which can be seen through its seromuscular wall. At this point, the endoscope may need to be repositioned to keep the light at the desired position. It is also important that the monitor to the endoscope remain clearly visible to the surgical team because termination of the procedure is determined when the lower esophageal sphincter is seen to be relaxing and the gastric lumen comes into view.

Using the grasping forceps, both sides of the pleura covering the distal esophagus are grasped and the myotomy is begun by making an incision with the scissors (Figs. 23-5 and 23-6). This has to be done carefully because the greatest risk of perforation into the esophageal

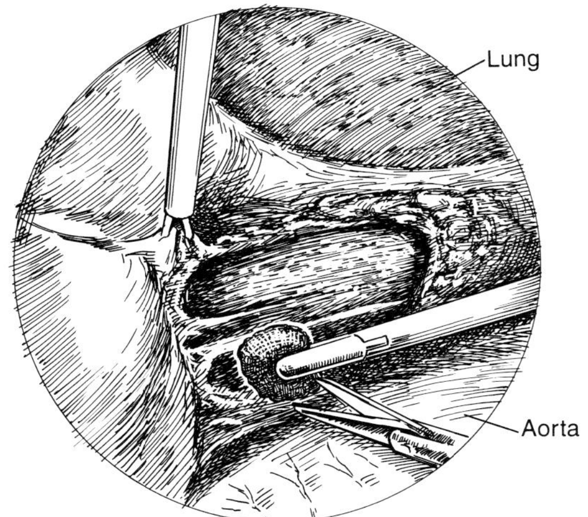

FIGURE 23-4. The esophagus is mobilized to the gastroesophageal junction, the most distal aspect of the myotomy.

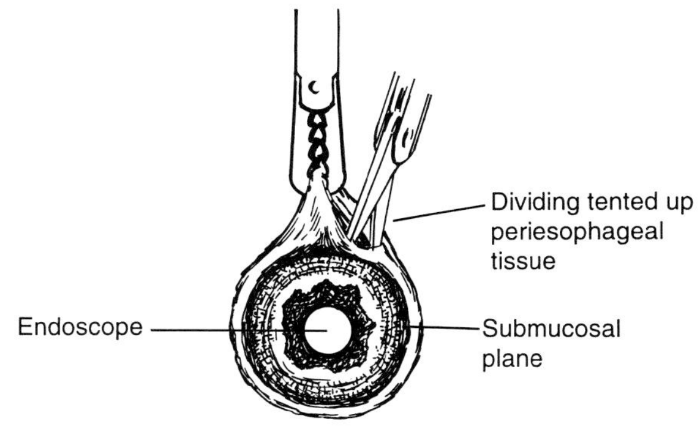

FIGURE 23-5. Cross section of the esophagus, in which the periesophageal tissue is divided and the dissection carried to the submucosal plane.

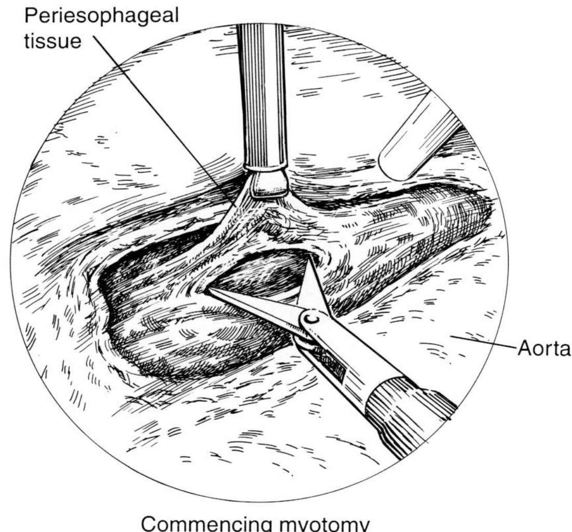

FIGURE 23-6. The myotomy is begun by incising the tented periesophageal tissue (as seen in Fig. 23-5) and taking it down to the submucosal plane, where the mucosa bulges out.

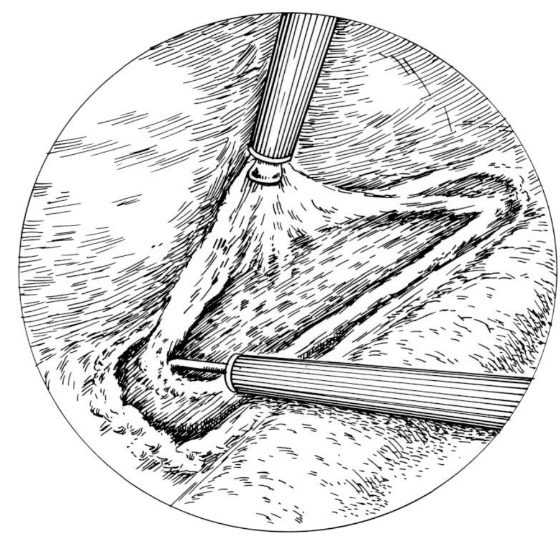

FIGURE 23-8. The myotomy is extended toward the diaphragm at the gastroesophageal junction.

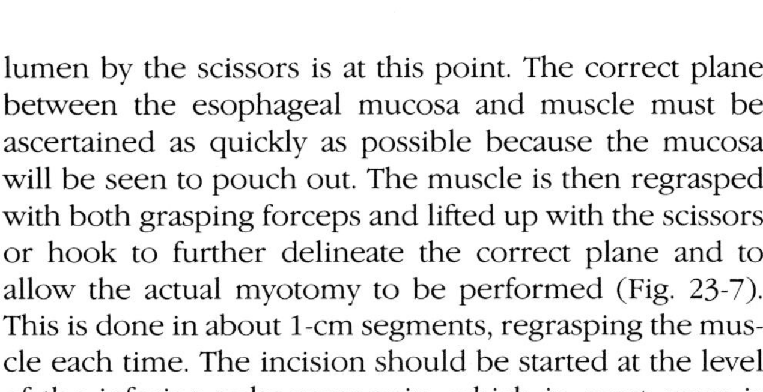

lumen by the scissors is at this point. The correct plane between the esophageal mucosa and muscle must be ascertained as quickly as possible because the mucosa will be seen to pouch out. The muscle is then regrasped with both grasping forceps and lifted up with the scissors or hook to further delineate the correct plane and to allow the actual myotomy to be performed (Fig. 23-7). This is done in about 1-cm segments, regrasping the muscle each time. The incision should be started at the level of the inferior pulmonary vein, which in most cases is the most proximal extension. The myotomy is continued inferiorly to the diaphragm. The grasping forceps become even more important as the dissection nears the diaphragm (Fig. 23-8). The cut edges of the muscle must be retracted proximally to keep the esophagus in view or the diaphragm obscures the most distal portion of the myotomy. It is important not to proceed too far onto the gastric fundus because gastroesophageal reflux can result from too generous a myotomy. Using the thoracoscopic technique, however, proceeding too far distally with the

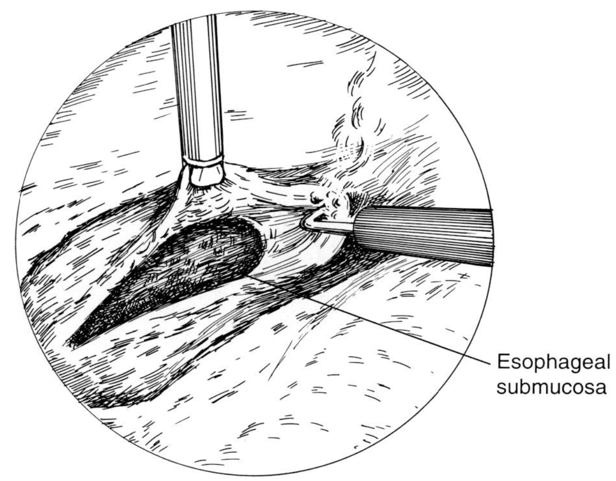

FIGURE 23-7. The esophageal wall is grasped and the muscle divided with a hook.

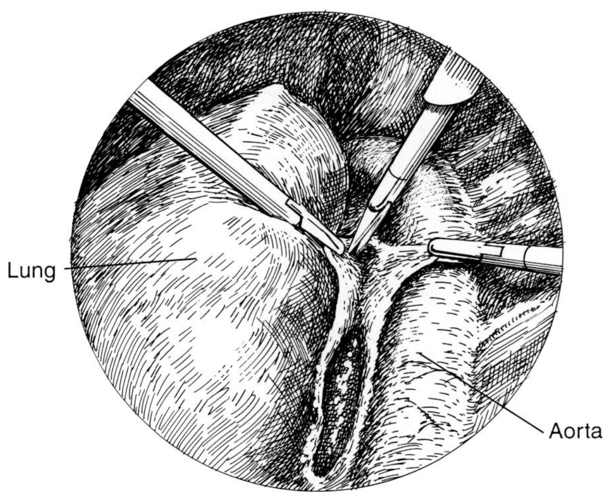

FIGURE 23-9. The myotomy is extended as far cephalad as possible for diffuse esophageal spasm.

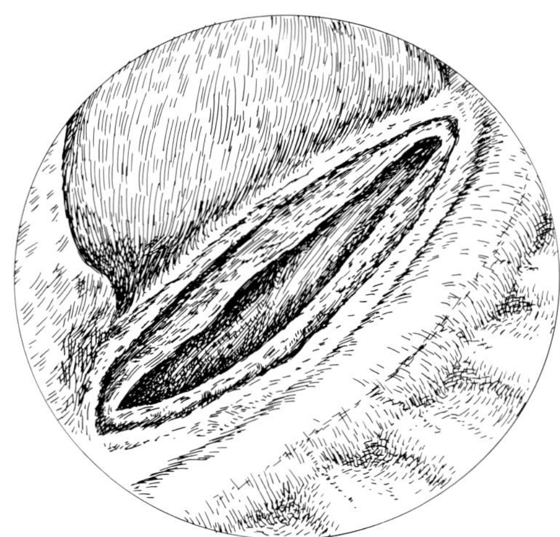

FIGURE 23-10. Completed long esophageal myotomy, from gastroesophageal junction to the aortic arch.

myotomy is usually not a problem because it is hard to visualize the stomach through the thoracoscope. Secondly, the moment the last important hypertrophic esophageal muscle is cut, the gastric lumen appears through the endoscope and the dissection is then terminated. For patients with diffuse esophageal spasm, the procedure is performed in the left pleural cavity, and the myotomy is extended to the upper thoracic esophagus (aortic arch) as far as possible (Fig. 23-9).

Normal saline is placed in the thoracic cavity and the endoscope withdrawn while insufflating air into the esophageal lumen to make sure there is no air bubbling, which would indicate a breach of the esophageal mucosa (Fig. 23-10). If there is any question of a perforation, contrast media can be instilled through the endoscope and a radiograph taken while the patient is on the operating table. The area is then irrigated, hemostasis achieved with electrocautery, and a chest tube placed low, toward the area of the myotomy through the inferior 10-mm trocar. The other trocars are removed, and the skin is closed with interrupted absorbable subcuticular sutures. The left lung is then reinflated and a chest tube is placed to pleurovac suction. A chest radiograph is obtained in the recovery room to make sure that the lung has been reexpanded. The patient is started on a clear liquid diet the following day and is slowly advanced over the next several days to a regular diet. Meats should not be allowed for 1 week. Patients often rapidly regain lost weight over the first 3 to 4 weeks after the procedure because of resolution of dysphagia.

Chapter 24

Laparoscopic Surgery: An Atlas for General Surgeons, edited by
Gary C. Vitale, Joseph S. Sanfilippo, and Jacques Perissat.
J. B. Lippincott Company, Philadelphia, © 1995.

Laparoscopic Surgery for Adhesiolysis

Harry Reich

Intra-abdominal adhesions are usually the sequelae of general surgical or gynecologic operations, pelvic inflammatory disease (gonococcal or chlamydial), appendicitis, or endometriosis. Adhesions occur after abdominal surgery in more than 60% of cases, although fewer than 30% are symptomatic.

Adhesions may be responsible for chronic persistent abdominal pain without associated pelvic pathology. Clinically, adhesions present as chronic or acute abdominal or pelvic pain, partial or complete mechanical bowel obstruction, or infertility. Although adhesions probably cause pain by entrapment of expansile viscera, the relation of adhesions to abdominal pain is still controversial. In contrast, mechanical small bowel obstruction after previous surgery demonstrates unequivocally the most severe effect of adhesions.

Patients with chronic or recurrent abdominal pain and a history of numerous abdominal surgical procedures are often denied treatment if they are not obstructed or symptomatic of intermittent bowel obstruction. While surgical therapy is withheld, multiple abdominal diagnostic procedures (including abdominal computed tomography scan) are frequently ordered. These patients are then sent to chronic pain clinics for evaluation. Although few studies exist, a report suggests that women with severe, dense, vascularized bowel adhesions have a significant reduction in pain after adhesiolysis.[1]

Patients with symptomatic adhesions usually desire minimally invasive therapy. If given the choice between a laparoscopic surgical procedure and laparotomy, they rarely choose the latter. This choice is seldom offered, however, although most adhesiolysis procedures performed using laparotomy can be accomplished through the laparoscope. Although the advantages of laparoscopic enterolysis over classic laparotomy have not been proved, it is possible with laparoscopy to diminish peritoneal mesothelial cell ischemic damage from trauma, drying, talc, packs, and delayed bleeding. Laparoscopic surgery is clearly the preferred method of access for many surgical procedures because of the decreased risk of de novo adhesion formation.[2,3] Similar surgical outcomes have been demonstrated when compared with laparotomy in the management of extensive adhesions.[4,5] Surgical advantages of laparoscopy include panoramic pelvic visualization and magnification, techniques similar to microsurgery, and documentation of absolute hemostasis by underwater examination. The patient enjoys simultaneous diagnosis and treatment and all the advantages of minimally invasive surgery in terms of cosmetics and rapid recuperation. Ileus is rare after laparoscopic surgery. At this time, the onus should be on the surgeon to prove that laparotomy results in better outcome than laparoscopy, not vice versa.

This chapter discusses advanced laparoscopic equipment, techniques, and their application relative to chronic adhesiolysis procedures—primarily omentolysis and enterolysis. Acute lysis of adhesions to prevent the formation of chronic adhesions has been reviewed previously.[6–8] The general aim is to provide discussion of the most appropriate application of state-of-the-art laparoscopic surgical techniques.

EQUIPMENT

Laparoscopes

Four different laparoscopes are used for adhesiolysis: a 10-mm, 0°, straight viewing laparoscope; a 10-mm operative laparoscope with 5-mm (or less) operating channel; a 5-mm straight viewing laparoscope for introduction through a 5-mm trocar sleeve; and an oblique-angle laparoscope (30° to 45°) for upper abdominal procedures—especially when operating directly beneath the umbilicus. A HydroLaparoscope (Circon-ACMI, Stamford, CT) is available with a built-in lens-washing and irrigation system that cleans the distal lens during surgery and rinses the operative site.

High-Flow Carbon Dioxide Insufflators

The ability to maintain a relatively constant intra-abdominal pressure between 10 and 15 mmHg during long laparoscopic procedures is essential. High-flow carbon dioxide (CO_2) insufflation up to 15 L/minute compensates for the rapid loss of CO_2 during suctioning.

Gasless Laparoscopy

Abdominal wall subcutaneous emphysema occurs frequently during anterior abdominal wall adhesiolysis because peritoneal defects result in free communication with the rectus sheath. This compromises the peritoneal cavity operating space. A useful technique is to insert a Laparolift anterior abdominal wall retractor (Origin Medical Systems, Menlo Park, CA) once the umbilicus has been cleared of adhesions.

Thirty-Degree Tiltable Operating Room Table

The steep Trendelenburg's position (20° to 40°), with shoulder braces and arms at the patient's sides, is useful. Operating room tables capable of a 30° Trendelenburg's position are necessary for advanced laparoscopic surgical procedures, especially when the deep pelvis is involved. The hand-controlled Champagne model 600 (Affiliated Table Company, Rochester, NY) is used; an electronically controlled table capable of this degree of body tilt is also available (Skytron Model 6500, Grand Rapids, MI).

Rectal and Vaginal Probes

A sponge on a ring forceps is inserted into the posterior vaginal fornix, and an 81-French rectal probe (Reznik Instruments, Skokie, IL) is placed in the rectum to define the rectum and posterior vagina for lysis of pelvic adhesions when there is a significant degree of cul-de-sac obliteration. This facilitates opening of the posterior vagina (culdotomy). Whenever rectal location is in doubt, it is identified by insertion of the rectal probe.[4]

Trocar Sleeves

Trocar sleeves are available in many sizes and shapes. For most cases, 5.5-mm cannulas are adequate. Laparoscopic stapling is performed through 12/13-mm ports. U.S. Surgical (Norwalk, CT) 12.5-mm trocar sleeves with adjustable locking retention collars (Reich screw grid design) hold their position well for stapling but their trap makes extracorporeal suturing cumbersome.

Short, trapless 5-, 10-, and 12-mm trocar sleeves with retention screw grids around their external surfaces are used in most cases (Richard Wolf, Medical Instruments, Vernon Hills, IL; Apple Medical, Bolton, MA). Once placed, their portal of exit stays fixed at the level of the anterior abdominal wall parietal peritoneum, permitting room for instrument manipulation.[9] These trocar sleeves facilitate efficient instrument exchanges and evacuation of tissue while allowing unlimited freedom during extracorporeal suture tying.

TECHNIQUES

The advanced laparoscopic surgical techniques include scissors dissection, aquadissection, electrosurgery, laser, and suturing. Aquadissection and scissors dissection are used in preference to thermal energy sources.

Scissors Dissection

Blunt or round-tipped 5-mm scissors with one stable blade and one movable blade are used to divide thin and thick bowel adhesions sharply. Scissors that cut represent new laparoscopic instrumentation. Sharp dissection is the primary technique used for controlling adhesiolysis to diminish the potential for further adhesion formation. Electrosurgery and lasers are usually reserved for hemostatic dissection of adhesions where anatomic planes are not evident or vascular adherences are anticipated. Blunt-tipped sawtooth scissors (Richard Wolf Medical Instruments, Vernon Hills, IL), and curved scissors cut well without cautery. U.S. Surgical (Norwalk, CT) disposable scissors function best with a combination of cutting and electrosurgery. Hook scissors are not useful for adhesiolysis.

Scissors are the best instrument to use to cut avascular or congenital adhesions and peritoneum. Loose fibrous or areolar tissue is separated by inserting closed scissors and withdrawing them in the open position. Pushing tissue with the partially open blunt tip is used to develop natural planes.

Surgeons should select scissors that feel comfortable in their hands. To facilitate direction changes, the scissors should not be too long or encumbered by an electrical cord. This author prefers to control bleeding by making rapid exchanges between scissors and microbipolar forceps through the same portal instead of mainly using electrosurgery with the scissors.

Aquadissection

Aquadissection is the use of hydraulic energy from pressurized fluid to aid in the performance of surgical procedures.[10] The force vector is multidirectional within the volume of expansion of the noncompressible fluid; the force applied with a blunt probe is unidirectional. Instillation of fluid under pressure displaces tissue, creating cleavage planes in the least resistant spaces. Aquadissection into closed spaces behind the peritoneum or adhesions produces edematous, distended tissue on tension, with loss of elasticity, making further division easy and safe using blunt dissection, scissors dissection, laser, or electrosurgery.

Aquadissectors (suction-irrigators with the ability to dissect using pressurized fluid) should have a single channel to maximize suctioning and irrigating capacity and a solid distal tip to perform atraumatic suction-traction-retraction, irrigate directly, and develop surgical planes (aquadissection). Small holes at the tip impede these actions and spray the surgical field without purpose. The shaft should be specially treated by bead blasting to provide a dull finish to prevent CO_2 laser beam reflection, allowing it to be used as a backstop.

The Aqua-Purator (WISAP, Sauerlach, Germany, or Tomball, TX) was the first of the aquadissection devices. It delivers fluid under 200 mmHg pressure at a rate of 250 mL/10 seconds. One liter can be instilled in 35 seconds. The market is crowded with many aquadissection devices.

Electrosurgery

Monopolar electrosurgery should be avoided when working on the bowel unless the surgeon is well-versed in this modality. The expert laparoscopic surgeon can use monopolar electrosurgery safely to cut or fulgurate tissue but desiccation (coagulation) on the bowel should be performed with bipolar techniques.[11,12]

Monopolar cutting current is safe. Cutting current is used to both cut or coagulate (desiccate), depending on the portion or configuration of the electrodes in contact with the tissue. The tip cuts, whereas the wide body tamponades and coagulates. The voltage is theoretically too low at pure cutting power to arc or spark 1 mm.

Monopolar coagulation current with conventional electrodes and electrosurgical generators can arc or spark about 1 to 2 mm and is used in proximity to but not in contact with tissue to fulgurate diffuse venous and arteriolar bleeders. It takes 30% more power to spark or arc in CO_2 than in room air; thus, at the same electrosurgical power setting, less arcing occurs at laparoscopy than at laparotomy. Coagulation current is modulated so that it is on only 6% of the time and uses voltages more than 10 times that of cutting current.

Electrosurgical injury to the bowel from electrode insulation defects or capacitive coupling can occur beyond the surgeon's field of view during laparoscopic procedures. While the surgeon views the tip of the electrode, electric discharge may occur from its body (insulation failure) or from metal trocar cannulas surrounding the electrode if they are separated from the skin by plastic retention sleeves. These problems can be eliminated by using the Electroshield EM-1 monitor system (Electroscope, Boulder, CO), which consists of a reusable sheath that surrounds the laparoscopic electrode and the Electroshield EM-1 monitor to detect any insulation faults and shield against capacitance coupling.

The argon beam coagulator uses argon gas at 2 L/minute and high-voltage coagulation current to increase the amount of spark or arc that is possible with conventional fulguration while penetrating the tissue superficially. It is rarely used during adhesiolysis. Bipolar desiccation for large vessel hemostasis was first reported in 1986.[13,14] A cutting current is used to obtain a uniform bipolar desiccation process. Large blood vessels are compressed and bipolar cutting current passed until complete desiccation is achieved (i.e., the current depletes tissue fluid and electrolytes until it ceases to flow between the forceps, as determined by an ammeter or current-flow meter [end point monitor: Electroscope EPM-1, Boulder,CO]). Coagulating current is not used because it may rapidly desiccate the outer layers of the tissue, producing superficial resistance, which may prevent deeper penetration.

Finally, when discussing electrosurgery, it is important to emphasize that cautery, thermocoagulation, or endocoagulation refer to the passive transfer of heat to tissue from a hot instrument heated by electric current. The temperature rises within the tissue until the cell proteins begin to denature and coagulate, with resultant cell death. No electric current goes through the patient's body. The term "cautery," when referring to electrosurgery, should be abandoned.

Teamwork for Hemostasis

When active bleeding is encountered, the surgeon irrigates and suctions at the bleeding site until the source is identified. The suction-irrigator is replaced with bipolar forceps by rapid instrument exchange while the surgeon continues to observe the vessel (on the video screen). The surgeon removes the suction-irrigator, and the assistant immediately inserts the bipolar forceps through the trapless trocar sleeve. The surgeon—without much arm movement—releases the suction-irrigator and grasps the bipolar forceps, without taking his eyes off the bleeding vessel on the video screen. This maneuver takes practice and teamwork but it reduces remarkably the number and size of secondary sites necessary to perform the procedure. With practice, a good laparoscopic surgical team makes fast instrument exchanges, so that little pneumoperitoneum is lost. In operating rooms where this teamwork is not available or cumbersome trocar sleeves are used, it is best to tamponade the vessel after locating it, usually with the tip of the suction-irrigator, and to introduce the bipolar forceps through a third lower-quadrant cannula while using the second lower-quadrant cannula for retraction at the operative site.

Laser Dissection

Use of the CO_2 laser through the operating channel of the laser laparoscope allows the surgeon a panoramic field of vision, with the ability to cut or ablate tissue perpendicular to and in the middle of the field. In addition, a CO_2 laser, with its 0.1-mm depth of penetration and inability to traverse through water, allows the surgeon some security when working around the bowel, ureter, and major vessels. Backstops are rarely necessary because of the superficial depth of penetration of this laser, complemented by the wet surgical field. When working around the bowel, the CO_2 laser is set between 10 and 20W in superpulse or ultrapulse mode to allow tissue cooling between pulses by reducing thermal conduction.

The major problems encountered when using a CO_2 laser through the operating channel of an operating laparoscope are jumping, blooming, and loss of the beam. If the laser laparoscope coupler does not connect with the laparoscope at precisely 90°, asymmetric beam passage through the channel occurs. This beam energy heats the CO_2 purge gas unevenly, causing it to act as an asymmetric lens, refracting the CO_2 laser energy to a spot different from where the aiming helium neon (HeNe) beam was located. New laser couplers correct the problem.

The passage of CO_2 gas through the laparoscope lumen (a necessity to purge this channel of debris) results in a decrease in both power delivered to the tissue and power density at the tissue. This occurs because the 10.6-μm wavelength of the laser beam is absorbed and thus is heated by the CO_2 purge gas, which has the same wavelength. Power to tissue is reduced by 30% to 50% with a 7.2-mm laparoscopic operating channel (12-mm scope) and by 60% with a 5-mm operating channel (10-mm scope). Although it is desirable to operate at high-power density for a short time to minimize damage to surrounding tissue, heating of CO_2 gas in the laparoscope lumen results in an increase in spot size and thus a reduction in power density (the concentration of laser energy on the tissue) at higher power settings. At higher power settings with the CO_2 laser (80 to 100 W), a large spot size (3 to 4 mm) is obtained, which is extremely coagulative and provides hemostatic cutting.[15]

The Coherent 5000L laser introduces the ^{13}C isotope of CO_2 with an 11.1-μm wavelength beam to circumvent absorption of laser energy by the CO_2 purge gas in the operating channel of the laparoscope. A 6-mm beam enters the coupler from the end of the laser arm and emerges as a 1.5mm spot 350 to 400mm away. The 1.5mm spot size is maintained at all settings. At high-power settings, the power density at impact is 10 times more than at similar settings, with a 10.6-μm wavelength beam that results in a 4-mm spot from heating of CO_2 purge gas.

Heraeus LaserSonics maintains a small spot size by inducing rapid flow of gas through the operating channel of the operating laparoscope by suctioning the peritoneal cavity through the sleeve surrounding the laparoscope. The gas is exchanged faster than it can be heated, and smoke generated from the laser is evacuated as it is made.

Fiber lasers (KTP, argon, and YAG) are not used because they lack the versatility of electrosurgical electrodes for cutting, coagulation, or fulguration. The energy from these lasers is converted to heat in the tissue, due to absorption by the tissue protein matrix. A larger volume of tissue is involved in the laser thermal effect, with coagulation initially and vaporization only after protein is heated to greater than 100°C. In contrast, energy from the CO_2 laser is totally absorbed by water and rapidly converted to thermal energy, with a smaller volume of tissue involved in the laser thermal effect as cutting proceeds.

Suturing

An excellent technique for laparoscopic suturing was developed in 1970 by Clarke, using a knot pusher (Marlow Surgical, Willoughby, OH) to tie in a manner similar to the way one would hand-tie a suture at open laparotomy.[16] The surgeon applies the suture to the tissue, pulls the needle outside, and while holding both strands, makes a simple half hitch. The Clarke knot pusher is put on the suture, held firmly across the index finger, and the throw is pushed down to the tissue. A square knot is made by pushing another half hitch down to the knot to secure it while exerting tension.

Suturing with large curved needles requires a technique to put them into the peritoneal cavity without a large incision (i.e., through a 5-mm lower-quadrant incision).[17] To suture with a CT-1 needle, a trocar sleeve placed lateral to the rectus sheath is taken out of the abdomen and loaded by (1) introducing a needle holder through the sleeve to grasp the distal end of the suture, (2) pulling the suture through the trocar sleeve, (3) reinserting the instrument into the sleeve, and (4) grasping the suture about 2 to 3 cm from the needle. The needle driver is inserted into the peritoneal cavity through the original tract; the needle follows through the soft tissue and thereafter, the trocar sleeve is reinserted. Even large needles can be pulled into the peritoneal cavity in this manner. At this stage, the Semm straight-needle holder (WISAP) is replaced with a Cook oblique curved-needle driver (Cook OB/GYN, Spencer, IN) and the needle applied to tissue. Afterward, the needle is stored in the anterior abdominal wall parietal peritoneum for later removal after the suture is tied. The suture is cut, the cut end of the suture is pulled out of the peritoneal cavity through the trocar sleeve, and the knot tied with the Clarke knot pusher. To retrieve the needle, the trocar sleeve is unscrewed. The needle holder inside the trocar then pulls the needle through the soft tissue while grasping the suture remnant that is attached to it. The trocar sleeve is easily replaced, with or without another suture.

Adhesion Prevention

Peritoneal regeneration after ischemic damage or denudation occurs from mesothelial or reserve cell growth from the bottom of the defect or injured area.[18] Adhesion-prevention regimens that are more expensive than Ringer's lactate solution should be used only at the centers doing clinical research. Hulka said in 1988 that "Reich's solution to pollution is dilution"; that opinion has not changed (Hulka, personal communication, 1988). This author believes that adhesion reduction requires minimal thermal damage to tissue, absolute hemostasis, clot evacuation, copious irrigation to dilute fibrin and prostaglandins arising from operated surfaces and bacteria, and leaving 2 to 3 L of Ringer's lactate in the peritoneal cavity at the end of each operation to physically separate normal and compromised structures.

Many surgeons use intraperitoneal Ringer's lactate solution to prevent adhesions but prospective studies are rare. Rose and coworkers determined by weighing the patients that lactated Ringer's solution is absorbed over 2 to 3 days.[19] A study in 1992 found that Ringer's lactate was superior to Gore-Tex Surgical Membrane (WL Gore, Flagstaff, AZ) and Interceed (Johnson & Johnson Medical Inc., Arlington, TX) in adhesion prevention.[20]

The Gore-Tex Surgical Membrane is a nonabsorbable inert barrier of expanded polytetrafluoroethylene, with pore size less than 1-mm. It is used after division of severe adhesions by overlapping the defect by at least 1 cm and suturing in place to ensure a reasonably flat implant.

Short-interval second-look laparoscopic adhesiolysis (2 to 4 weeks) may be considered to diagnose and treat adhesions that develop immediately postoperatively. Many studies in the literature document the efficacy of second-look laparoscopy after pelvic reconstructive surgery.[21–23] Second-look laparoscopy ideally should be performed between the time of serosal healing (8 days) and established adhesion fibrosis (21 days).

Aquadissection techniques are ideal in this situation, and the aquadissector is often the only instrument needed. Adhesion interfaces are readily identifiable with laparoscopic visualization, and serosal cleavage planes are created by aquadissection. Second-look laparoscopy after extensive laparoscopic adhesiolysis should be considered, although patient acceptance of a second laparoscopic procedure after a 2- to 4-hour first case is limited.

LAPAROSCOPIC PERITONEAL CAVITY ADHESIOLYSIS

Both laparoscopic and laparotomy extensive adhesiolysis can be time-consuming and technically difficult and are best performed by an expert surgeon. Despite lengthy laparoscopic procedures (2 to 4 hours), most women are discharged on the day of the procedure. They avoid major abdominal incisions, experience minimal complications, and return to full activity within 1 week of surgery.

Classification

Extensive peritoneal cavity–adhesion procedures need a classification system. The single best indicator of the degree of severity and expertise necessary for adhesiolysis is the number of previous laparotomies. The frequency of symptoms of small bowel obstruction indicates the need for surgery.

Peritoneal adhesiolysis is classified as enterolysis, which includes omentolysis and female reproductive reconstruction (salpingo-ovariolysis and cul-de-sac dissection, with excision of deep fibrotic endometriosis). Bowel adhesions are divided into upper abdominal, lower abdominal, pelvic, and combinations. Adhesions surrounding the umbilicus are upper abdominal because they require an upper abdominal laparoscopic view for division. The extent, thickness, and vascularity of adhesions vary widely. Intricate adhesive patterns exist, with fusion to parietal peritoneum or various meshes. Adhesions cause pain by entrapment of the organ they surround. The surgical management of extensive pelvic adhesions is one of the most difficult problems facing surgeons.

Preoperative Preparation

Patients are informed preoperatively of the high risk for bowel injury during laparoscopic procedures when extensive adhesions are suspected. They are encouraged to hydrate and eat lightly for 24 hours before admission. A mechanical bowel preparation (GoLYTELY or Colyte) is administered orally the afternoon before the surgery to induce brisk self-limiting diarrhea to cleanse the bowel without disrupting the electrolyte balance.[24] The patient is usually admitted on the day of surgery. Patients are encouraged to void on call to the operating room. A Foley catheter is inserted only if the bladder is distended or a long operation is anticipated. A catheter is inserted near the end of the operation and removed in the recovery room when the patient becomes aware of its presence to prevent bladder distention. Use of prophylactic antibiotics should be considered preoperatively.

When extensive small bowel adhesions are expected, 90 cm^3 or six tablets of charcoal are administered the night before surgery. Should accidental small enterotomy occur, identification and repair are simplified by the presence of intraluminal charcoal.

Positioning of Patient

All laparoscopic surgical procedures are performed under general anesthesia, with endotracheal intubation and an orogastric tube in place. The routine use of an orogastric tube is recommended to diminish the possibility of a trocar injury to the stomach and to reduce small bowel distention. The patient's position is flat (0°) during umbilical trocar sleeve insertion and upper abdominal adhesiolysis but a steep Trendelenburg's position (20° to 30°), reverse Trendelenburg's position, and side-to-side rotation are used when necessary. Lithotomy position, with the hip extended (thigh parallel to abdomen) is obtained with Allen stirrups (Edgewater Medical Systems, Mayfield Heights, OH) or knee braces, which are adjusted to each individual patient before the patient is anesthetized.

Incisions

In most cases, a vertical midline incision on the inferior wall of the umbilical fossa, extending to and just beyond its lowest point, is used. Veress needle insufflation is continued until a pressure of 20 to 25 mmHg is obtained, usually after 4 to 6 L. It is not necessary to lift the anterior abdominal wall during trocar insertion after establishment of a 4- to 6-L pneumoperitoneum at 20 to 25 mmHg because the parietal peritoneum and skin move as one. The palmed trocar is positioned with moderate pressure in the incision to the peritoneum at a 90° angle and upturned to about 30° in one continuous thrusting motion, with the wrist rotating nearly 90°. The result is a parietal peritoneal puncture directly beneath the umbilicus. The high-pressure setting used during initial insertion of the trocar is lowered thereafter to diminish the development of vena caval compression and subcutaneous emphysema. A relatively constant intra-abdominal pressure between 10 and 15 mmHg is maintained during long laparoscopic procedures.

Special entry techniques are necessary for patients who have undergone multiple laparotomies, have lower abdominal incisions traversing the umbilicus, or who have extensive adhesions, either determined clinically or noted in another physician's operative record. Open laparoscopy or microlaparotomy both carry the same risk

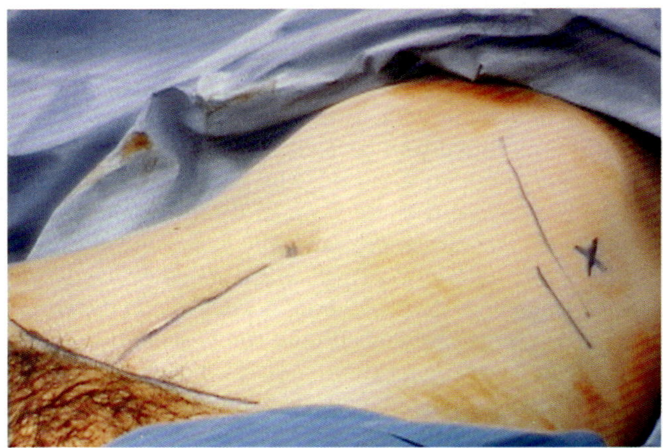

FIGURE 24-1. Draped anterior abdominal wall, with pubis in lower left corner. Previous lower abdominal midline and transverse incisions are marked. Veress needle insertion site in the left ninth intercostal space, anterior axillary line, is denoted by an X. The costochondral junction is marked below it (i.e., the tenth rib).

for bowel laceration if the bowel is fused to the umbilical undersurface.

If CO_2 insufflation is not obtainable through the umbilicus, a Veress needle puncture is performed in the left ninth intercostal space, anterior axillary line (Figs. 24-1 through 24-5). Adhesions are rare in this area and the peritoneum is tethered to the undersurface of the ribs, making subcutaneous insufflation unusual. The Veress needle tip is then inserted at a right angle to the skin but at a 45° angle to the horizontal anterior abdominal wall between the ninth and tenth ribs. A single pop is felt on penetration of the peritoneum. Pneumoperitoneum to a pressure of 20 to 25 mmHg is obtained. A 5- or 10-mm trocar is then inserted at the left costal margin in the

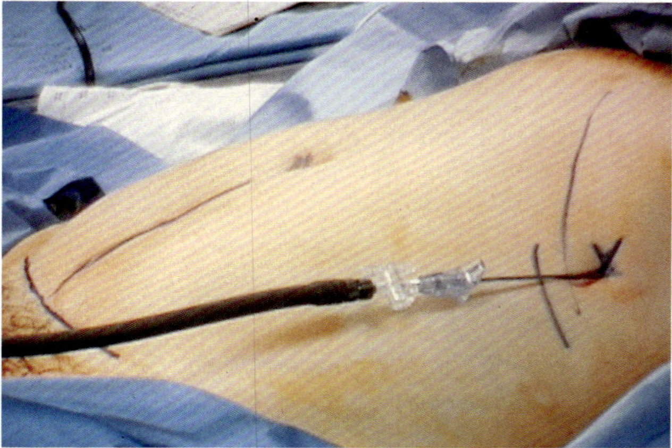

FIGURE 24-2. Surgineedle (U.S. Surgical) has been inserted into ninth intercostal space. Establishment of pneumoperitoneum pulls the needle tip upward as the anterior abdominal wall expands.

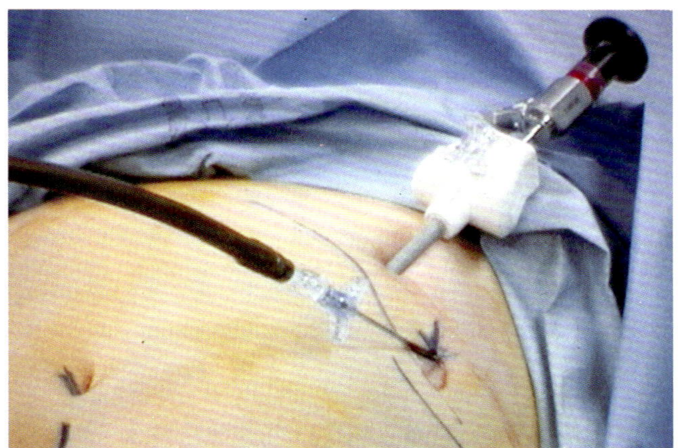

FIGURE 24-3. A 5-mm trocar with laparoscope is inserted just below the costochondral margin in the left mid-clavicular line.

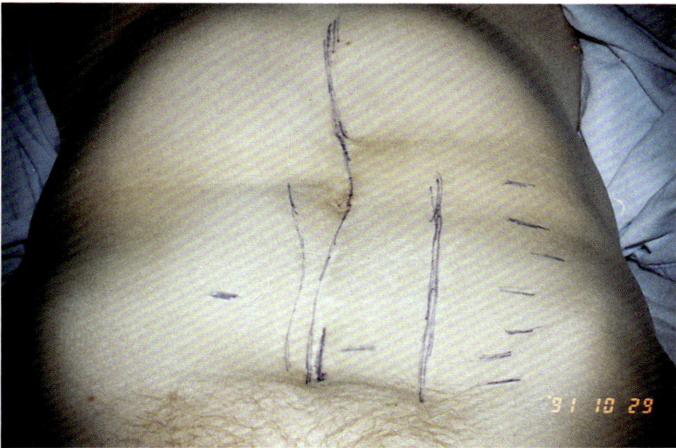

FIGURE 24-5. Anterior abdominal wall, with sites of previous surgery marked. Patient had undergone over 10 laparotomies.

mid-clavicular line, giving the surgeon a panoramic view of the entire peritoneal cavity.

When extensive adhesions are encountered surrounding the umbilical puncture, the surgeon should immediately seek a higher site. Thereafter, the adhesions can be freed down to and just beneath the umbilicus, where an umbilical portal can be established safely for further work.

Other laparoscopic puncture sites are placed as needed, usually lateral to the rectus abdominis muscles and always under direct laparoscopic vision. When the anterior abdominal wall parietal peritoneum is thickened from previous surgery or obesity, the position of these muscles is judged by palpating and depressing the anterior abdominal wall with the back of the scalpel; the wall appears thicker where the rectus muscle is enclosed, and the incision site is made lateral to this area near the anterior superior iliac spine.

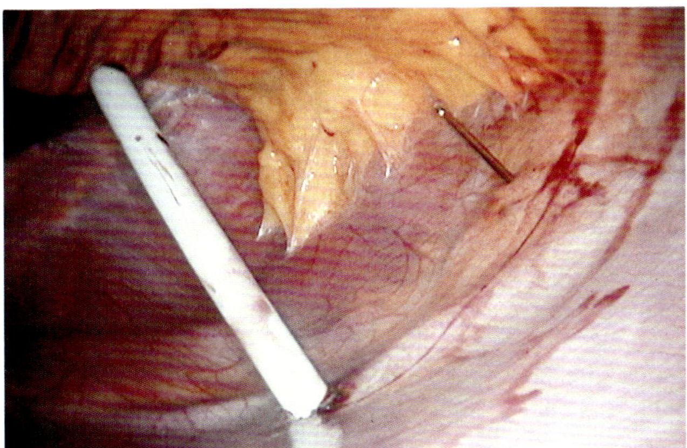

FIGURE 24-4. Laparoscopic view of upper abdominal trocar sleeve and Surgineedle after undersurface of umbilicus was freed of adhesions and umbilical site established.

If an umbilical insertion is possible and extensive adhesions are present close to but below the umbilicus, the operating laparoscope with scissors in the operating channel is the first instrument used. If a left upper quadrant incision is necessary, there is usually room for another puncture site to perform initial adhesiolysis with scissors.

Surgical Plan for Extensive Enterolysis

A well-defined strategy is important for small bowel enterolysis. For simplification, this is divided into three parts:

1. Division of all adhesions to the anterior abdominal wall parietal peritoneum. Small bowel loops encountered during this process are separated, using their anterior attachments for countertraction instead of waiting until the last portion of the procedure (running of the bowel).
2. Division of all small bowel and omental adhesions in the pelvis. The rectosigmoid, cecum, and appendix often require some separation during this part of the procedure.
3. Running of the bowel. With use of atraumatic grasping forceps and usually a suction-irrigator for suction traction, the bowel is run. Starting at the cecum and terminal ileum, loops and significant kinks are freed up to the ligament of Treitz in the high upper abdomen.

General Adhesiolysis, Including Enterolysis

Adhesions that are encountered initially involve the anterior abdominal wall parietal peritoneum. These consist

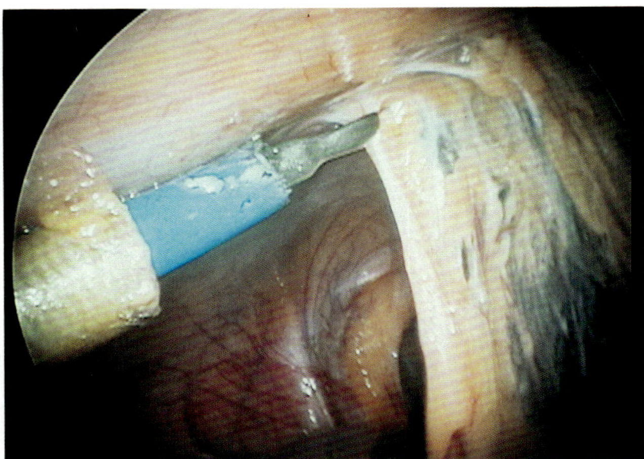

FIGURE 24-6. Spoon electrode, used to divide vascular omental adhesions (100-120 W cutting current results in cutting with coagulation). These adhesions must be taken down to beneath the level of the umbilicus before dividing pelvic adhesions. Photograph is taken through a 5-mm laparoscope inserted at the left costochondral margin in the mid-clavicular line.

of omentum and small bowel attachments, with varying degrees of fibrosis and vascularity. Small bowel adhesions to the anterior abdominal wall are released. If these adhesions extend from above the level of the umbilicus, another incision is made above the level of the highest adhesion, and the laparoscope is inserted there. Adhesions are easier to divide when working from above them than from below because an acute angle usually exists between the omentum or bowel and the parietal peritoneum, allowing gravity to help delineate the plane of separation.

Adhesions are taken down with scissors, electrosurgery, or CO_2 laser. In most cases, the initial adhesiolysis is performed with scissors. If the adhesions are close to the trocar insertion, using CO_2 laser through the laparoscope results in reflection, with loss of precision. Electrosurgery (cutting current) through a knife, spatula, or scissors electrode is used only when the surgeon is certain that the small bowel is not involved in the adhesion (Figs. 24-6 through 24-10).

Initially, blunt-tipped or hooked scissors in the operating channel of an operating laparoscope are inserted into the interface between the anterior abdominal wall parietal peritoneum and the omentum. Rotating the laparoscope so that the scissors exit at 12 o'clock instead of 3 o'clock facilitates early adhesiolysis. First, blunt dissection is performed by inserting the scissors at the interface, spreading, and withdrawing them. This maneuver is repeated many times to delineate the thin avascular adhesions from thicker vascular fibrotic attachments, which are individually coagulated and divided. Frequently, adhesions can be bluntly divided by grasping the adhesion in the partially closed scissors and pushing.

After initial adhesiolysis, more space is created to allow better access and exposure for further adhesiolysis. Safe entry sites for secondary trocars become visible (Figs. 24-11 through 24-13). After their insertion, an electrosurgical spoon or knife electrode is used to divide the remaining omental adhesions. If the small bowel is involved or intermingled with the omental adhesions, dissection proceeds with scissors through the second puncture site, aided by traction on the small bowel from an opposite placed puncture site (Figs. 24-14 through 24-25). Rarely is a CO_2 laser used through the operating channel of the operating laparoscope. When using a CO_2 laser, the adhesive interface is distended with fluid by aquadissection before vaporizing individual adhesive layers (Fig. 24-26). Aquadissection of adhesions may be nec-

(text continues on page 236)

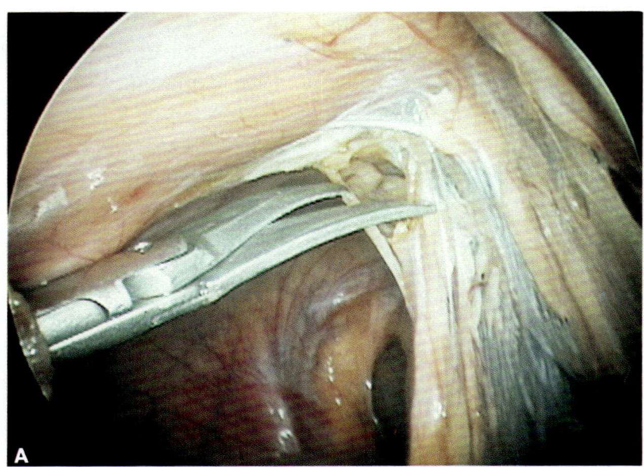

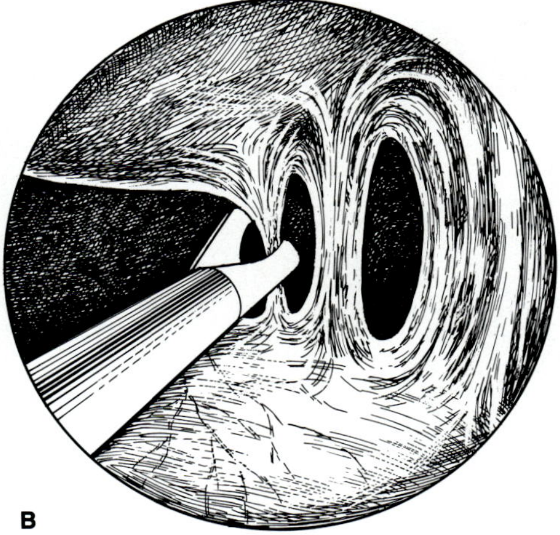

FIGURE 24-7. (**A**) Avascular adhesions are divided with scissors without electrosurgical attachment. (**B**) Schematic of scissors being used for adhesiolysis.

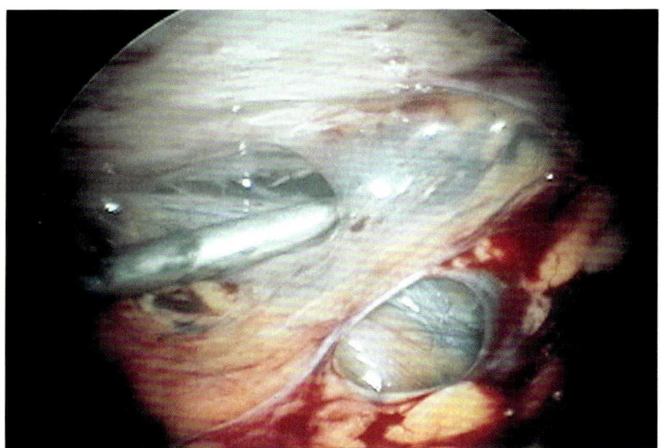

FIGURE 24-8. Suction irrigator is inserted to instill fluid, which distends the adhesions, making their interface with the parietal peritoneum easier to identify.

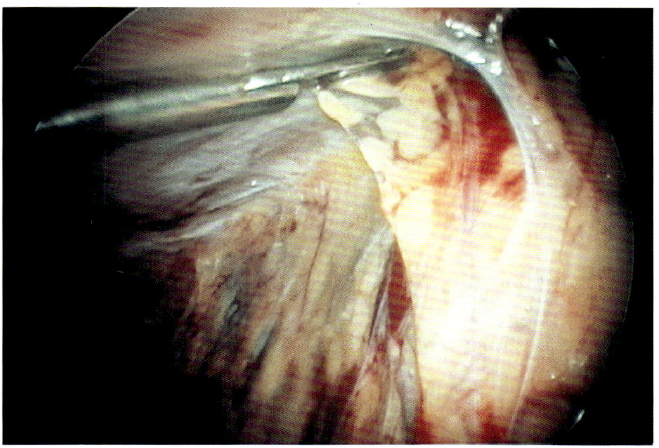

FIGURE 24-9. Scissors dissection of adhesions continues.

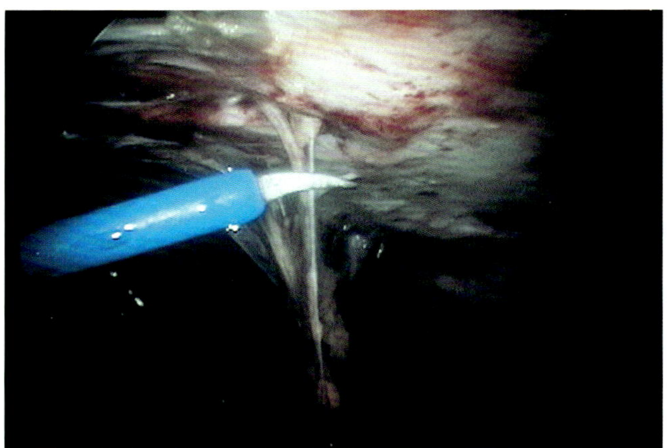

FIGURE 24-10. Some adhesions are divided with a curved knife electrode at a setting of 60 W cutting current.

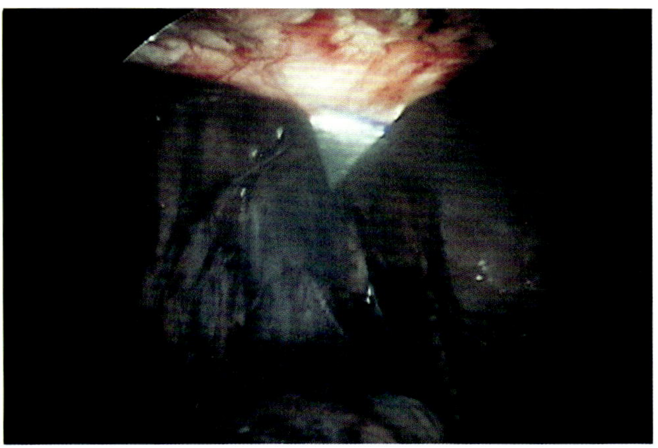

FIGURE 24-11. When umbilical area is freed of all adhesions, an umbilical trocar is inserted so that further visualization can be through a 10-mm 0° laparoscope. This provides the surgeon with a closer view of the pelvic adhesions for further adhesiolysis.

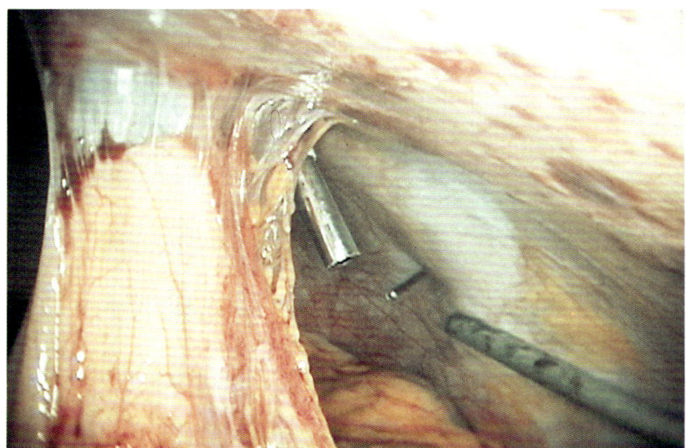

FIGURE 24-12. View of upper abdomen with small bowel loop adhesion. Note Veress needle through ninth intercostal space anterior axillary line and also position of 5-mm laparoscope inserted just beneath the costochondral margin in the mid-clavicular line.

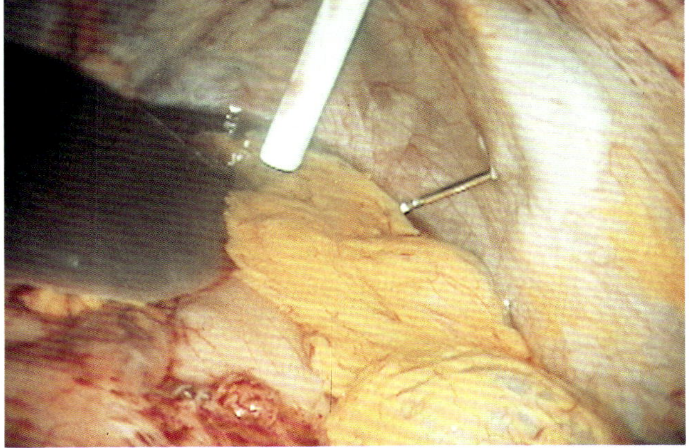

FIGURE 24-13. All upper abdomen bowel adhesions have been divided and a clear view obtained of upper abdominal Veress needle and 5-mm trocar sleeve.

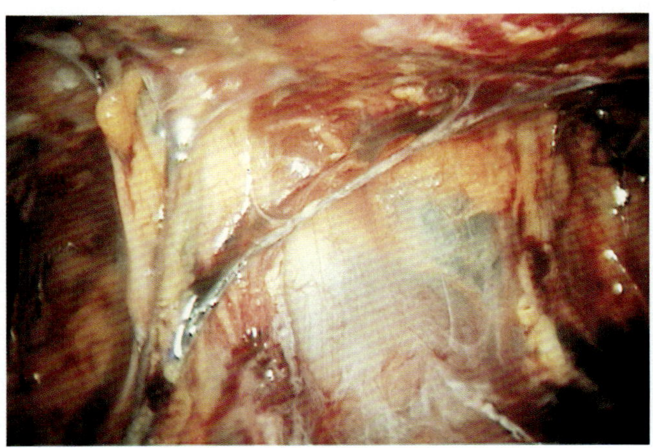

FIGURE 24-14. View of lower abdominal omental and small bowel adhesions.

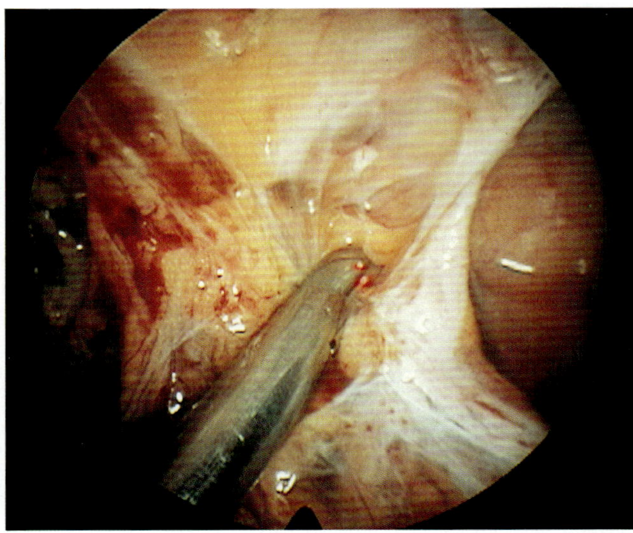

FIGURE 24-15. Carbon dioxide (CO_2) laser HeNe beam can be seen in center of visual field, near tip of aquadissector, which is being used to suction and to retract omental and small bowel adhesions.

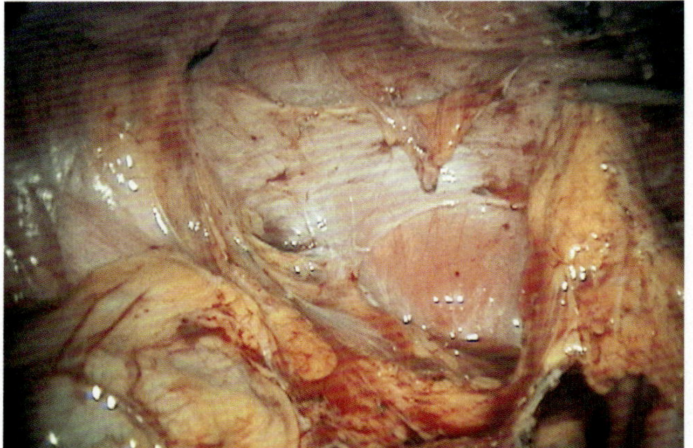

FIGURE 24-16. Finally, all anterior abdominal wall parietal peritoneum adhesions are freed. Note the small triangular flaps of anterior abdominal wall parietal peritoneum that has been created during the dissection. The rectosigmoid has been partially mobilized from the left pelvic sidewall.

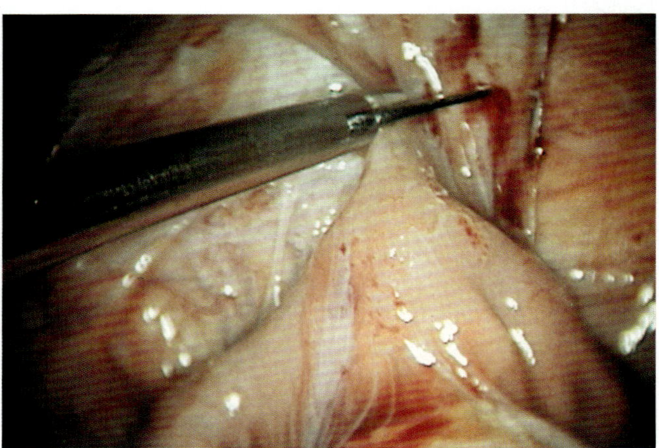

FIGURE 24-17. Scissors are used to divide small bowel adhesions. Note transillumination of the fixed blade of the scissors is transilluminated before the adhesion was divided.

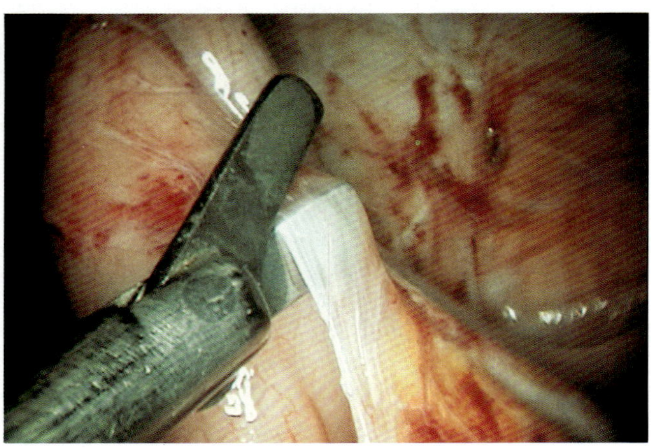

FIGURE 24-18. Scissors division of bowel adhesions after transillumination.

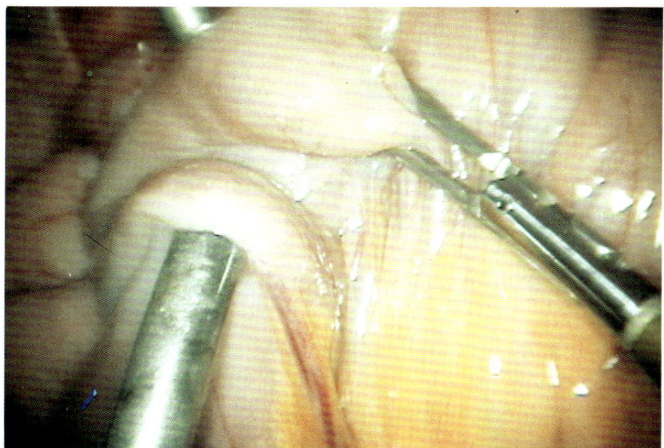

FIGURE 24-19. Running the bowel. Bowel traction demonstrated, using atraumatic Babcock clamp and suction-traction from the aquadissector with solid distal tip.

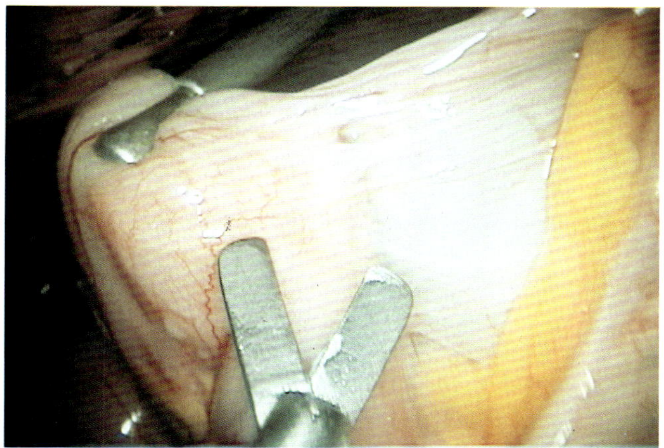

FIGURE 24-20. Again, traction helps delineate adhesions before scissors division.

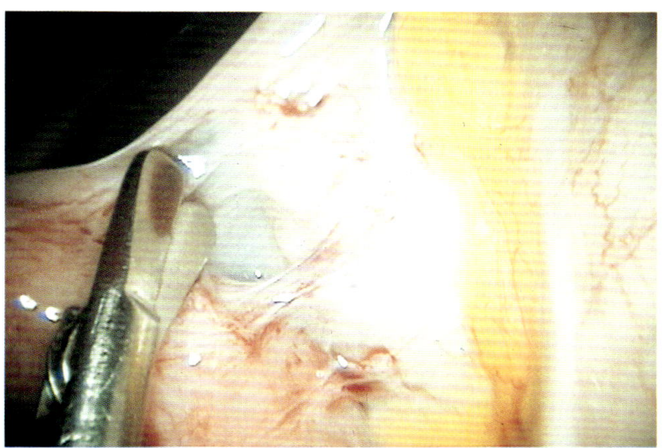

FIGURE 24-21. Careful scissors division continues.

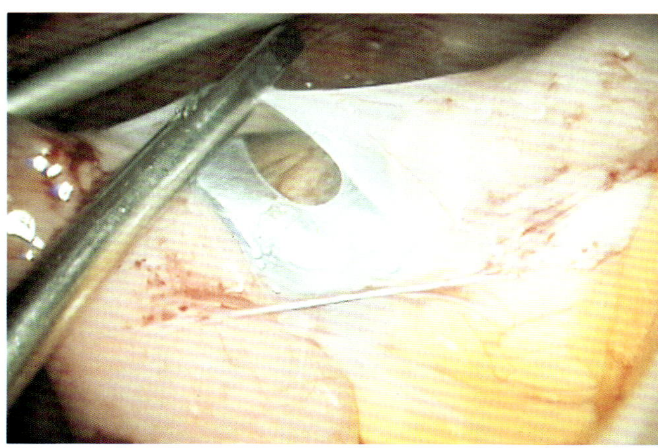

FIGURE 24-22. Scissors division.

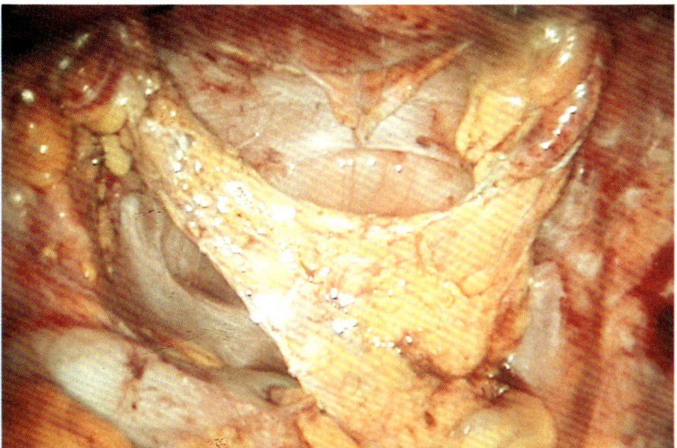

FIGURE 24-23. Large redundant omentum free near end of procedure.

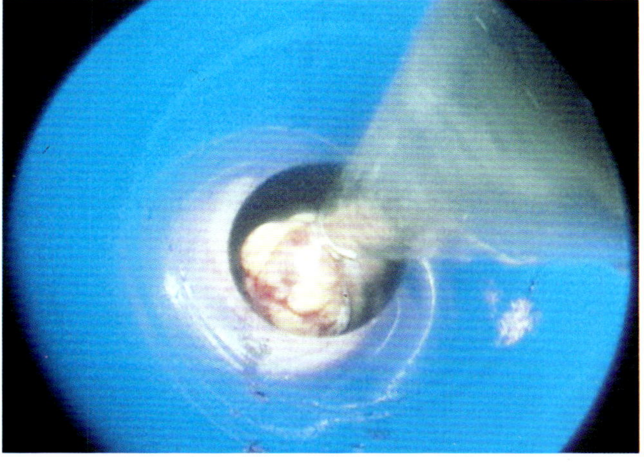

FIGURE 24-24. Omentum is pulled into umbilicus after partial omentectomy by placing Endoloop around its base.

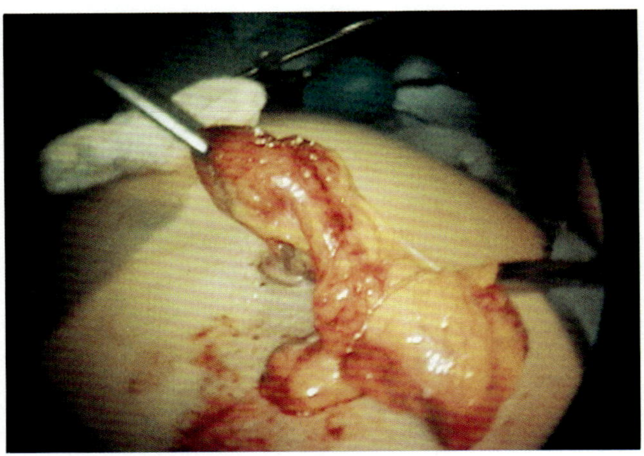

FIGURE 24-25. Omentum is pulled out through umbilicus.

essary because it is often impossible to identify small bowel serosa enmeshed in the adhesions. After freeing small bowel segments, denuded areas of bowel muscularis may be closed with a transversely placed seromuscular suture of 3-0 polyglactin 910 (Vicryl, Ethicon Endo-Surgery, Cincinnati, OH) on an ST needle. With perseverance, essentially all anterior abdominal wall parietal peritoneum adhesions can be released.

It is best to control even slight bleeding immediately. A possible advantage of the laparoscopic route is the necessity for meticulous hemostasis as the procedure continues because bleeding can hinder the next step. Sources of bleeding are more difficult to locate at the end of the procedure. If a vessel is injured, the laparoscope is retracted, so that the pumping blood does not obstruct visualization during bipolar desiccation of the vessel. The suction-irrigator is used to clean the laparoscopic lens, which is then wiped on the serosa (e.g., bowel) before continuing.

Postoperative Care

Same-day discharge is common, even after long procedures. Physical motility of the bowel is encouraged by early ambulation and ingestion of a clear liquid diet for 2 to 4 days. Patients are instructed to return gradually to their normal activity during the week after surgery.

Partial small bowel obstruction during the week after surgery is usually due to ileus and is treated by intravenous hydration and the insertion of a nasogastric tube if vomiting is present. In general, surgical exploration should be avoided in these cases.

If peritonitis occurs in the first few days after the operation, it must be assumed that an injury to the bowel has gone unnoticed, and a laparotomy is indicated. If an abscess forms postoperatively, it can be drained percutaneously under sonographic guidance or possibly by means of laparoscopy. Recurrent adhesions may occur, even with atraumatic techniques.

CLINICAL EXPERIENCE

Between 1984 and 1992, a total of 364 laparoscopic enterolysis procedures were performed; 236 were extensive. Concomitant pathology included severe endometriosis (94) and pelvic abscess (10). One of the 364 was male; he had pelvic lymphadenectomy for staging of recurrent prostate cancer. Left ninth intercostal space entry was first used in 1991; since then, it has been utilized in more than 50 cases, without complications.

In this high-risk group, there were 11 small bowel perforations.[24] Management approach was laparotomy (four patients) and laparoscopy (seven patients). In all 11 instances of bowel perforation, each woman had a significant laparotomy history (average, four; range, two

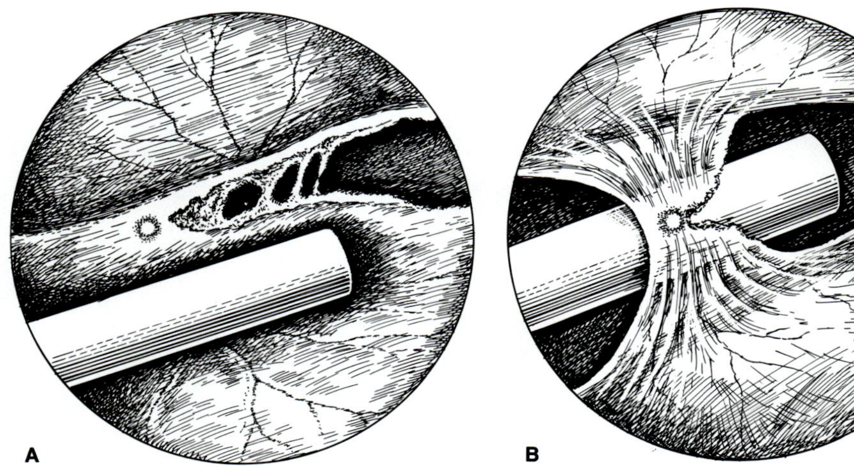

FIGURE 24-26. (**A**) Laserlysis of adhesions, with use of suction-irrigator, depressing tissue. (**B**) Laserlysis of adhesions using an irrigator as a backstop.

to nine). Eight had a history of bowel surgery. No large bowel perforations occurred during adhesiolysis.

CONCLUSION

No longer can the surgeon ignore the benefits of minimally invasive surgery for adhesiolysis. Although these techniques and procedures are not without risk, patients should not be denied their inherent advantages. Astute clinicians must work together to discern the most appropriate use(s) for this therapy.

References

1. Peters AA, Trimbos-Kemper GC, Admiraal C, Trimbos JB, Hermans J: A randomized clinical trial on the benefit of adhesiolysis in patients with intraperitoneal adhesions and chronic pelvic pain. Br J Obstet Gynaecol 1992;99:59.
2. Postoperative adhesion development after operative laparoscopy: evaluation at early second-look procedures. Operative laparoscopy study group. Fertil Steril 1991; 55:700.
3. Luciano AA, Maier DB, Koch EI, Nulsen JC, Whitman GF: A comparative study of postoperative adhesions following laser surgery by laparoscopy versus laparotomy in the rabbit model. Obstet Gynecol 1989;74:220.
4. Reich H, McGlynn F, Salvat J: Laparoscopic treatment of cul-de-sac obliteration secondary to retrocervical deep fibrotic endometriosis. J Reprod Med 1991;36:516.
5. Reich H: Laparoscopic treatment of extensive pelvic adhesions, including hydrosalpinx. J Reprod Med 1987;32:736.
6. Reich H, McGlynn F: Laparoscopic treatment of tubo-ovarian and pelvic abscess. J Reprod Med 1987;32:747.
7. Henry-Suchet J, Soler A, Loffredo V: Laparoscopic treatment of tuboovarian abscesses. J Reprod Med 1984;29:579.
8. Reich H: Endoscopic management of tuboovarian abscess and pelvic inflammatory disease. In: Sanfilippo JS, Levine RL, eds. Operative gynecologic endoscopy. New York: Springer-Verlag, 1989:118.
9. Reich H, McGlynn F: Short self-retaining trocar sleeves for laparoscopic surgery. Am J Obstet Gynecol 1990;162:453.
10. Reich H: Aquadissection. In: Baggish M, ed. Laser endoscopy, the clinical practice of gynecology series. Vol 2. New York: Elsevier, 1990:159.
11. Odell R: Principles of electrosurgery. In: Sivak M, ed. Gastroenterologic endoscopy. New York: WB Saunders, 1987:128.
12. Reich H, Vancaillie T, Soderstrom R: Electrical techniques. Operative laparoscopy. In: Martin DC, Holtz GL, Levinson CJ, Soderstrom RM, eds. Manual of endoscopy. Santa Fe Springs: American Association of Gynecologic Laparoscopists, 1990:105.
13. Reich H, McGlynn F: Laparoscopic oophorectomy and salpingo-oophorectomy in the treatment of benign tubo-ovarian disease. J Reprod Med 1986;31:609. Abstract.
14. Reich H: Laparoscopic oophorectomy and salpingo-oophorectomy in the treatment of benign tubo-ovarian disease. Int J Fertil 1987;32:233.
15. Reich H, MacGregor TS, Vancaillie TG: CO_2 laser used through the operating channel of laser laparoscopes: in vitro study of power and power density losses. Obstet Gynecol 1991;77:40.
16. Clarke HC: Laparoscopy—new instruments for suturing and ligation. Fertil Steril 1972;23:274.
17. Reich H, Clarke HC, Sekel L: A simple method for ligating with straight and curved needles in operative laparoscopy. Obstet Gynecol 1992;79:143.
18. Robbins GF, Brunschwig A, Foote FW Jr: Deperitonealization: clinical and experimental observations. Ann Surg 1949;130:466.
19. Rose BI, MacNeill C, Larrain R, Kopreski MM: Abdominal instillation of high-molecular-weight dextran or lactated Ringer's solution after laparoscopic surgery. A randomized comparison of the effect on weight change. J Reprod Med 1991;36:537.
20. Pagidas K, Tulandi T: Effects of Ringer's lactate, Interceed (TC7) and Gore-Tex Surgical Membrane on postsurgical adhesion formation. Fertil Steril 1992;57:199.
21. Jansen RP: Early laparoscopy after pelvic operations to prevent adhesions: safety and efficacy. Fertil Steril 1988; 49:26.
22. Diamond E: Lysis of postoperative pelvic adhesions in infertility. Fertil Steril 1979;31:287.
23. McLaughlin DS: Evaluation of adhesion reformation by early second-look laparoscopy following microlaser ovarian wedge resection. Fertil Steril 1984;42:531.
24. Reich H: Laparoscopic bowel injury. Surg Laparosc Endosc 1992;2:74.

Chapter 25

Laparoscopic Surgery: An Atlas for General Surgeons, edited by Gary C. Vitale, Joseph S. Sanfilippo, and Jacques Perissat. J. B. Lippincott Company, Philadelphia, © 1995.

Laparoscopic Pelvic Lymphadenectomy

Thierry G. Vancaillie

In the ongoing attempt to improve the rate of survival of patients undergoing surgery for malignancy of the lower urogenital tract, the emphasis has shifted. Originally, it was believed that the more radical the surgery and the more extensive the pelvic lymphadenectomy, the better the outcome would be. This belief persisted for several decades, yielding crippling and morbid procedures due to efforts to remove all affected tissue.[1,2] Surgeons and radiotherapists both claimed to have developed the best approach to the treatment of malignancy of the lower genitourinary tract in both men and women. Neither approach has demonstrated any clear advantage, however, apart from differences in distribution of recurrent disease.

Among the various approaches, it is clear that survival depends on the extent and aggressiveness (grade) of the tumor at the time of diagnosis. As a result, the emphasis on early detection of malignancy has increased through education of the public and through screening methods, such as the cervical Papanicolaou smear and transrectal ultrasound examination of the prostate. Pelvic lymphadenectomy is still important in the staging of malignancy of the lower urogenital tract, however. In 1980, Grossman and coworkers reported on the prognostic importance of even a single microscopic focus of lymphatic spread.[3] Lymphadenectomy by laparotomy, however, produces significant morbidity—sometimes even death. The early postoperative complication rate for lymphadenectomy alone varies from 12% to 24% in patients with prostatic cancer (Table 25-1).[4–8] Not unexpectedly, this complication rate rises slightly (17% to 33%) when combined with radical prostatectomy.

Can one justify using a procedure that is noncurative, given the rate of complications? Arguments can be made for either side. To devise a therapeutic approach, encompassing the full array of brachytherapy, teletherapy, surgery, hormone therapy, and cytostatic therapy, the information gained from pelvic lymphadenectomy can prove extremely valuable. Nonetheless, it remains a staging operation, which may require a hospital stay of 6.8 days (average), with the possible need for blood transfusion and the risk of thromboembolic accidents, wound infections, or lymphocele.[8] It is a small wonder that there is a constant and consistent search for alternative methods to detect lymphatic spread of malignant cells.

The least invasive line of investigation involves the various imaging methods—computerized tomography, magnetic resonance imaging, and lymphography. As performed, all of these methods are unsatisfactory because none allow visualization of microscopic invasion of the lymph nodes. As screening methods become more extensive and the opportunity for diagnosis at early stages increases, the detection of microscopic lymphatic disease becomes vital.

More invasive imaging procedures, such as guided-needle aspiration for cytology, yield information that is more valuable because of the tissue sample obtained. The morbidity of guided-needle aspiration is extremely low; however, it is estimated that the false-negative index may be 5% to 15%.[9] This makes a negative result relatively worthless.

A third approach, pelvioscopy, was developed in Denmark in the 1970s and consisted of lymphadenectomy by insertion of a mediastinoscope through a small incision medial to the iliac crest.[10,11] This procedure imitates the retroperitoneal open procedure but avoids the large incision and incurs fewer complications than does the standard lymphadenectomy. Hald and Rasmussen reported a series of 12 patients with prostate or bladder cancer, in which this technique was used.[10] The main advantage was the short duration of the operation (average, 20 minutes). The authors investigated only one pel-

TABLE 25-1
Early Postoperative Complication Rates of Surgical Interventions in Patients with Prostatic Cancer

	Lymphadenectomy	Lymphadenectomy Plus Prostatectomy
Study	N(%)	N(%)
Lieskovsky, et al[4]	2/17(12)	13/65(20)
McCullough, et al[5]	6/30(20)	9/30(30)
McLaughlin, et al[6]	7/30(23)	10/30(33)
Nicholson, et al[7]	—	8/47(17)
Ray, et al[8*]	12/50(24)	—

* *Transperitoneal approach.*

vic sidewall, however. The chief disadvantage of pelvioscopy is that it is based on sampling palpable lymph nodes. In the study above, no nodal tissue was obtained in four of 12 patients. In France, Salvat and Dargent* developed a modification of this technique for use in women with cervical malignancy. They make a single incision in the midline, suprapubically, to gain access to both pelvic sidewalls. Because of the midline incision, accessibility to the proximal part of the iliac vessel is limited. The advantages of the procedure include a short operating time and the avoidance of general anesthesia. It is not a complete resection, however, but only a sampling technique.

In 1985, Fuerst reported an animal experiment in which a dye, isosulfan blue, was injected interstitially to "mark" the lymph nodes.[12] The dye, through lymphatic absorption, marked the nodes of fatty tissue and enabled directed biopsy. Unfortunately, further data have been published on this technique.

Another procedure, laparoscopic pelvic lymphadenectomy, was developed to retain the advantages of pelvioscopy, avoid the morbidity and complications of classic lymphadenectomy by laparotomy, yet attain the same objective as classic surgery—the excision of complete chains of lymph nodes. Querleu** in France was the first to use this procedure in systematic fashion for use in women with cervical malignancy.

There is little difference between the technique of lymphadenectomy in men and in women. In the United States, there is less interest in it among gynecologic oncologists because the standard treatment for cervical malignancy in its earliest stages is abdominal hysterectomy combined with lymphadenectomy. In Europe, where there is more experience with vaginal surgery for cervical malignancy, surgeons are more interested in performing laparoscopic pelvic lymphadenectomy before vaginal hysterectomy or radiation (whichever is appropriate). The benefit for the patient is lower postoperative morbidity.

PROCEDURE

Although laparoscopic lymphadenectomy is an endosurgical procedure, it should not be considered minor surgery. General surgeons and urologists have historically little training in laparoscopy, in contrast to gynecologists, for whom it is likely to be the first procedure performed as an intern. A positive aspect of this lack of experience, however, is that general surgeons and urologists may have little prejudice regarding the difficulty of laparoscopy.

The practice of endosurgery is complex; it relies heavily on highly developed technologic advances that dramatically enhance the surgeon's skills. Because no single individual can be responsible for all the essential variables—light intensity, carbon dioxide (CO_2) absorption, water pressure, and laser safety, to name only a few—it is essential that such surgery be undertaken by a well-coordinated team. This team consists of a circulating nurse, a surgical technician, a surgeon, an assistant, an anesthesiologist, a radiologist, and a pathologist—the last because the goal of the entire procedure is to provide a specimen for the pathologist to examine. The importance of a team approach cannot be overemphasized.

Anesthesia

It is not the purpose of this chapter to discuss anesthesia in depth, but certain aspects relevant to particular types of surgery warrant discussion. Specific to laparoscopy is the use of CO_2, of which large volumes are used. There must be constant monitoring of both pulmonary and vascular CO_2 partial pressures and of the patient's temperature. To avoid interference of respiratory movements with the surgery, a low tidal volume is required. Hyper-

**Free communication presented at the American Association of Gynecologic Laparoscopists, Baltimore, MD, August 11–13, 1988.*

***Free communication presented at 13th Annual Workshop on Reconstructive Pelvic Surgery in Gynecology, Leuven, Belgium, August 31-September 2, 1989.*

ventilation is therefore routinely used with this type of operative laparoscopy.

Certain factors, such as changes in the patient's position to achieve optimal access and the increased intra-abdominal pressures resulting from insufflation, interfere with venous return and diastolic filling pressures. The anesthesiologist is better able to respond to hemodynamic variations by close surveillance of the patient's heart by liberal use of arterial and central venous lines.

Instrumentation

The instruments used in laparoscopy are highly specialized and compared with the instruments used for open surgery are extremely delicate. Because they are elongated and have tiny joints, they are more easily damaged than instruments used in conventional surgery. For these reasons and because the technique totally depends on optimal instrumentation, special care must be taken to ensure that damage to instruments is minimal. Our surgical team finds that assigning one member of the team to care for the instruments greatly reduces damage and frustration. This person often spots malfunctioning equipment and replaces it before it breaks down and he or she often assists during surgery.

Circulating Nurse

Anyone who studies the amount and complexity of the equipment used in laparoscopy understands the need for a plan relative to the organization of the hardware. In addition to the many switches, dials, and regulators that must remain accessible and within reach, there are floor pedals, hoses, electric lines, and cables that must be kept from underfoot. Truly, the operating room for laparoscopy is proof of the adage "a place for everything and everything in its place." The setup in our operating suite is depicted in Figure 25-1. The circulating nurse must know how to connect the various cables and hoses before the procedure is started. Every person in the room should understand the function of each piece of equipment and how it is set up.

Positioning the Patient

Because of the nature of endoscopic surgery, physical and technical restrictions on the number and movement of ancillary instruments abound. Specifically, the operative field must be presented to the surgeon in a fashion that limits extreme lateral movement. To compensate for the restrictions of the technique, proper initial positioning of the patient and constant adjustment of that position are absolutely essential. The operating table can be adjusted to include the Trendelenburg's, reverse Trendelenburg's, and lateral tilt positions. The ideal position for the patient undergoing endoscopic pelvic lymphadenectomy is dorsal recumbent, with elevation of the pelvis. A roll of towels placed beneath the patient's buttocks before scrubbing with an antibacterial agent produces the necessary pelvic forward tilt. To permit maximal mobility for the surgeon and assistants, it is important that the patient's arms be aligned along his or her trunk. The anesthesiologist must become accustomed to the use of long intravenous lines that once established are hidden under the drapes for the rest of the procedure. The ideal position for lymphadenectomy of the right obturator chain is a 10° Trendelenburg's with a 30° left lateral tilt. The surgeon standing to the left of the patient has the most direct approach to the right obturator fossa. The patient must be secured to the operating table with re-

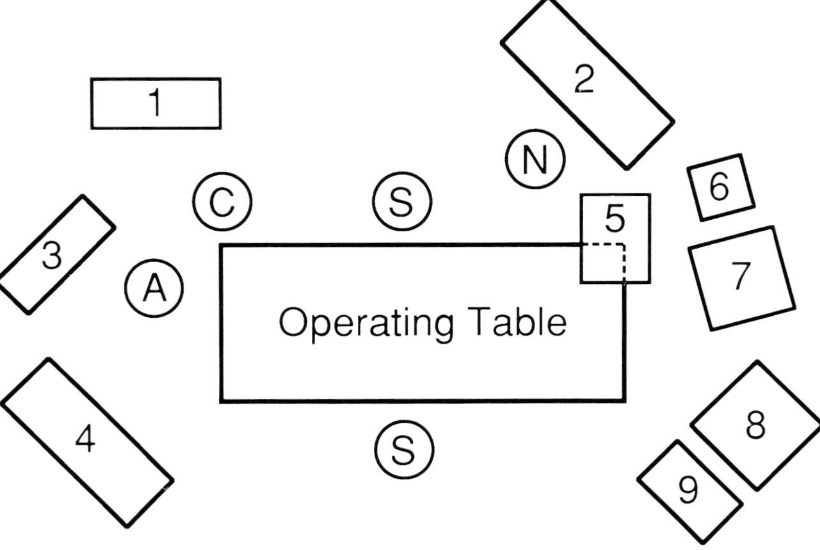

FIGURE 25-1. Laparoscopy operating suite. *1,* Operating table, with the instruments for emergency laparotomy; *2,* operating table with the laparoscopy instruments; *3,* anesthesia cart; *4,* anesthesia machine; *5,* Mayo stand, with most frequently used laparoscopic instruments; *6,* equipment to preheat endoscopes; *7,* hardware cart with TV monitor; *8,* hardware cart with TV monitor; *9,* laser; *A,* Anesthesiologist; *C,* Camera holder/assistant; *N,* Surgical technician; *S,* Surgeons.

straining straps at the level of the shoulders and upper thigh.

Preparing the Patient

Because introducing the Veress needle and positioning the first-puncture trocar are both "blind" procedures, the risk of complications such as bowel perforation exists. A gastric tube should be placed routinely to reduce the risk of inadvertent intragastric insufflation. Visualization is improved if the patient's stomach is empty because this reduces the volume of the abdominal contents.

The use of a mechanical bowel prep (e.g., GoLYTELY or magnesium sulfate, and Reglan) and air instead of nitrous oxide (N_2O) for anesthesia also improves visualization. Nitrous oxide accumulates in the bowel lumen, resulting in reduced intra-abdominal operating volume. Intraluminal gas can be reduced by having the patient abstain from dairy products for 2 days before surgery. These seemingly insignificant details can result in greatly improved access and visualization of the operating field—a factor that is far from insignificant.

Incisions

Insufflation is accomplished with a Veress needle introduced through an incision inside the umbilicus, not beneath it. In patients who have had a previous operation, with a resultant midline scar, insufflation must be performed away from the scar, along the mamillary line, either left (preferably) or right, depending on the location of the scar. Insufflation is continued until the intra-abdominal pressure reaches about 15 mmHg. The amount of gas needed to reach this pressure varies from 2.5 to 7.0 L. Pressures higher than 15 mmHg cause excessive compression of the large veins, interfering with the hemodynamic homeostasis of the patient. The best indicator that the Veress needle is well positioned is a lack of resistance to insufflation. The main trocar (i.e., first-puncture trocar or trocar for telescope) is inserted through the umbilicus at the same site where the Veress needle was introduced. Under certain circumstances (e.g., umbilical hernia, plastic surgery, scar), the trocar may be inserted elsewhere. It is wise, however, to insert the trocar close to the umbilicus to visualize the two pelvic sidewalls properly.

Second-puncture trocars are introduced halfway between the umbilicus and pubis or iliac spine along a semicircular line (Fig. 25-2). The operator should be alert to the possibility of injuring the epigastric vessels and can avoid this complication by visualizing them directly through the laparoscope. Three or four ancillary trocars are required to perform the surgery. There are several combinations possible. The distance between trocars must be as far as possible to allow optimal use of the ancillary instruments. In slender patients, it may be

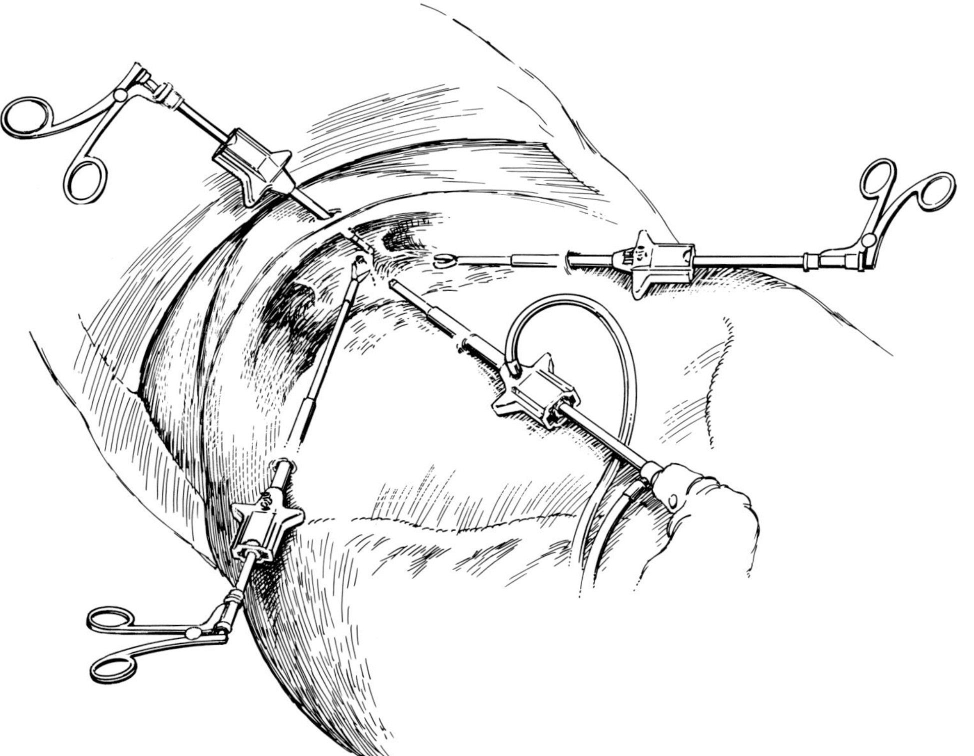

FIGURE 25-2. Placement of trocars for laparoscopic lymphadenectomy: umbilicus, suprapubic, left lateral, and right lateral. Alternatively, the surgeon may choose to place two lateral trocars on each side.

difficult to use four trocars. When three trocars are used, one is inserted in the midline and the others are inserted lateral from the epigastric vessels, at the level of the anterior superior iliac spine. The sizes are 10 mm for the midline trocar and 5 mm for the lateral trocars.

The use of four trocars allows some flexibility in the site of insertion. If they are inserted too far from the midline, the surgeon may have difficulty reaching across the patient. As a result, the risk of injury to the epigastric vessels is greater when using two trocars on each side. Usually, the lower of the two trocars is pierced through the wall lateral from the epigastric vessels and the upper one is placed at or above the level of the umbilicus at the edge of the rectus muscle. The size of the trocars varies. Most commonly, one of four trocars will be 10 mm and the three others will be 5 mm in diameter. The availability of at least one 10-mm or 12-mm trocar allows the use of a clip applicator or other mechanical device, occasionally used to complete the surgery.

Landmarks

The umbilical ligament is a "laparoscopy-specific" landmark. Intra-abdominal insufflation makes the umbilical ligament stand out but during laparotomy, little attention is paid to this anatomic structure. In patients who have had previous operations, the suprapubic course of the ligament may be distorted. To retrieve this valuable landmark, the surgeon probes for the pubic bone and is able to recover the ligament at that level in most patients. Some readjustment in spatial representation of the pelvic anatomy is required. The abdominal distention, combined with the craniocaudal angle of view, shows the pelvis in a way dissimilar from its appearance at laparotomy. It may be said that years of experience in performing tubal ligation do not prepare the surgeon to undertake procedures in the retroperitoneal space.

The second most valuable landmark is the pubic bone. It is valuable because the surgeon can "feel" it. Palpation as a surgical aid is severely curtailed in laparoscopy. This represents a significant handicap to the surgeon because it is one of the main roadblocks in mastering laparoscopic techniques. One factor that plays a major role in the making of an experienced laparoscopist is the recovery of the tactile sense that is lost in procedures performed by laparoscopy. The surgeon intuitively discovers the difference between manual palpation of various structures and palpation with an instrument that connects his hand to structures several inches away. For the neophyte laparoscopist, the anatomic structure most easily recognized by palpation is the pubic bone.

Other landmarks, such as the ureter and the iliac vessels, play a secondary role. The ureter is most readily found at the level where it crosses the common iliac artery. It is also at this level that accidental ligation is most likely to occur because of its proximity with the infundibulopelvic ligament. Early isolation of the ureter is recommended in all procedures that involve the retroperitoneal space of the pelvic sidewall.

Limited Lymphadenectomy

When performing limited lymphadenectomy (resection of the obturator chain), the surgeon standing on the left side of the patient begins operating on the right pelvic sidewall. In the surgeon's left hand (if right-handed), a grasping forceps is introduced through the subrapubic port. In the right hand, a cutting instrument is operated through the left lateral trocar. Because the cutting instrument is the one the surgeon is most familiar with, there is no advantage in using a device such as a laser. The assistant standing on the right of the patient improves exposure by manipulating a probe or grasping forceps. The peritoneum is initially incised lateral to the umbilical ligament, beginning at the level of the internal inguinal ring, which lies in a plane above the pubic bone (Fig. 25-3). In women with uterus in situ, the initial surgical cut may be the transection of the round ligament, which is more readily accessible than the umbilical ligament. In men, the vas deferens is transected once it is positively identified. This greatly improves access to the obturator fossa.

The incision of the peritoneum is then carried laterally to the course of the ureter or the infundibulopelvic ligament (Fig. 25-4). In some patients, the ureter can be visualized through the peritoneum, which makes it easier for the surgeon to delineate the distal portion of the incision line. The ureter is most readily identified at the level where it crosses the common iliac artery. Next, the

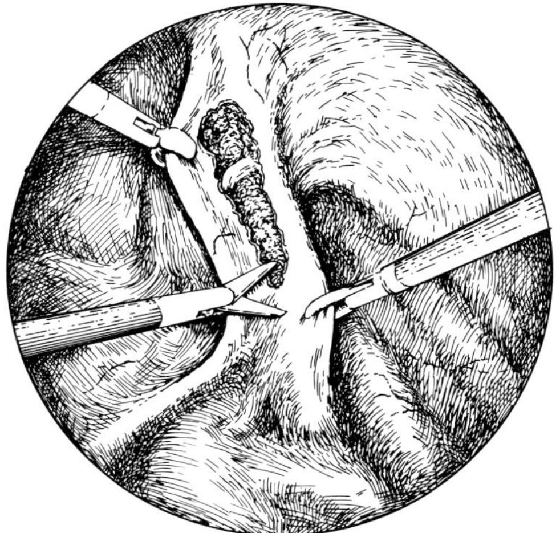

FIGURE 25-3. Extended pelvic lymphadenectomy on the right side. The peritoneum is incised lateral from the umbilical ligament and the ureter, between the pubic bone and the pelvic brim.

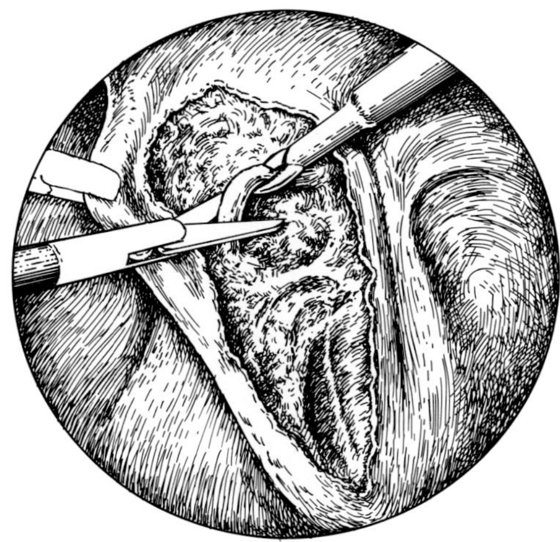

FIGURE 25-4. The dissection is carried further, including transection of the vas deferens (or round ligament in the female). The soft tissues at this level can be easily bluntly divided to reach the obturator fossa.

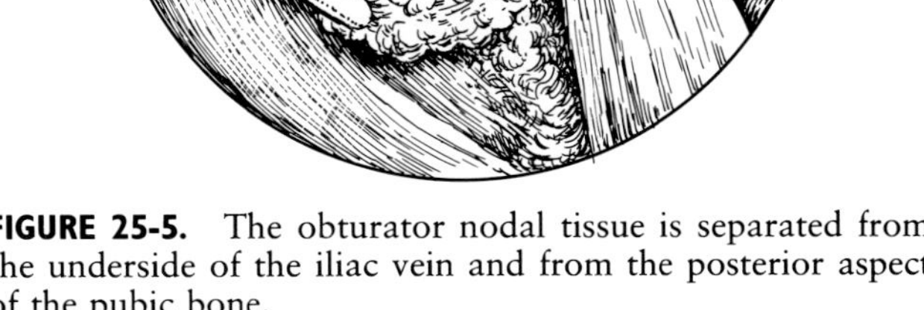

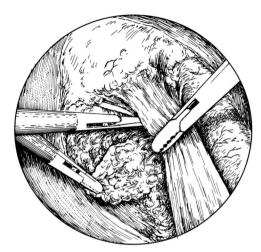

FIGURE 25-5. The obturator nodal tissue is separated from the underside of the iliac vein and from the posterior aspect of the pubic bone.

peritoneum should be bluntly dissected off the sidewall to expose the obturator fossa and the iliac vessels. The operator then locates the pubic bone by placing a forceps along the umbilical ligament and gently probing the paravesical space. It is helpful to identify other anatomic structures to facilitate dissection at the bone, at least early in the procedure.

The operator, after identification of the pubic bone, directs the dissecting forceps downward and slightly laterally to unroof the obturator fossa. As long as the dissecting instrument is kept away from the sidewall, no vital structure is at risk. This maneuver may not seem important at first but it facilitates later resection of the nodal tissue out of the obturator fossa because the peritoneum is already detached from the tissue bundle. During this part of the procedure, it may appear that some fibrous and even vascular bands cross over the iliac vessels at the level of the vas and below it (toward the hypogastric vessels). Sections of these strings after coagulation further benefit dissection of the area, especially at the level of the iliac bifurcation. This maneuver requires the most profound knowledge of the pelvic anatomy, and a tense moment may ensue when the surgeon works in the area of the hypogastric vessels when these vessels are not highly visible.

Once this part of the dissection is accomplished, the surgeon should be able to distinguish the vital structures of the sidewall: the external iliac vein and artery and the obturator nerve, between which lies the lymphatic chain. The assistant should retract the external iliac vessels to give the surgeon better access to the lymphatic tissue. The nodal tissue should be grasped about 3 cm proximal to the pubic bone because there is less risk of injuring the circumflex vein or an aberrant obturator vein at this level (Fig. 25-5). The operator then continues dissection along the medial aspect of the external iliac vein, until the obturator nerve is visualized, and then detaches the nodal tissue from the iliac vein and the pubic bone. Usually, an aberrant obturator vein can easily be identified during this process. In about half of the patients, the vein can be spared; in the remainder, it must be coagulated or clipped and then transected. At this point, the lymphatic chain can be further dissected off the sidewall or first transected at the level of the pubic bone. The obturator nerve must be positively identified before transection.

Next, the surgeon performs the cephalad transection of the lymphatic chain at the junction of the external iliac vein and obturator nerve (Fig. 25-6). This is a particularly delicate procedure because the area is difficult to reach and is near the hypogastric vein. A technical difficulty particular to endosurgical lymphadenectomy exists when the surgeon is unable to sustain a strong grasp on the nodal tissue during blunt dissection at the proximal end. This marks the end of the so-called limited pelvic lymphadenectomy. The nodal tissue should be left in the obturator fossa until the opposite side is completed.

The left side should be completed as described above, except that the surgeon and assistant exchange places, with the surgeon on the right side of the patient and the assistant on the left. We prefer to operate with two surgeons, each alternating as principal surgeon and assistant. This eliminates the need for changing sides during the operation, which can be extremely disorienting because it changes the optical perspective. Note that certain differences are routinely found between the right and left sides. There are frequently (indeed, almost always) adhesions between the sigmoid colon and the left pelvic sidewall, probably resulting from subclinical diverticulitis. These adhesions must either be dissected

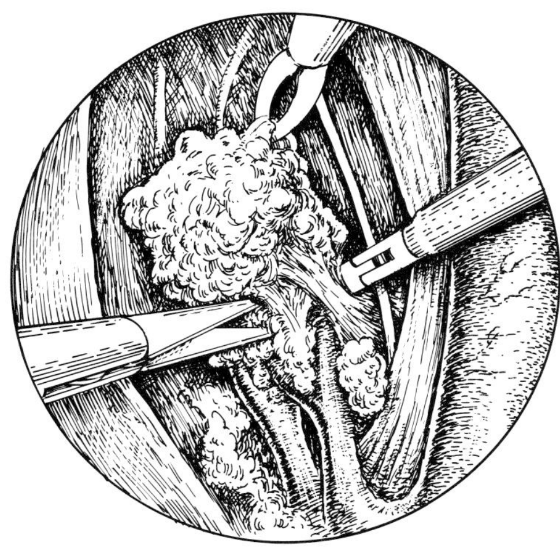

FIGURE 25-6. The obturator node bundle is further dissected free from underlying structures, such as the obturator vessels and nerve.

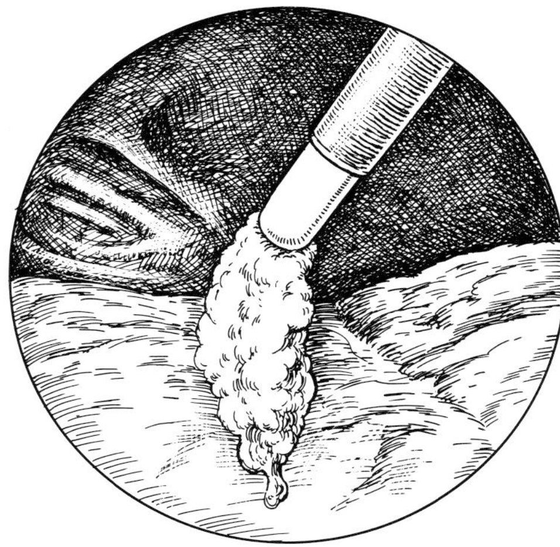

FIGURE 25-7. The laparoscope has been introduced through a lateral port. A 10-mm cup biopsy forceps is introduced through the umbilical port. The lymphatic tissue is grasped and carefully extracted. Alternatively, one can insert the specimen in a plastic bag, which is then retrieved at the umbilicus.

free before opening the peritoneum or the peritoneum incised above the pelvic brim and folded downward and medially, thus separating the sigmoid colon from the sidewall.

When the dissection is completed on both sides, the tissue is removed through a 10-mm incision, using either the first-puncture trocar or an ancillary trocar (Figs. 25-7 and 25-8). If the surgeon uses the first-puncture trocar to remove the tissue, visualization can be accomplished by inserting a 5-mm 0° endoscope through an ancillary trocar. The operator grasps the nodal tissue with either a large spoon forceps or with a regular grasping forceps introduced through a reducing sleeve. When the specimen appears to be too large, it is appropriate to use an endosurgical container for storage of the specimen, which can then be removed after slight enlargement of one of the 10-mm incisions.

Extended Lymphadenectomy

Extended lymphadenectomy (obturator and iliac chain) is defined as the resection of all nodal and fatty tissue from the iliac bifurcation to the pubis between the ureter and the genitofemoral nerve. In addition to the dissection previously described, the external iliac artery, external iliac vein, hypogastric artery, and ureter must be meticulously dissected. We began using this extended dissection of the right side with our 31st case, as part of a prospective study evaluating the diagnostic value and morbidity of extended lymphadenectomy.

The anatomy of the pelvic sidewall, as well as the location of the iliac and hypogastric vessels and the ureter, can be more clearly identified once the obturator nodal tissue has been removed.

Dissection of the obturator nerve defines the bottom of the surgical field. The lateral limits must be delineated. These lateral limits are furnished by the ureter and the genitofemoral nerve, which form a "V," the angle of which is located at the bottom of the common iliac artery. The pubic bone defines the distal border.

At this point, the fourth branch of the hypogastric artery offers a helpful landmark. The artery may be differentiated from the ureter by applying gentle traction on the ligament. Arterial pulsations are more easily distinguished palpably than visually, partly because of the atherosclerosis that is present in virtually every older patient. Once the surgeon has identified the ureter and

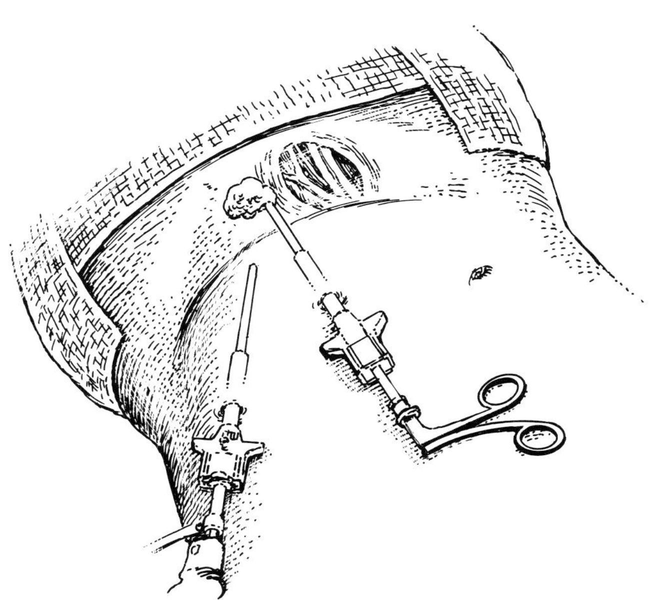

FIGURE 25-8. Different view of Figure 25-7.

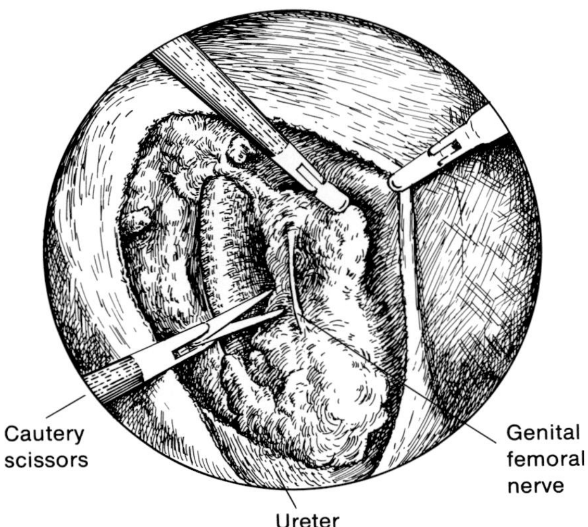

FIGURE 25-9. Dissection of the external iliac lymphatic chain. The area is bordered laterally by the genitofemoral nerve and medially by the lower border of the iliac artery. The distal end of this lymphatic chain is transected at the level of the circumflex vein.

hypogastric artery, the peritoneal incision is extended cephalad to 1 to 2 cm beyond the common iliac artery, dissecting the peritoneum off the external iliac vessels, forming a flap that the assistant then holds and retracts (Fig. 25-9). The fatty tissue lateral to the iliac vessels is bluntly divided until the genitofemoral nerve can be identified. The operator carries this dissection along the entire length of the external iliac artery. Great care must be taken at the distal end to avoid injuring the epigastric and circumflex vessels (Fig. 25-10). Cloquet's ganglion can sometimes be identified when the lymphatic chain is grasped and traction exerted in a cephalad direction. Removal of the ganglion probably adds little to the prognostic value of the procedure, and it represents an additional surgical risk because it is well-vascularized and located near the epigastric and circumflex vessels. We usually leave the ganglion in place, limiting resection to those patients in whom we are able to dissect it completely from the surrounding vascular structures. After completion of the lateral and distal dissection, the operator gives attention to the iliac artery. Using scissors, the surgeon incises the adventitia of the iliac artery over the entire exposed length and retracts fatty tissue medially (Fig. 25-11). Next, blunt dissection of the groove between artery and vein is undertaken, with the artery being held gently to one side to facilitate the dissection (Fig. 25-12). The adventitia of the hypogastric artery is then dissected, down to the insertion of the umbilical ligament (Fig. 25-13). The medial lateral border, delineated by the ureter, is bluntly dissected. This represents the end of the extended lymphadenectomy on one side (Fig. 25-14). We do not routinely denude the ureter.

Samples are removed as previously described. We do not close the peritoneal incisions because the edges of the incisions approximate once the abdomen is deflated. Formation of a lymphocele during healing may even be prevented by the incomplete closure of the peritoneal incision.

The peritoneal cavity is deflated and the 10-mm incisions closed, using a single stitch through the fascia. An advantage to subcutaneous absorbable suture material is that it need not be removed. Simple approximation of the smaller incisions suffices. The patient may be extubated and transferred to the recovery room.

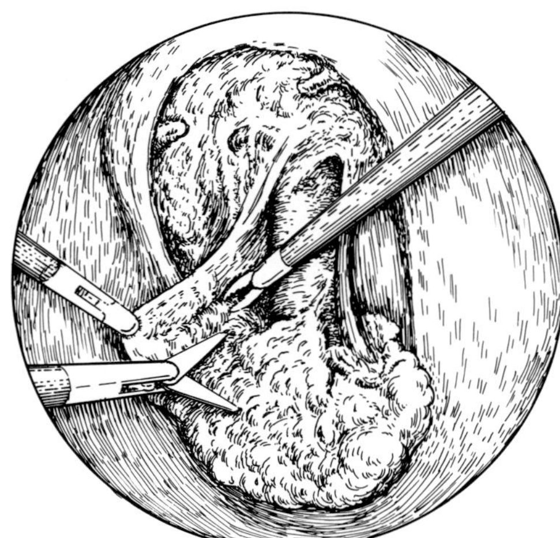

FIGURE 25-10. The dissection of the external lymphatic chain, after transection of its distal end, is carried up to the level of the crossing of the ureter.

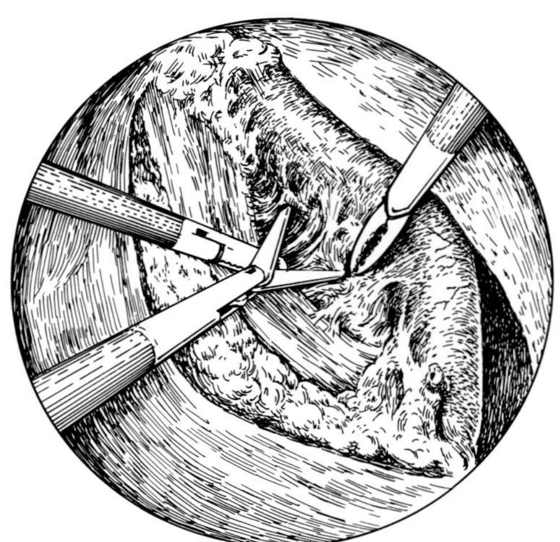

FIGURE 25-11. The nodal tissue from the obturator fossa is detached from the external iliac vessels. Here, the tissue is separated from underneath the external iliac artery.

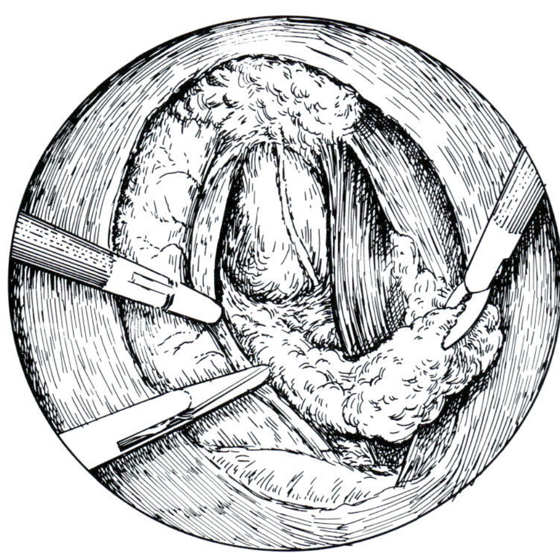

FIGURE 25-12. The lateral aspect of the obturator node bundle can be more easily accessed between the psoas muscle and external iliac vessels.

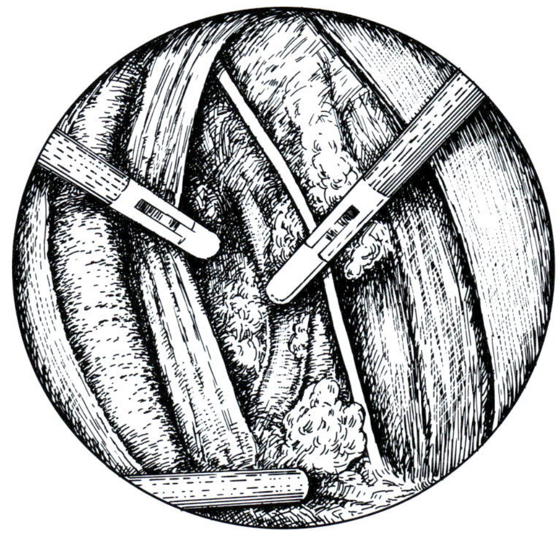

FIGURE 25-14. End view of the extended right pelvic lymphadenectomy.

It must be emphasized that although there are no large surgical dressings in evidence, the patient has just undergone a procedure that represents major surgery; the postsurgical monitoring should reflect this fact. The need for strict monitoring of vital signs is underlined because many patients who undergo surgery for lower genitourinary tract malignancy are older. Postoperative therapy includes administration of antibiotics and restriction of physical activities for about 1 week. The patient may be allowed to return home after 24 hours of observation but depending on his or her general status, this period may be extended. A follow-up visit to the surgeon should be scheduled to take place 4 to 5 days after surgery to discuss further treatment.

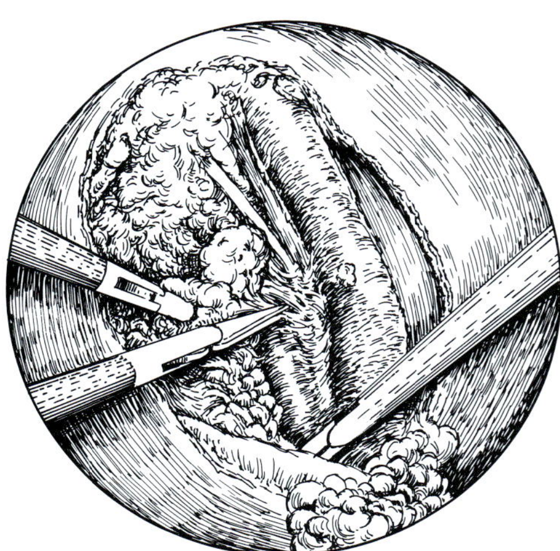

FIGURE 25-13. The most difficult time of the dissection is during the separation of the nodal tissue from the iliac vessels at the level of the bifurcation of the common iliac. Extreme care is taken in this area because of the vicinity of the iliac veins.

COMPLICATIONS

We have found intraoperative morbidity for this procedure to be extremely low. No patient required laparotomy for inadvertent damage, and perioperative blood loss did not exceed 100 mL in any individual. The procedure had to be terminated early in two out of 220 patients because of hypercarbia that could not be corrected by hyperventilation. We do not know, however, whether this problem was the result of instrument malfunction or represented a true complication.

Five patients suffered postoperative hemorrhage, requiring repeat laparoscopy and blood transfusions. Only one actually presented with bleeding from the operative site; in the four other patients, a trocar was the culprit.

Two major complications occurred: one patient had a small bowel injury followed by peritonitis, and one patient had inadvertent resection of a portion of the ureter. Both these patients required laparotomy to repair the injury. A lymphocele or lymphedema was found in nine of 220 (4%) patients, a low rate when compared with that reported for lymphedema in patients undergoing an open procedure. Other factors such as postoperative adjuvant therapy with radiation probably play a major role in the genesis of lymphedema.

No patient in our series has experienced a thromboembolic accident, probably because our patients are mobile soon after surgery. They report little postoperative pain, and oral medication sufficed for analgesia as soon as 4 hours after surgery. Because most of the patients are older and a fall could be disastrous, early ambulation is restricted but patients are encouraged to exercise in bed. Although we apply thrombosis-prevention devices routinely to patients 60 years of age or older, we have not yet been able to evaluate their efficacy.

References

1. Correa RJ Jr, Kidd CR, Burnett L, Brannen GE, Gibbons RP, Cummings KB: Percutaneous pelvic lymphnode aspiration in carcinoma of the prostate. J Urol 1981;126:190.
2. Gervasi LA, Mata J, Easley JD, et al: Prognostic significance of lymph nodal metastases in prostate cancer. J Urol 1989; 142:332.
3. Grossman IC, Carpiniello V, Greenberg, Mallo TR, Wein AJ: Staging pelvic lymphadenectomy for carcinoma of prostate. J Urol 1980;124:632.
4. Lieskovsky G, Skinner DG, Weisenburger T: Pelvic lymphadenectomy in the management of carcinoma of the prostate. J Urol 1980;124:635.
5. McCullough DL, McLaughlin AP, Gittes RF: Morbidity of pelvic lymphadenectomy and radical prostatectomy for prostatic cancer. J Urol 1977;117:206.
6. McLaughlin AP, Saltzstein SL, McCullough DL, Gittes RF: Prostatic carcinoma: incidence and location of unsuspected lymphatic metastases. J Urol 1976;115:84.
7. Nicholson TC, Richie JP: Pelvic lymphadenectomy for stage B, adenocarcinoma of the prostate: justified or not? J Urol 1977;117:199.
8. Ray GR, Pistenma DA, Castellino RA, Kempson RL, Meares E, Bagshan MA: Operative staging of apparently localized adenocarcinoma of the prostate: results in fifty unselected patients. I. Experimental design and preliminary results. Cancer 1976;38:73.
9. Schuessler WW, Vancaillie TG, Reich H, Griffith DP: Transperitoneal endosurgical lymphadenectomy in patients with localized prostate cancer. J Urol 1991;145:988.
10. Hald T, Rasmussen F: Extraperitoneal pelvioscopy: a new aid in staging of lower urinary tract tumors. A preliminary report. J Urol 1980;124:245.
11. Iversen P, Bak M, Juul N, et al: Ultrasonically guided I125 seed implantation with external radiation in management of localized prostatic carcinoma. Urology 1989; 34(4):181.
12. Fuerst D: Laparoscopic examination of pelvic lymph nodes. Urology 1985;26(5):482.

Index

Page numbers in *italic* indicate figures; those followed by *t* indicate tables.

D

Q

R

S

T